# Nursing Home Administration

Edited by

**Stephen M. Schneeweiss, Ed.D., F.R.S.H.**
Vice Provost, Research Administration
Ithaca College

and

**Stanley W. Davis, Ph.D.**
Professor of Psychology and
Hotel Administration
School of Hotel Administration
Cornell University

**UNIVERSITY PARK PRESS**
Baltimore · London · Tokyo

**University Park Press**
International Publishers in Science and Medicine
Chamber of Commerce Building
Baltimore, Maryland 21202


Copyright © 1974 by University Park Press


Printed in the United States of America

**Library of Congress Cataloging in Publication Data**

Schneeweiss, Stephen M
  Nursing home administration.

  1. Nursing homes—Administration. I. Davis,
Stanley W., joint author. II. Title. [DNLM: 1. Hos-
pital administration—U.S. 2. Nursing homes—U.S.
WX150 S358n]
RA997.S36     658'.91'3626116     74-13498
ISBN 0-8391-0658-0

# Contents

# Contributors

**Justin Alexander, Ph.D.** Director and Professor, Division of Physical Therapy, Ithaca College and Director and Assistant Professor of Physical Therapy, Albert Einstein College of Medicine, New York

**Peter Cayan, M.S.** Chairman, Division of Business Management, State University Agricultural and Technical College, Delhi, New York; licensed nursing home administrator

**Stanley W. Davis, Ph.D.** Professor of Psychology and Hotel Administration, School of Hotel Administration at Cornell University, Ithaca, New York

**Louis DiCarlo, Ed.D.** Professor and Acting Dean, School of Allied Health Professions, Ithaca College, Ithaca, New York (retired)

**V.N. Ferrante, O.T.R.** Practicing Occupational Therapist, A. Holly Patterson Home, Uniondale, New York

**Verna Gillis** Director, Continuing Education, Frederic D. Zeman Center for Instruction, The Jewish Home and Hospital for the Aged, New York, New York

**Bernice Hopkins, R.D.** Lecturer, Human Nutrition and Food, New York State College of Human Ecology, Cornell University, Ithaca, New York

**Alvin Jacobson, Ph.D.** Director and Professor of Environmental Health, Center for Allied Health Professions, Illinois State University, Illinois

**Ralph W. Jones, M.S.** Professor of Speech Pathology and Audiology, Ithaca College, Ithaca, New York (deceased)

**Thomas Kavazajian, Ph.D.** Professor of Psychology, Nassau Community College, Garden City, New York

**Martha Mackay, B.S., R.N.** Administrator, Auburn Nursing Home, Auburn, New York

**Monroe Mitchel, M.S.** Administrator, A. Holly Patterson Home, Uniondale, New York

**Albert C. Neimeth, J.D.** Assistant Dean, Cornell Law School and Practicing Attorney, Ithaca, New York

**Florence Olsson** Director of Activities, Isabella Geriatric Center, New York

**Alan Schachter, C.P.A.** Partner, Lester Witte and Company; lecturer, Ithaca College; licensed nursing home administrator

**Stephen M. Schneeweiss, Ed.D., F.R.S.H.**  Vice Provost, Research
Administration and Director of Graduate Studies, Associate Professor,
Health Care Administration, Ithaca College; Former Education Director,
York State Nursing Home Association; Fellow, Royal Society of Health;
licensed nursing home administrator

**Norma Wasmuth, B.S., R.N.**  Instructor, Administration of Health Services
Program, Ithaca College, Ithaca, New York

**Gordon Wheeler, M.S.**  President, Accounting and Management Systems, Inc.,
Syracuse, New York

# Preface

As the population of our nation and the life expectancy of the individual simultaneously increase, the number comprising our elderly population steadily expands. The nursing home in America, for many years a viable alternate life-style for a variety of reasons, today has the capacity to play a major role in the lives of elderly citizens. It is the intent of this book to present an overview of the structure and potentialities of the modern nursing home with emphasis on the current responsibilities of nursing home administrators. We hope that a thorough reading of this book will stimulate innovative programs, generate new ideas by challenging old ones, and provide an actual theoretical basis from which to develop concrete operational programs.

*Nursing Home Administration* is aimed at the proprietary segment of the industry and the framework and codes by which it operates. We have tried to provide its administrators and staff with a series of goals to be implemented by dedicated administrators. It is the moral and ethical obligation of the administrator to provide competent care for all persons entrusted to his charge, be they ill, senile, or infirm.

To keep up with the ever-changing practices and procedures within the discipline of nursing home administration, the professional administrator must prepare for the higher levels of knowledge and education necessary for the operation of the non-static nursing home. With the introduction of third-party payment programs for long-term health care, licensure and the steady expansion of the nation's elderly population, administrator education is a major factor in determining the future of the nursing home industry and profession.

The material presented in this book was used by more than 500 currently licensed administrators for instructional purposes. This book is a synthesis of and response to our years of experience, involvement, and immersion in the nursing home industry which now is emerging into a new era of professionalism. It is also a point of departure for further study of the professional development of the administrator and the improvement of nursing home facilities.

We wish to express our sincere appreciation to the contributing authors for providing material for each of the chapters. We are also indebted to the New York State Nursing Home Association and to Ithaca College for their foresight and support of the production of the television series that prompted the writing of this book.

We deeply feel that this volume contributes to improved care in our nursing home system.

*Ithaca, New York*                                    Stephen M. Schneeweiss
*June 1974*                                            Stanley W. Davis

# Introduction
# The Nursing Home Industry: An Overview

*Alan Schachter*

## HISTORICAL SURVEY

Caring for the aged infirm has been a problem of mankind dating back to ancient times. In order to fully understand the problems of the various institutions concerned with caring for the aged, it is necessary to study the evolution of these establishments. Early vestiges have been traced back to the ruins of ancient cities. As time progressed the medieval church became the major proponent of health care. Hospitals were erected in most cathedral cities in Europe. During the Renaissance the first almshouses appeared. The almshouse was a catch-all institution that housed orphans, diseased prostitutes, epileptics, the blind, the aged infirm, and many other unfortunates; thus, there was a wide variation in the state of health, age, mental capacity, and moral sensibility of the residents within its population. The living conditions were subhuman, and the chances of survival for a prolonged period were almost nil. Yet, the almshouse was a product of the moral fiber of the times. It was widely believed that poverty was directly proportional to one's moral shortcomings.

The English Poor Laws imposed the first legal responsibility on society to care for the aged and infirm. These harsh laws were created with a spirit of repression. They were intended to instill a fear of the lack of financial prudence in carrying out one's affairs.

Why institutional care for the aged had less than an auspicious beginning within the original thirteen colonies in America is evident. The settlers established the almshouse for the care of undesirables and unfortunates of early American society. It is interesting to note that some differentiation was made as to the treatment of those people who suffered economic losses caused by Indian raids. These unfortunates were not placed in the almshouse but were given financial help through channels within the community. This differentiation was a significant step in reversing the horrors of the alms-houses.

By the 1800's, growing concern about conditions in the almshouses mounted. Women such as Dorothea Dix created waves of moral indignation that led to the establishment of specialized institutions to care for certain segments of the almshouse population. Orphanages, homes for the blind, residences for occupational classes (e.g., seamen), and homes for disabled veterans were all products of this wave of social conscience. With the advent of modern medicine, many persons with communicable diseases were cured. These individuals were freed from the almshouses, leaving behind the aged and semi-feeble who were suffering from chronic and degenerative diseases. As each group of unfortunates was siphoned off to a specialized institution, its members met with more understanding and better living conditions; yet, these improved conditions never filtered back to the source institutions, the almshouses. Society had literally turned its back on its aged and infirm.

It was not until the passage of the Social Security Act of 1935 that any inroads were made into the solution of the problem. This act relieved local governments of a good part of the financial burden of caring for the aged infirm. The act was passed during the depression years when many people who had large amounts of capital frozen in their spacious living quarters chose to subdivide them into homes for the elderly rather than lose them entirely. The system established to compensate proprietors did not offer incentives to develop high standards of care. The facilities could provide only the barest minimum level of care; they were not capable of administering any sort of rehabilitative care. These homes were the forerunners of today's nursing homes which provide custodial care, the third level of care (see next page).

The concept of the extended care facility had the same basic roots as that of the nursing home, but its fruition arose from a different set of circumstances. When the orphan group was removed from the almshouse population, a theory was espoused that, "in the removal of external pressures by the provision for adequate food and rest, and in the development of 'good habits' of body and mind, improvement would accrue automatically."[1]

During World War I, an active approach was taken in regard to the rehabilitation of the wounded in order to get the men back to battle as rapidly as possible. Teams of trained specialists actively intervened in the recuperation process. The theories evolving from the orphan and disabled soldier groups coupled with the realization that "there are unrealized potentials for independence existing in every human being, regardless of age and economic usefulness"[2] formed the foundation of what is now known as the extended care facility.

## PROFILE OF TODAY'S MARKET

Present-day health-care facilities for the aged offer varying levels of care, and it is important to differentiate among these levels because each has a different ultimate price to the consumer. The three basic levels are:

Level I: Extended Care. This level is an extension of hospital nursing care—high-intensity care with potential for rehabilitation. It is not "extended" in time, and, in fact, lasts only a few weeks. The facility providing this level of care would be an extended care facility.

Level II: Skilled Nursing Care. This level represents long-term care. It is of medium intensity and does not focus on rehabilitation. Very often the condition of the patients receiving this care will be of a terminal nature. The facility providing this care would be a nursing home.

Level III: Minimal Nursing Care (H.R.F.–Health Related Facility). This level is also known as long-term care, but the patient receiving this type of care will be semi-ambulatory or, in most instances, ambulatory. The care is custodial in nature, although restorative activities are also available. The facility providing this level of care would be a health-related facility.[3]

These levels of care exclude mental health patients who need twenty-four hour non-nursing supervision and residents of domiciliary homes who are not considered patients. Depending on the level of care, the daily charges for each patient can range from fifteen to fifty dollars. Since nursing salaries account for more than 50 percent of the operating expenses of an institution, one can materially alter the cost of care by varying the level of nursing care administered.

When one speaks of the "nursing home industry," one includes extended care facilities, nursing homes, and health-related facilities. In recent years, this industry has undergone a tremendous growth rate that has been paralleled by an even greater increase of governmental funds spent for institutional care.

It is estimated that 75 percent of today's aged-care institutions of the proprietary nature are corporations.[4] It is also estimated that the overall rate of occupancy of all institutions is 92 percent.[5] Newly constructed institutions usually range in size from 150 to 200 beds.

The two main problems of the industry today are:

1. Adverse publicity. The public image of the nursing home industry has been far from bright (e.g., Nader's Raiders). Owing to poor national publicity, the public, government, and even health-care professionals have been somewhat suspicious of the industry.

2. Providing quality care at a reasonable cost. The industry faces many administrative challenges in defending its costs as measured against govern-

ment reimbursement formulas. This problem is twofold because, in many cases, the formulas as well as the actual costs appear to be somewhat out of line with reality.

## CONDITIONS OF PARTICIPATION

The secretary of Health, Education, and Welfare (HEW) issued a group of regulations entitled the *Conditions of Participation, Extended Care Facilities,* which was comprised of two basic components: the first being a legal definition established in the Social Security Act—Public Law 89–97, Section 1861J (which follows)—and the second being a group of additional requirements established by the HEW after extensive consultations with experts in the field of hospital and nursing home care. Section 1861J[8] defines the term "extended care facility" to mean:

An institution (or a distinct part of an institution) which has in effect a transfer agreement . . . with one or more hospitals having agreements in effect under Section 1866 and which . . .
1. is primarily engaged in providing to inpatients (A) skilled nursing care and related services for patients who require medical or nursing care, or (B) rehabilitation of injured, disabled, or sick persons;
2. has policies, which are developed with the advice of . . . a group of professional personnel, including one or more physicians and one or more registered professional nurses, to govern the skilled nursing care and related or other medical services it provides;
3. has a physician, a registered professional nurse, or a medical staff responsible for the execution of such policies;
4. (A) has a requirement that the health care of every patient must be under the supervision of a physician, and (B) provides for having a physician available to furnish necessary medical care in case of emergency;
5. maintains clinical records on all patients;
6. provides 24-hour nursing service which is sufficient to meet nursing needs in accordance with the policies developed in paragraph (2), and has at least one registered professional nurse employed full-time;
7. provides appropriate methods and procedures for the dispensing and administering of drugs and biologicals;
8. has in effect a utilization review plan. . . ;
9. in the case of an institution in any State in which State or applicable local law provides for the licensing of institutions of this nature, (A) is licensed pursuant to such law, or (B) is approved, . . . as meeting the standards established for such licensing;

10. meets such other conditions relating to the health and safety of individuals who are furnished services in such institution or relating to the physical facilities thereof as the Secretary may find necessary. . . .

To be a certified extended care facility, a nursing home must comply with all the statutory provisions of Section 1861J and must have no significant deficiencies in meeting all the other "Conditions of Participation." If there are deficiencies, they must exist in areas other than those covered by Section 1861J, and the facility must have plans to correct them. The Department of Health within each state, operating under agreement with the secretary of the HEW, is designated to certify whether a facility is in compliance with the "Conditions." Certifications are in effect for one year; however, those facilities having deficiencies must meet the standards of certification within nine months.

Some of the major areas covered in the "Conditions"[9] are:

1. There must be an effective governing body, a suitable full-time administrator, and approved policies.
2. There must be a twenty-four hour nursing service and a full-time professional registered nurse. Each nursing tour must have a charge nurse who is either a licensed practical or a registered nurse.
3. The dietary service must be directed by a qualified individual (either a dietician or someone acting under the guidance of a dietician consultant) and must meet daily dietary needs of the patients.
4. Restorative services must be provided under medical direction.
5. The nursing home must have an arrangement for obtaining clinical laboratory, x-ray and other diagnostic services.
6. Medically related social needs of the patients must be provided for.
7. Diversional, recreational, and religious activities must be provided for the patients.
8. Several requirements concerning housekeeping, sanitation, and other environmental factors are defined in detail.

Two other areas are of special importance. One requires that a written transfer agreement with a local hospital that has been approved for Medicare must be obtained. The transfer agreement is a written document providing for appropriate transfer of patients and relevant information between the extended care facility (ECF) and the hospital. The second area provides for a utilization review plan by two or more physicians of the admissions to the institution, the duration of the stays, and professional services rendered. It is the purpose of the utilization committee to insure that each patient receive the proper level of care. If the committee fails to perform critically, the intent of the program will be undermined. I have observed instances in which the committees have failed to screen the patients carefully; the Medicare Program was then paying for patients not in need of extended care. It was not until the fiscal intermediaries developed an inhouse review as an adjunct to the regular ECF utilization review committees that many lapses came to the public eye. The facilities in which lapses occurred were faced with the problem of repaying sizeable sums of money to the program. These types of unprofessional lapses have led to an untold amount of bad publicity and suspicious reactions by government officials. The only hope for continued Federal support of extended care facilities lies in the industry's realization that compliance with the "Conditions of Participation" is mandatory.

## NOTES
1. McArthur R., 1970. The historical evolution from almshouse to ECF. Nursing Homes. 19:14.
2. *Ibid.,* p. 15.
3. Sherman, J., 1967. Categories of care. Nursing Homes. 16:24.
4. Coleman and Company. 1968. The nursing home industry. p. 13. Coleman and Company, New York.
5. *Ibid.*
6. *Ibid.,* p. 2.
7. *Ibid.,* p. 10.
8. Conditions of participation: Extended care facilities. 1968. Federal Health Insurance for the Aged CFR Title 20, Chapter III, Part 405. p. 1. U.S. Government Printing Office, Washington, D.C.
9. *Ibid.,* pp. 23—24.

# The Administrator as Coordinator of Health-Care Services

*Monroe Mitchel*

**1** Dramatic gains in medical science, development of miracle drugs, and the marvels of electronic equipment have been impressed on the public's imagination during the past thirty years, while concurrent progress in the field of long-term care has been less than significant. Nursing homes generally have not enjoyed a good reputation and too often have been thought of as places where people have been sent to die. Happily, the introduction of Medicare and the concurrent upgrading of standards have helped to change this image to a much more positive one, with the public gradually becoming more aware of the enormous strides made in recent years in the programming of long-term care. Today, American nursing homes have the potential to restore feelings of self-worth and human dignity to their aged residents.

Similarly, the nursing home administrator, once thought of as completely untrained, has now been forced to upgrade his preparation for the role and broaden his understanding of long-term care activities as a result of the new nursing home administrator's licensure requirements, which were introduced nationally as part of the Medicare amendments several years ago. This legislation was enacted after years of criticism of nursing home administrators.

As recently as 1965, a large percentage of nursing home administrators had not received any formal college training and were traditionally considered unsophisticated in the delivery of health-care services. Also, it was often alleged that nursing home operations frequently generated large profits, ostensibly at the expense of the aged patient. This high-profit pattern surfaced dramatically during the stock market boom of publicly held stocks in the nursing home field during the mid-1960's.

The corollary to the profit motive criticism was that the administrators involved were unconcerned about their patients and did not appear to have feelings for the individual. Another charge still prevalent today focuses on the do-nothing, unavailable nursing home administrator. In many, he was un-known and was never seen on the premises. Neither the patients nor the staff knew him. In short, he was an absentee manager. The charge of absentee management, I believe, served as one of the greatest indictments in the field of nursing home administration, and led directly to the necessity of the licensure law.

The administrator's personal influence on the health-care environment is directly related to his visibility. The subsequent formation of attitudes and establishment of rapport greatly affect his ability to establish policies, recog-nize problems, and inspire solutions. One requisite for control in a nursing home situation is that all individuals in positions of authority be recognizable personalities, whose goals and ambitions for the organization are clearly demonstrated by their own example and performance. In short, the adminis-trator is the catalyst for the development and implementation of all services.

## THE ADMINISTRATOR AND THE PHYSICIAN

The administrator initially must focus his attention on the physician, who is obviously a key person on the health-care team. The physician places the individual in a nursing home and is responsible for the patient's treatment. The administrator must establish rapport with the physicians in the commu-nity so that he can convey to them an accurate understanding of the services and capabilities of his particular nursing home. In certain areas of the country, there are a large number of nursing homes. Some are better than others. Some are big, some are small. Some are capable of providing rehabili-tative services, others are not. Some have a speech therapist, others do not. Some have a very definite motivational activities program, others simply have television. The average physician does not have the time to learn about the various services available in each nursing home by personal investigation. This means that the administrator must be able to describe to a physician in an accurate and definitive fashion the capabilities of his agency to provide required services. All too often, neither the physician nor the family has investigated the nursing home's capacity to meet the particular needs of a special patient, often a member of the family who is in distress and needs extended or long-term care. Perhaps a course of therapy that involves a great deal of psychological trauma is required. If the physician and the family have not investigated the facilities available to them in their respective commu-nities, they probably do not know where to turn to meet their special needs or problems. This, of course, can create unnecessary distress, and often leads to an indictment against the nursing home in general.

The physician is the major clinical professional resource available to the family. If he advises placement in a given nursing home, the family will usually follow his advice. Therefore, the physician must know the advantages and disadvantages of the various nursing homes in his community since he establishes the clinical eligibility of the patient for admission, and prescribes a course of follow-up therapy. If he is skilled in geriatric medicine, he recognizes the need to give strong personal support to his patient; therefore, he will allow himself to be drawn into the total spectrum of patient services in the nursing home, thereby aiding the administrator and nursing home in achieving their goals. The administrator must never lose sight of the vital role played by the physician in the nursing home.

## CATEGORIES OF LONG-TERM CARE FACILITIES

Since there are numerous categories of facilities licensed to provide services to the aged, it is necessary for the family confronted with placing an aged member in a nursing home and the physician who is caring for the patient to identify and define the types of services offered by the various agencies. The facilities available can be grouped as Domiciliary Care Facilities, Health-Related Facilities, Extended Care Facilities (or Nursing Homes), and Senior Citizens' Hotels.

### Domiciliary Care Facilities for Adults

Domiciliary Care Facilities include Homes for the Aged, Public Homes, Homes for Adults (proprietary or nonprofit), and Residences for Adults. They may be more specifically defined as follows.

*Residence for Adults or an Adult Home.* A facility other than a Nursing Home, Health Related Facility, Home for the Aged, or Public Home which holds itself out, advertises, or otherwise represents itself as providing living quarters, central dining, housekeeping services, and activities programs for adult persons, who, because of age of disability, require such services on a continuing basis.

*Proprietary Home for Adults.* A private facility, operated for compensation and profit, for the purpose of providing suitable services to two or more adult persons, unrelated to the proprietor, who, though not requiring medical or nursing care, are in such condition by reason of their age, infirmities, or disabilities to require, in addition to lodging and board, the services of attendants to assure their safety and comfort and to enable them to be bathed, dressed, or fed, or to move about.

*A Public Home.* A residence for adults administered by a unit of a local department of social services, and typically operated without an infirmary.

*Home for the Aged.* A proprietary or voluntary nonprofit facility for the care of the aged, operated without an infirmary, and organized to provide services similar to those offered by an Adult Home as described above.

In New York State, for example, as in many other states, all Domiciliary Care Facilities are inspected and approved by the State Department of Public

Welfare. If the number of beds in the home is less than five, the local Department of Social Services conducts inspections and grants approval to operate. If the home cares for five or more people, the State Board of Social Welfare has jurisdiction and serves as the inspecting and approving agency. It should be noted that the "non-nursing" type facilities, broadly listed above under the heading of Domiciliary Care Facility, are virtually alike in actual function, despite their licensure under different titles.

### Health-Related Facility (Intermediate Care Facility)

A Health-Related Facility is an intermediate care facility that provides lodging, board, social activities, social services, and minimal physical care to include the services of at least one professional nurse on a daily basis. Intermediate care facilities typically do not admit non-ambulatory patients unless a pre-admission evlauation determines that the facility can appropriately care for such individuals.

### Extended Care Facility or Nursing Home

An Extended Care Facility or Nursing Home is an agency that provides 24-hour skilled nursing care and rehabilitative or restorative services, along with other health services, under the supervision of a licensed physician. Facilities certified as Extended Care Facilities are approved to operate under the Federal Medicare Program and the State Medicaid Program. Facilities certified solely as Nursing Homes are typically not approved to participate in the Federal Medicare Program.

### Senior Citizens' Hotel

Other types of facilities have proliferated throughout the country. Of these, the senior citizens' hotels are generally not recommended for chronically ill people. However, many people who are quite aged but do not suffer from chronic illness, who can get about easily and do not require any type of drug therapy or similar treatments, can do very well in senior citizens' hotels and are often quite happy to be among their own peer group. As a health-care facility, however, senior citizens' hotels certainly leave a great deal to be desired.

### THE RELATIONSHIP OF THE PHYSICIAN TO THE NURSING HOME UNDER MEDICARE

Emphasis is placed on the role of the physician in the nursing home under the conditions of participation for an extended care facility under Medicare, whose requirements are that the extended care facility admit patients in need of skilled nursing care "only upon the recommendation of a physician."[1] Therefore, the physician must be the individual in the community who knows or should know what the nursing home and the community are capable of doing. If he is satisfied that a specific nursing home can provide the type of services necessary for his patient, he will make the selection and place the individual in that nursing home.

A second point stressed in the conditions of participation for Medicare is that health care must be provided under the continuous supervision of a physician, with each facility having a physician available to furnish special medical service in case of an emergency. Apart from these regulations, it must be obvious that a nursing home cannot function adequately without medical supervision.

To expand further on the physician's role, the New York State Nursing Home Code, for example, stipulates that in proprietary nursing homes "the patient, next of kin, or sponsor, must designate a personal physician for that patient and obtain from that personal physician confirmation that he will visit the patient not less often than once every thirty days and at such other times when an emergency exists or when a rapid change in the patient's clinical condition warrants."[2]

A definition of emergency or rapid change in the patient's condition is typically left to the judgment of the director of nursing services. New York State Code requirements are typical of those of most states in the nation, namely, that the physician must see his patient who is in a nursing home at least once every thirty days. The administrator, of course, is involved in making sure that the physician does provide this care. Another section of the New York State Code dealing with patient services states that "the operator of a proprietary nursing home shall require that the personal physician, the patient, next of kin or sponsor, designate an alternate physician to attend the patient for periodic or emergency visits, whenever the personal physician is not available."[2] This requirement is vital also, because, if the physician who has admitted the individual to the home goes away for a month or more, or becomes ill, or is otherwise unable to attend his patient, provision must be made for another physician to attend the patient. This is particularly vital in an emergency situation.

One more example from the New York State Nursing Home Code, that is representative of other state codes is that "the nursing home administrator, or his designee, must record in writing in the patient's chart the name, address, and telephone number of the personal physician and his alternate physician."[2] He must also "record confirmations of the agreement with the physician for the provision of medical care to the patient."[2] The administrator must notify the physician if a regular visit has been omitted, and similarly must contact him promptly when an emergency exists in order to assure the patient of appropriate medical care at all times.[2]

In simple terms, this means that the administrator is required to maintain surveillance over the accessibility and delivery of physicians' services, thereby assuring the provision of appropriate medical care in the nursing home.

The New York State Code provides that the operator or administrator be responsible for the "establishment and maintenance of written medical policies satisfactory to the department,"[3] in this case, the Department of Health of the State of New York. The operator must also "appoint a medical advisory committee or a consulting physician with the following responsibilities: (1) to develop and amend medical policies, (2) to supervise medical services, (3) to advise the operator regarding medical and related problems, (4) to establish procedures for medical matters such as physicians' visits, medical records, consulting services, and rehabilitative services."[3] In short, the administrator should utilize an advisory committee of physicians to help him supervise medical care. This committee should be concerned with the preparation and utilization of medical records, the establishment of specific clinical services, and the relationships with other institutions and agencies such as general hospitals, rehabilitation centers, and the like.

It is interesting to note that the New York State Code differentiates between nursing homes operated under proprietary auspices [the majority of all homes in the United States (approximately 70 percent) and those administered under voluntary or public auspices (approximately 30 percent)]. In the proprietary nursing home, every individual must have his own physician and the private physician-patient relationship is carefully maintained. In this situation, the physician is charged with the responsibility of instructing the nursing home staff in the implementation of his prescribed plan of medical and motivational activities.

In the public or voluntary nursing home, an allowance is made for the home to hire physicians and to provide medical services directly. The New York State Nursing Home Code provides that "the operator of a public or voluntary nursing home shall appoint a New York State licensed physician as medical director or chief of staff to (1) direct and supervise the health and medical care program of the nursing home, (2) to develop medical policies including medical staff by-laws and rules and regulations in cooperation with the medical board or medical advisory committee, and (3) to submit these policies to the administration for approval."[4] Finally, the New York State Code stipulates that "the medical staff of a public or voluntary nursing home shall (1) be sufficient to meet the medical needs of the patients, and (2) meet the requirements and abide by the medical policies including medical staff by-laws, and rules and regulations established by the nursing home."[4]

Medicare requirements and various State codes spell out the general responsibilities of physicians. Obviously, the nursing home administrator expects more of the physician than simple conformity to law. All too often, nursing homes complain that they just did not know enough about the patient when he was admitted. If only they had known some specific hidden facet, it would have made all the difference in the world. Too frequently, the nursing home admits a patient on the basis of a simple, and very inadequate, description of his true condition. The home frequently does not find out what his real problem is until after admission. Therefore, the physician must assume the responsibility of advising the nursing home in detail of the individual's complexities and infirmities. He must also provide information about the environment from which the patient came if it is pertinent to the patient's care. A description of the family situation in general, and its relationships to the patient, are frequently critical in the psychological handling of an individual patient.

Naturally, the physician's admitting diagnosis and regular prognosis statements with follow-up changes of order must be concise and clearly stated. When this pertinent information is not provided, the home unnecessarily struggles in its attempt to provide maximum care. In short, the physician must direct the patient's care in a manner that clearly establishes his ongoing responsibility and sincere concern.

I have dwelled on the role of the physician and his importance to the nursing home environment because of the oft-repeated, generalized allegation that physicians, as a group, spend too little time in the nursing home caring for their individual patients, and contribute little or nothing to the enrichment of many homes' multi-disciplined team approach to long-term care programming.

Frequently, the physician appears to concern himself simply with the basic requirement that the home be functionally comfortable and safe for his patient, while being adequately staffed with appropriate professional and nonprofessional personnel on all shifts to carry out his orders. However, the unfortunate reality is that the demand for nursing home beds in many parts of the nation still exceeds the supply, and, therefore, many physicians find themselves compromising even these modest standards.

Despite the fact that virtually every state code today emphasizes safety and patient care, the newspapers still carry headlines about the inadequacy of care in certain homes, along with vivid descriptions of the horrifying results of nursing home fires in facilities all too often minimally comforming to safety standards. It is imperative that we concern ourselves with fire and general operating safety. It is the moral obligation of every nursing home administrator to have his facility suitably staffed and maintained to preclude accidents resulting from negligence of employees or accidents caused by patients as a result of the debilitating nature of chronic diseases.

Additionally, reports are frequently heard that, in many nursing homes, there are too few registered nurses on duty in the daytime, less professional nursing in the evening, and virtually no professional nursing staff at night. The physician cannot be concerned with the administrator's problem in obtaining the staff. It is no secret that the demand for professional nurses far exceeds the supply. On a national scale, there are far more positions available for nurses than there are nurses to fill these positions. However, these circumstances do not excuse the nursing home and the nursing home administrator from trying to obtain the largest possible number of professional nurses who can, in a competent and professional manner, provide the "round-the-clock" care needed.

The physician has every right to expect an appropriate staffing complement to be ready on a 24-hour basis to carry out his instructions for routine and emergency treatment. It is the administrator's responsibility to provide that staff and have available adequate services, particularly for the patient whose condition changes radically. The needs of the individual must be met; the physician cannot accept an answer that there was no one to deliver care to his patient when it was required.

## NURSING SERVICE

Since the physician in a nursing home is not present to observe his patient continually as he would in a hospital, the nurse is clearly his "eyes and ears," and must have the experience and ability to observe changes that take place as a result of the administration of drugs or therapeutic procedures. A professional nurse in the long-term care setting must, of necessity, carry a broader range of professional responsibilities than the acute hospital nurse. In addition to her normal hospital duties, she often serves as part-time diagnostician, occupational therapist, psychologist, recreation worker, and friend. She must also be able to recognize and respond to a clinical emergency.

In terms of percentage of total personnel payroll costs and critical nature of service, nursing care is clearly the predominant feature of nursing home activities. The conditions of participation for Medicare state that "the extended care facility should provide 24-hour nursing service sufficient to meet the nursing needs of all patients. There should be at least one registered professional nurse employed full-time and responsible for the total nursing service."[5] As an added condition, "there should be a registered professional or a licensed practical nurse who is a graduate of a state approved school of practical nursing in charge of activities during each tour of duty."[5]

Obviously, one nurse is a minimum standard. Since nursing is the major activity in terms of services and personnel, it would seem that more description than the phrase "necessary service" ought to be provided. The New York State Nursing Home Code is an example of one state code that attempts to itemize more closely how much nursing care is necessary. It also defines the "objective of the nursing service to be: (1) to provide nursing care for patients' illnesses and for the restoration and protection of their physical and emotional well-being, and (2) to plan, administer, and provide nursing care in conformance with the stated general purposes and policies of the nursing home along with the physician's plan for the medical management of each patient."[6]

The New York State Nursing Home Code charges the nursing home administrator with the following responsibility: "he shall employ and have on duty registered professional nurses, licensed practical nurses, and nursing aides sufficient in number to provide an average of not less than two and one half hours of nursing care time for each patient for each 24-hour period, or for each patient for each twenty-four hour period a combined average of nursing care time approved by the Department of Health and computed on the basis of an average of not less than 1 hour for each ambulatory self-care patient, 2 hours for each semi-ambulatory partial self-care patient, and 4 hours for each bed and chairbound patient."[6] Under terms of the regulations in effect in various states, or in the absence of regulations more specific than Medicare regulations, it is the duty of the nursing home administrator to make sure that sufficient nursing care is provided for patients under his jurisdiction (see your state's code in reference to this area).

## OTHER COMPONENTS OF GOOD-QUALITY NURSING HOME CARE

In addition to medical and nursing care, each home should have the ability to provide, in an individualized and dignified atmosphere, a total program that contributes actively, in every way, to the well-being of its residents. Restoration of physical functioning in the form of a comprehensive rehabilitation program should be stressed, along with a strong health-maintenance program designed to prevent avoidable secondary crippling diseases. The total climate of the home must be geared to create a healthy atmosphere and incentives for living. The patient must be motivated to participate, within the limitations of his own debilities, within the nursing home community. In effect, the nursing home must be literally a second home for the individual under care. He must feel that he is a person, not a thing. All too often, patients are treated as if they were inanimate objects. When a cleaner comes into a room and sweeps around the patient without acknowledging the patient's presence, when a nursing aide or food service worker places food on the table in front of a patient and it remains untouched, yet no one lifts a finger to find out why the individual has not eaten, there is obviously lack of understanding and concern for the genuine human needs in the long-term care environment. Staff members who act in such a way deny the whole concept of individualized care and concern for the specific needs of the patient.

In order to provide a well-rounded program of health care and motivational activities for a patient so that he will gain "incentives for living," additional components are necessary. Rehabilitation and restorative services are critical to the nursing home environment and have helped change the once poor image of long-term care to a hopeful and positive outlook for many. Restorative services for extended care facilities typically include modalities such as physical therapy, occupational therapy, speech and audiological services, and assistance in the activities of daily living, all prescribed by the physician and carried out under medical direction. In addition, restorative nursing care should be provided to maintain function or improve the patient's ability to carry out the activities of daily living. "When an extended care facility provides restorative services, beyond restorative nursing care, whether directly or through cooperative arrangements with appropriate agencies such as hospitals, rehabilitation centers, state or local health departments, or independently practicing therapist, these services should be given by qualified therapists."[7]

A good-quality nursing home program should include dental services since care of the teeth is a very important aspect of the care of the aged. Ophthalmology and podiatry services should be available since failing eyesight and various problems of the feet represent complicating problems for the aged patient. Diagnostic, radiologic, and laboratory programs are essential for adequate care. Good social services and excellent motivational activities programming are also essential to good quality care.

Utilization review should also be included as a component in nursing home care. Utilization review, in essence, implies that the extended care facility has a plan that allows review of the services provided by the agency and that makes certain that individuals receiving care receive all the benefits they are entitled to under the law. Utilization review keeps the nursing home focused on treating the people who need to be treated.

Finally, a transfer agreement with an acute general hospital is essential in order to guarantee rapid hospitalization to a patient who suddenly becomes acutely ill. Every extended care facility under the Medicare program must have a transfer agreement so that it can provide acute hospital care when necessary.

Add to this list the necessary institutional "hotel" services that maintain a conducive living environment and sustain good health-care practices, and you will have a well-oriented nursing home.

## THE ROLE OF THE ADMINISTRATOR IN
## THE NURSING HOME

Tying all the foregoing together must involve high-quality administration. The administrator is the captain of the team and is essential for a smooth-running organization. His work is a major component of high-quality care.

Good administration can be defined as the accomplishment of clearly established goals and objectives by a team of individuals working together in a health-care environment conducive to the achievement of maximum results. This means that the primary role of the administrator of the nursing home is to get people representing various disciplines to carry out what they have been hired to do in the most efficient manner possible. The administrator does this by creating a favorable working environment. He imbues the staff with a feeling of confidence in one another, and improves their individual and group competence. He makes each job meaningful to the individual, and instills the feeling in his employees that each is doing something worthwhile. He teaches the employees to recognize that they are part of the health-care team, and therefore their personal performance is vital to making this concept work.

In order to direct his agency effectively, the administrator must establish clearly desirable goals and objectives that can be easily communicated to his staff. If the staff members in turn are properly motivated, they will work to their fullest capacity to achieve them. If the administrator has set up a good working environment, his staff will be encouraged to be innovative and to implement new ideas. If he inhibits their freedom to act, he may create a sterile environment that may defeat the agency's overall goals and objectives.

One illustration of an appropriate nursing home goal would be focused on the administration's concern for the individual worth and dignity of each patient. The objective can be simply stated as *the desire to protect the individuality of each patient while making every effort to meet the patient's specific personal needs with a broad spectrum of services and programs.*

In addition to clearly established goals, the administrator must strive to establish a strong team orientation. The nursing home team is comprised of health-care personnel who must work together. They must depend on one another. Consider the ramifications of not working together. Take the case of the partially paralyzed stroke victim who is being taught to ambulate. A physical therapist works with that individual in rehabilitation 30 minutes a day, with effective results on the parallel bars. But after the 30-minute session, the patient is put back in his wheelchair, wheeled back up to his room, and then put to bed with no follow-up on the part of the nursing personnel. When this happens, there is no team orientation. All the gains made in rehabilitation and physical therapy are lost if the individual is not encouraged to take advantage of the progress made in therapy. Similarly, consider a therapist who is working with an individual and trying to bolster his morale and build up his independence. This individual is suffering from loss of eyesight. If the team member who delivers the food is untrained to the problems of blindness and does not identify the type of food or its position on the plate for the patient, he may unwittingly cause the patient to spill the food all over himself producing embarrassment and destroying the individ-ual's self-esteem and motivational gains made through a variety of other disci-plines. If such unpleasantness occurs, team orientation has broken down. The individual has not been treated appropriately. Without everyone moving in the same direction, team objectives cannot be carried out.

The administrator, in my judgment, is a vital professional on the nursing home health-care team. He is the individual who molds the staff into a harmonious group, all working within an environment designed to enhance good patient care. He must be an intelligent, sensitive human being who clearly understands the debilitating nature of chronic disease and the impor-tance of the service his home has been licensed to render. He should be the type of person who recognizes that the long-term care patient also requires long-term concern. He recognizes the need to motivate staff and patient alike. He must be someone who is visibly interested in the needs of the patient. He cannot be hidden in his office, but must make himself available to patients and staff.

Ideally, the administrator is a dynamic, energetic individual who is sensi-tive to the needs of his patients, and whose unwavering dedication inspires his staff members to maintain the highest possible standards.

## NOTES

1. Conditions of Participation, ECF Regulations, 405.1123.
2. Codes and Rules and Regulations of the State of New York, 10 Health (C) 731.lh.
3. Codes and Rules and Regulations of the State of New York, 10 Health (C) 731.1A-C.
4. Codes and Rules and Regulations of the State of New York, 10 Health (C) 731.1e.
5. Conditions of Participation, ECF Regulations, 405.1124 (e).
6. Codes and Rules and Regulations of the State of New York, 10 Health (C) 731.2.
7. Conditions of Participation, ECF Regulations, 405.1126 (c).

# Personnel Selection and Training

## S. Davis and P. Cayan

2   This chapter and the one that follows are designed to give a brief summary of personnel management and related problems in the management of nursing homes. To do this effectively a great deal of information and concepts pertaining to nursing home management, but which were originally used successfully in other institutions and industries, must be covered. In order that the reader follow the process in an orderly fashion and also be able to apply the concepts discussed to his own situation, we have introduced the "System Concept." A nursing home is a man-machine system (this will be defined later). All man-machine systems are similar in many ways. In discussing the system we can start with problems of people entering the system (hiring), helping these people to improve within the system (training), and then continue on through the entire process including the management of the system, creating the appropriate climate, and the like. In other words, we use the system concept to define a general framework within which all of the functions of personnel management are carried out in their proper place. In this way we hope that we can give you a basis for understanding the basic thoughts of people working in the field of personnel management in such a way that you may readily apply the information to nursing home management.

### THE MAN-MACHINE SYSTEM CONCEPT

Originally machines were conceived as extensions of man's capacity for perceiving and manipulating the environment. Lights enable one to see in the dark, jacks help lift heavy weights, and lift trucks move heavy objects; they are tools. In recent years, however, it has become apparent that the potentialities of machines as tools are overshadowed by the possibilities demonstrated when machines are embedded in a complex organization or system. This concept is particularly true when machines are designed, men trained, and groups organized with the notion that they are part of a total system. Thus, the electric light bulb is not just a single tool to provide light to read by, but rather is part of a total lighting system that functions as one of the many uses of power. The light is part of a total power system, and the power system is part of a total power distribution system. The point is to design machines and train the men working with them not just to perform a simple function, but to perform as part of a total system.

As a system, the telephone becomes not just a tool for transmitting the human voice, but part of a total communications system that requires the invention of new devices, new materials, and the acquisition of new skills by the people participating in the system. For example, originally most of the switching that occurred when one placed a phone call was done manually by operators. The caller would ask the operator to ring a particular number in his city, perhaps that of his neighbor or the doctor nearby. The operator actually connected wires physically by means of "jacks" to complete the call. Then came the dial system. One of the limits of this system is the time required to operate a set of relays set in motion by the dialing operation. It has also been proven that the dial method is very cumbersome. The time to dial the number one takes one tenth of the time it takes to dial zero because of the relative location of these two digits on the dial, and yet most of the popular numbers—the ones that are easy to remember—have zeros in them. For example, you may remember the old Glenn Miller hit "Pennsylvania 6-5000." Pennsylvania 6-5000 takes thirty times longer to dial than Pennsylvania 6-5111 because of the position of the 0's in relation to the 1's. The recent introduction of the push button system has now increased the efficacy of the telephone as part of the total communications system. Push buttons take less time to operate than do dials, and Pennsylvania 6-5000 can be called in the same amount of time as Pennsylvania 6-5111. Thus, the original tools become part of the total system.

What is a system anyway? In particular the kind of system we have been talking about is a man-machine system. The long-term care facility is a man-machine system; General Motors Corporation is a man-machine system; the U.S. Government is a man-machine system; and when driving your car you are a man-machine system. A man-machine system is an organization whose components are men and machines working together. Now what are they working together for? They are working together to achieve a common goal. How do they work together to achieve this common goal? They work together by means of a communications network. Thus, a man-machine system is any organization whose components are men and machines working together to achieve common goals and tied together by a communications network.[9]

As systems have become larger and more complex, they have created serious economic, political, social, psychological, and other problems. The most important psychological problems in the system arise from the necessity to: (1) identify qualified persons, (2) select, acquire, classify, and train these individuals to keep them working for system goals, and (3) organize them into a working team. What we are going to be concerned with is the individual in the system. We are concerned with how to train workers, how to acquire them, how to move them about within the system. To do this intelligently, we must add the concept that within a system there are sub-systems, that is, pieces, portions, or hunks within a system that can be pulled out and made separate from the rest and thus studied separately.

A total system can be divided in many different ways. A convenient one for study is to think of tools and hardware or machines as a sub-system. The human being in the system or the personnel sub-system is another portion of the system. Management and organization can be thought of as still another sub-system. Our concern is how management can affect the total system, and how management influences the personnel sub-system in particular.

## APPLICATION OF MAN-MACHINE CONCEPT TO NURSING HOMES

Why is the system concept important to those who are interested in administering nursing homes? We would like to help you to conceive of a complex set of interrelationships that comprise any organization or any system. A man doing a simple task such as scrubbing the floor can be thought as being part of a total system. If you can think of your facility as a total system, then some of the interrelationships that start to appear can be handled more easily. The various parts of an organization cannot any longer be thought of simply as tools for the extension of man's capacities, but, instead, must be designed in such a way as to integrate with the other parts of the system. To do what? To accomplish the system purposes which constitute another factor when thinking about systems. The system purposes or goals are important because without some purpose in mind, some goal for the organization, the system itself won't operate. It is senseless to even talk about an organization that does not have organizational goals. In other words, both system's components—that is, *men* and *machines*— must be planned from the very beginning, with the system's goals as the point of reference.

The system you operate embraces several assumptions and it is these assumptions that are important for us to look at seriously in greater detail. First of all, in any system, people are entering and leaving the system constantly. In between entering and leaving, these people can be organized into operating the man-machine system. Secondly, these people are in the system for different periods of time. Lastly, but extremely important, these people differ individually. With these factors in mind, it cannot be assumed that once a system has been established it will be a stable and unchanging one; rather, we must realize that positional turnovers are inevitable. We assume that positions are held for different lengths of time. Some are short-hitch summer positions; others are filled by people planning to make this type of work their career (some may do so well at your facility that they remain a lifetime); also there is a general turnover of individuals who are dissatisfied, find better paying positions, or leave for personal reasons.

## HOW MAN AND MACHINES DIFFER

In our study of the man-machine system as applied to the nursing home, we will, of course, emphasize the man in the system, but it is important to indicate some of the differences between the man and the machine. In this way, perhaps, we can see clearly the demands placed on the individual by the system.

Gagne[7] stated that there are several different types of characteristics in which man and machines differ. One set he called functional characteristics— that is, characteristics in which man and machines differ in terms of the kinds of functions that they perform.

*Man and machines differ in their versatility.* Man can perform many more diversified tasks than machines can perform. Think, for a moment, of man and his versatility when a sudden snowstorm lashes out. Man becomes a snow shoveler, a food hoarder, a television watcher, and performs many different kinds of functions as a result of the demands placed upon him. A snow shovel can only be a snow shovel. It might be an inadequate dirt shovel or a poor coal shovel, but basically a snow shovel is a snow shovel.

*One man can do a certain task better than another man whereas machines generally are about the same in their ability, depending upon their design and functional range.* Now the problem for the psychologist in industry arises in part from this lack of correspondence between the relative ability of man for different kinds of work or different kinds of activities. That is, because a person may be able to do a particular task better than his neighbor is just the reason that the psychologist, in worrying about care facilities, has to be concerned with the fact that individuals do differ. Machines are designed specifically with the only concern being that they perform their task inexpensively. One would not ordinarily use a pliers as a hammer since pliers do not make very good hammers. On the other hand, given an individual who fails to appear to carry out his assigned task, in many instances another individual, even an untrained one, can take his place. Stated differently, individual differences are the key to the personnel problem in any industry or any situation. For any action to be accomplished, there are great individual differences with respect to how man can carry out a specified performance. It is these differences that we are interested in studying.

Other ways in which man and machines differ will be mentioned briefly. *There are definite limits as to how well and how much a person can do.* Also there are definite limits to what a machine can do but these limits are different from those of man. The machine has a set of limits designed into it when it was built. Man, given various kinds of motivating forces, can be persuaded to exceed his normal limits or work nearer his capacity as a result of the kind of expectancies with which he is faced. Machines don't get angry and fail to perform their functions because they don't care to, and they don't refuse to work just because the foreman hasn't given them proper instructions. A machine won't try to make its operator think that it is doing a better job in order to get promoted. A machine won't fail to cooperate with another machine because it doesn't like the other machine or because it would prefer to receive from or give to another machine. Machine A won't spend most of its time trying to impress Machine B because Machine A is attracted by Machine B's measurements. It is obvious that we are discussing the types of problems that are quite often presented by people.

Another major difference between man and machines pertains to modifiability. In the kind of system that we are concerned with it becomes necessary at times to modify the components—both the man and the machines—of the system. While both components are modifiable the procedures to accomplish modification in man are very different from those in machines. To modify man requires retraining or, in some instances, replacement. Our ability to predict the product of our modification attempt is limited. You can see that while both man and machines work together intimately to perform the system's goals they are completely different in the kinds of work that are expected of them and the manner in which one must work with or administer them.

The functional differences between man and machines may also be viewed in terms of administrative factors.[7] For example, the problem of turnover or attrition differs between men and machines within the system. When machines wear out they must be replaced. Men typically aren't replaced in a system because they wear out, nor are they replaced because better types of men are designed. The outflow of personnel from a system occurs for different kinds of reasons, generally unfavorable ones. Faulty selection in the first place, for example, means that personnel must be removed. People leave one system and go to another system. Perhaps they feel that they are more urgently needed elsewhere or perhaps they get attracted by higher pay. Anyone looking at the employment section of Sunday's *New York Times* can see that it is filled with such blandishments. There are literally hundreds of advertisements trying to persuade talented people to leave one system and go to another.

Inflow of personnel into the system is also different from the inflow of machines. Inflow is used to replace outflow and also to expand or modify the system. In the case of machines, raw materials are generally available so that, in a reasonable time-frame, machines can be produced. With personnel, replacement presents quite a different problem. We cannot assume that the supply of personnel for a man-machine system is primarily one of selection and that the resources from which to draw are theoretically infinite. The military provides an example of this. At this moment the U.S. Army is several thousand men short of personnel with sufficient aptitude to learn to operate and maintain sophisticated electronic equipment. A sugar manufacturer in upstate New York chose to set up a new facility in a place where there were many handicapped people available because it was felt that the new facility provided an untapped personnel resource and a better chance of less turnover than if the facility were located elsewhere.

## INDIVIDUAL DIFFERENCES

All personnel problems require psychological understanding of the man within the system, and the important factor that must be understood is *individual differences.* Individual differences are the key to the problem of personnel management, to personnel evaluation, to why certain individuals are successful in your facility and why others are not, and why certain patients may be delighted to be a part of your facility while others are unhappy there. It may sound foolish to say that we are different one from another and that this difference is what causes problems, and yet the way most of us act and the attitudes most of us share in the relationship one to another demonstrate that we think of ourselves as being pretty much alike. We look alike in some ways—we all have ears, we all have eyes and noses, and we all love and hate—but yet we are not alike. The fact that we differ over a wide range of attributes is one of the keys to the problems of personnel placement, training, and management in your facility.

## MEASUREMENT OF INDIVIDUAL DIFFERENCES

The problem of individual differences was first recognized by the French psychologist, Binet.[4] Binet pointed out that despite the fact that children growing up in the same town, at the same time, are exposed to similar things—similar foods, similar games, similar language use, and the like—the reactions to and understanding of the things to which they are exposed differs from child to child. He deduced that mental ability might be estimated by observing how a child copes with tasks similar to ones that he faces in day-to-day life. Binet formulated a group of tasks that he thought to be representative of those encountered in normal life. He then asked youngsters to perform these tasks under specified conditions. The tasks included identifying familiar objects, naming coins, and unscrambling sentences. Binet then rated or scored each child according to how well he performed these tasks. The children tested were also rated independently by their teacher as to whether they were quick or slow learners, based on the teacher's experience with these pupils over a fairly long period. The teacher's ratings were then compared with the children's performance on the tasks that Binet had outlined for them. Binet was trying to devise some simple measure to determine the children who were fast learners and those who were slow learners. He set up the tasks and measured how well the children of the same age, say age ten, performed these tasks. He then ranked them from 0 to 100 according to their ability. However, this information all by itself has very little value. All we know is that Child C is more able to count coins or identify objects than Child B. But, when the teacher's rating of these children is added, another measure is provided. We thus have Binet's measures and the teacher's ratings of the same children. We now have a correlation between the measure that Binet made and the teacher's estimate. That is, the child whose performance was best according to Binet's measurements was estimated to be best by the teacher, while the least able child according to Binet's test was judged to be the poorest by the teacher. Thus, Binet's measurement predicted perfectly the teacher's estimates. Using statistics, we can actually compute mathematically the degree of relationship. In a similar fashion other tests have been developed which are samples of behavior, and which are used to predict behavior on the job or in school. The important fact is that because people do differ from one another, we must try to predict who is going to be successful and who is going to be unsuccessful in a given situation if our system is going to work efficiently. We must try to predict which kinds of abilities or skills are favorable to us and which kinds of skills are unfavorable to us. To do this, we try to correlate some measure (a test) that we can make with some independent measure of performance.

It is obvious that what we would like to do is to be able to hire all applicants for a position (or positions), and have them work for us, and then fire the ones who do not measure up to our standards. This, as it turns out, is really not very desirable because it is very expensive and most of us have neither the time nor the money to accept all applicants, train them, and then ask them to leave if they don't work out. What we then are forced to do is take measurements, like those Binet made, to obtain some estimate of the applicants' abilities to perform, and from these very short behavioral samples estimate how well they are going to perform in the system into which they propose to enter. To obtain measurements we must have a correlation. There must be a definite relationship between the measurements that we use and the performance on the task once the applicants are taken into the system. We have become a bit more sophisticated since Binet's time, although I might add that the test Binet devised is still used today and is called the Stanford-Binet. Recent statistical methods have enabled test designers to gain more information than formerly and a great many factors other than intelligence account for the tremendous range of individual differences among people. For example, Thurstone[10] argued that there are seven categories of measurable differences. These categories are: verbal comprehension, word fluency, number aptitude, inductive reasoning, memory, spatial aptitude, and perceptual speed. Other psychologists maintain that over sixty different traits can be measured by tests.

So far we have been concerned with mental skills and it is obvious to those who watch the golf classics or pro football that people also differ widely in motor skills. They differ, for example, in control precision, in reaction time, in finger dexterity, and in many other categories. Fleishman states that there are at least eleven different, identifiable motor skills that provide a range for individual differences:
1. control precision.
2. multilimb coordination.
3. response orientation.
4. reaction time.
5. speed of arm movement.
6. rate control.
7. manual dexterity.
8. finger dexterity.
9. arm-hand steadiness.
10. wrist-finger speed.
11. aiming.

The point demonstrated in the foregoing discussion is that these abilities can be measured and can be important to jobs and their performance. Thus, our ability to measure enables us to identify the individuals who are most likely to succeed in certain kinds of functions or jobs. That's not the whole story, however, because we still must determine what functions are important. All of us have been asked questions about our ability as we have applied for jobs only to say to ourselves, "but that isn't really important." A very simple question is one concerning height. Most of us have filled out application forms and have been asked: "How tall are you?" Also "How much do you weigh?" and "What is the color of your eyes?" Obviously these factors represent individual differences, but they have very little to do with ability to perform job-oriented tasks. The important point is to find out what properties of the job are important and then proceed to measure them.

The abilities that we have been discussing—verbal comprehension, word fluency, and motor skills—are what psychologist Lee Cronback[3] designates as maximum performance measures. That is, they are supposed to determine how well people perform these kinds of tasks. The psychologist and you, as administrators, must worry about another whole set of abilities in which people differ as individuals, and which are perhaps even more important to you. These are attitudes, interests, or personality. What is personality? Well, there are many definitions but one that we like to use is *"expectancy to behave in certain kinds of ways."* Cronback calls the measurements of attitude, interests, and personality *typical performance measures,* that is, measures of an individual's typical reaction to a particular kind of situation. This reaction is probably not solely a function of intelligence or motor skills. It is a function of attitudes, interests, and personality, developed as we have progressed and attained a certain age. Thus, individual differences can be thought of as being concerned with two different kinds of measurements: (1) measurement of maximum ability to perform certain kinds of skills and (2) measurement of typical performances of the behaviors in which all individuals vary, that is, personality, attitudes, interests, and the like. The problem, then, is how do you as an administrator select personnel, place them on the job, and then train them to take their proper place within the system. Another way of thinking of this problem is to consider the personnel problems in the system as constituting a personnel sub-system, complicated by a very complex problem, namely, that people differ from one another. In other words, you must cope with the problem of individual differences.

## PERSONNEL SELECTION

You must start by performing a job analysis. You cannot think of selection, placement, and training without first describing the job or defining the system task that needs to be done. To do this, you must analyze the job formally. A position is a group of tasks performed by one person. There are as many positions as there are workers. In other words, there is a position for each person within your long-term care facility. Each person holds a position. A *job* is a group of similar positions. For example, you may have several clerks in your office and many nurses or nurse's aides on your nursing floors. Each of these individuals holds a position; each has a different position, but together the nurses perform the job of nursing and the people in your office perform the job of clerk. An occupation is a number of allied jobs. Thus, we can speak of the position of typist within the job of clerk-typist and all of the office jobs—the job of clerk-typist, calculator operator, bookkeeper—fall within the occupation called "clerical." Job analysis refers to the procedures used to collect information about the nature and the conditions of work in a particular job. This analysis results in a job description that is the basis for many personnel decisions. First of all, the job itself is defined without reference to the worker who is going to perform that job. The job is defined in detail embracing a description of all of the functions the person doing that job would have to perform. You define exactly what must be done—make beds, clean rooms, bring in flowers, prepare vegetables, greet guests, clean floors, whatever. You define the job completely, and write it down.

After the job is defined you determine what *qualifications* an individual must possess if he is to perform this job in an adequate fashion. This results in a *worker description.* You then analyze the job description and from this create a worker description or worker specification. Each administrator should give serious consideration to the need for making job analyses and worker analyses and thereby formulate job descriptions and worker descriptions for each job in his facility. There are many reasons for doing this. First of all there is a lack of knowledge concerning jobs, because jobs are not constant, they change. You may start out with a certain job and a certain description, but within a very short time you will find that these jobs have changed. The product or service may be changed. That is, you may have a job description based on certain kinds of equipment. In the meantime, you replace that equipment and now the job is different. Employees themselves may enlarge on their duties or relinquish certain ones. They may even swap jobs and change them. Mary says to Jane: "I don't like this; would you mind doing it for me?" And Jane says: "No, I don't mind." As a result Jane is doing part of Mary's job and Mary annexes some part of Jane's job as compensation.

It is not easy to formulate a job description. Sitting behind a chair and guessing as to what the job entails is probably the worst way of doing it. Most people cannot do it adequately, the reason being that most jobs are quite complex, usually much more complex than we think.

Charters and Whitley[1] tried to discover the tasks that secretaries perform. There were 125 in the group studied. First of all, the secretaries were asked to record from memory all the tasks that their jobs entailed. The number found was 166. Then they were asked to keep a chart recording all of the tasks they performed over a period of a week. The number tabulated was 871—seven times that recalled from memory.

Another use for job and worker descriptions is the provision of common language for employment purposes. If you are calling an employment agency to help you find a particular employee, the more detail that you can furnish concerning the tasks which that individual is to perform the better the basis for the agency to react. If you have no specifications for the job, considerable confusion results.

In a study made by a milk-distributing company[2] the following question was asked: Are the delivery men who deliver milk door-to-door laborers, truck drivers, or salesmen? Job analysis showed that one-fourth of the men believed their job to be that of routine laborers. Another group felt that they were truck drivers. One third conceived of their job as that of salesmen. These men were all doing exactly the same thing—they were loading milk into the truck at the dairy and taking it out and delivering it to customers' homes throughout the city. The sales record of those who thought of themselves as salesmen was 80 percent higher than that of the other men. Clearly those who thought of their jobs as salesmen did the jobs of salesmen. As a result their record was much superior.

It is important to understand that people behave in the manner corresponding to their job description. If a man's job is described as that of a laborer and he believes it to be that of a laborer, he behaves as one. If he is convinced that he is a salesman, he will behave as salesman. As a result of their study, the milk company trained all of their route men to be salesmen. The sales of the company increased markedly as did the income of the men.

One of the aims of job and worker analyses is to develop measures of job proficiency. Using the job description as a base, one can develop means of measuring job success. Since all jobs within the system are related to one another, job descriptions provide you with some means of relating the various jobs functionally. Job descriptions can also be used to help set wage and salary scales. Also through them it is possible to improve your techniques for selecting new employees as well as to develop more effective methods of work. As you formulate a job description, you are very likely to note considerable waste. Many of the things people are doing aren't necessary or are being duplicated by someone else.

Where does one acquire the information necessary to do a detailed job analysis? The first thing, of course, is to observe the workers. This is one major source. Just because the worker does a job a particular way, however, does not mean that it is the way it has to be done. You must evaluate and choose, but certainly what the worker does is a basic source of information. Interviewing the workers in your facility is another source. Looking at the manuals, charts, and other material that they use quite often defines the job that they do and also provides descriptive insights. Finally, performing the job yourself is a good way to analyze it. In doing the job, you determine what the job actually requires of you. This then can be a good source of material for job analysis.

Having obtained a job description from your job analysis, it is then necessary to prepare a worker description. The function of worker analysis is to determine the *minimum requirement* for the job. We emphasize minimum rather than maximum. As soon as you set maximum requirements, you are perhaps setting requirements that are too high. This can mean that you are running the risk of hiring people who are overqualified for the job. A job can be overevaluated to the point where you are paying people too much to do something that is relatively simple. You should minimize the requirements for the job rather than maximize them.

The worker analysis should also indicate the relative importance of various traits, abilities, and the like, necessary to do the job. The worker description is estimated from your job description, plus your knowledge of what needs to be done. One of the most common dangers in preparing a worker description is that of tending to generalize too much, even to the point of being so nonspecific that the description is of little value. For example, if you say that a machinist requires manual dexterity, judgment, concentration, and the ability to plan, this is of no value because a cook requires the same kind of ability, so does a secretary. The machinist requires specific knowledge of certain machines which can be specified. The cook requires special knowledge of how to cook certain kinds of things. The minimum a cook should know how to do is to make gravy, even though gravy is a rather tricky thing to make. However, if a cook doesn't know how to make gravy, this means that he probably isn't a very good cook. Certainly, the knowledge of how to make gravy would provide the distinction between the machinist, the cook, and the secretary. Perhaps another minimum requirement for a cook would be the number of years of experience in this capacity.

Relatively recently in worker analysis, psychologists have been attempting to relate job requirements to specific behaviors. For example, instead of just stating the minimum requirements for a good secretary, you ask: "Who is the best secretary I ever had and how did she differ from the rest?" If you can define how she differed from the others, you are now setting specifications in detail for a secretary in your organization. Another way to put the question is: "Have you ever discharged a secretary?" If so, "Why?" If you discharged a secretary and can outline the reasons, these reasons will provide criteria of ability or performance that falls short of your minimum requirements. John Flanagan,[5] who developed the method known as the "critical incident technique," called those specific behaviors that have special meaning "critical incidents." In order to relate job requirements to specific behavior you must determine "critical incidents" for each job. What is the critical incident for a cashier? Some of you will say that it is the ability to count money quickly or the ability to add and subtract, but really the critical incident for a cashier is stealing; the critical requirement, honesty. You may have an employee who can add and subtract rapidly, but if he is not honest, he is not going to be a very good cashier.

Now let's assume that you have followed our advice and that you now have at your disposal job analyses and job descriptions, and a good worker analysis and worker description. These now define the system's positions that have to be filled. Most systems we talk about are operating and current, and therefore already have people working in them; however, tomorrow someone may leave and need to be replaced and hopefully your job description and worker description will be available to you. Thus, you can say: "O.K. Mrs. Smith has left us. She was a floor supervisor on the 3:00 to 11:00 shift and we are going to look for a replacement." You have the description and the minimum requirements of the job established. You place an ad in the paper, go to an agency, or ask your other employees if they know of anybody who could fill the position.

As people apply for the job you start acquiring information about them.

As mentioned previously, the information can be of two types. It can be acquired through typical performance measures, associated with attitudes, personality, and the like, and it can be gained by means of maximum performance measures, such as dexterity, word fluency, reaction time, and intelligence. What is the best way to obtain this information? One way, obviously, is to ask the prospective employee to fill out an application blank and report to you what he can do. At this point we would like to insert a word of caution. Most application blanks in existence are so long and wordy that they discourage applicants from the very beginning. You may remember applying for a simple job and being handed a three- or four-page application blank containing questions that seemed so farfetched as "How many teeth did your great grandmother have?" Look seriously at your worker description and your job description before making up an application blank. Then make sure that you are asking only for information that is relevant and important. How many brothers and sisters the person has probably has little relevance at all to his adequacy for your employment. His height and weight and most other related information have very little to do with it either. Certainly, color of hair, color of eyes, and similar characteristics do not affect his ability to perform. Look critically at each item and ask, "Do I really need to have that information?" You can probably eliminate many of the items if you examine the application blank critically.

You now have an application blank in front of you which you have created. It indicates, of course, that the person's name, address, and telephone number be given. Usually space will be provided for information concerning his education, previous places of employment, and what kind of jobs he has held. Probably inquiry will be made concerning how much money he earned in each of his previous jobs so that you can get some idea of the level of the positions that he has held. Based on the information gathered, you can begin to make a hiring decision. Most people, even though they could base their hiring decision on the information given in the application alone, will not hire someone at this point because of a very bad trait common to all of us. We all think that we are our own best psychologist. We want to see this individual who has applied and to talk to him. This involves conducting an interview. In spite of the fact that an interview is probably one of the poorest measuring devices that we can use—poorest in the sense of accuracy of measurement—we are not usually dissuaded from using it when we want to hire someone. It is a fact that generally we do not want to take someone into our system, the system we have nurtured and cared for and want to see flourish, without personally seeing and talking to the person. There is no question that the interview is used more frequently than any other single device or technique for personnel selection. An individual is seldom hired without having had one.

## The Interview

There are many kinds of interviews. The *unsystematic interview* is the kind of interview engaged in by most of us. It is casual and loosely organized. It is usually conducted on a spur-of-the-moment basis by someone who has worked his way up in the organization, who is dedicated, who likes people, who thinks he knows people, and who has pride in the organization—someone like ourselves perhaps. Don't conclude from these remarks that the interview is an unacceptable device; understand, rather, that placed in the hands of an inadequately trained, inexperienced person who doesn't use the proper procedural refinements, the interview cannot differentiate between individuals with high potential and those with low potential. In other words, there is no correlation between ranking based on a poor interview and performance on the job. Strong positive correlations can only be obtained if the interview can be systematized to increase the ability with which the interviewer manages to scale and rate a prospective employee.

We have introduced the word "systematic" as opposed to "unsystematic." "Patterned" is another word to use instead of "systematic." Systematic or patterned interviews have two essential characteristics: (1) they are planned in advance, and (2) the interviewers are technically proficient. Planning is necessary so that you can conduct the interview to collect the precise information with which you are concerned. You can't discover whether the individual fits your worker description if you ask, "Did you find it difficult to get here?" "What is your sister like?" "What did you do in high school?" or talk casually about world or local events. You must plan in advance to obtain the specific information desired. Needed information should evolve from the job and worker description that you have prepared ahead of time. You must have knowledge of the job to be filled and some notion of the worker performances on this job in order to understand the behaviors required by the job. You have to determine what information can best be obtained through the interview and what can best be obtained through other means. It makes no sense to ask the applicant how tall he is and what his education has been if that information has been given on his job application. The interview should be reserved for the special kinds of information obtainable only "on the spot." The interview actually is a performance sample. The individual you are thinking of bringing into your system, to do a certain kind of job, is sitting across the desk from you, or beside you on the sofa, perhaps sipping a cup of coffee. He is there behaving and you are collecting a sample, a very small sample, of his behavior. You want that sample to be the very best sample that you can possibly obtain and you want it to be related to the job that this person is going to do for you. Although you may find him charming and handsome, and observe that he uses good English and is capable of relating incidents well, he may be an incompetent worker at the job under consideration. You want to use this interview to obtain a sample of the kind of behavior that you expect of him when he is performing the job.

Now where does the technical training of the interviewer come in? First of all, we must counter the interviewer's bias. Each of us as individuals has certain attitudes, certain notions concerning people which are our biases. We may like redheads, we may like blondes; the various joke magazines are full of stories about why a certain secretary is hired and another is not. We all have some preconceived notions about certain types of individuals and their capabilities. We must somehow, as interviewers, make certain that we are objective and get rid of these biases. Another thing we must do is to make sure that the applicant is giving us information that we need and want. We can only do this to the extent that the individual being interviewed has confidence in the interviewer. The owners or managers of an organization are the toughest interviewers and probably the poorest. They tend to say: "What can you offer me? I am the boss here. I run this show. You show me what you can do for me." You must remember that the person being interviewed is probably scared stiff. You must motivate him to want to give you the kind of information that will help you decide whether or not to employ him. Pompousness or "standoffishnish," or making sure that he understands that you are the one in authority may not help at all. It may be that he is a very capable potential worker, but your attitude inhibits him. The manner in which the questions are asked can change his response. Remember that you are getting a sample of behavior and you want that sample to be as constant as possible. The nature of the questions asked, the arrangements of the questions asked, are they going from the general to the more specific or the other way around?

Not just anyone can be trained to interview, but most people can, particularly if they are willing to look at the person being interviewed as a human being who perhaps needs help, counsel, and assurance. One of the key functions of an interviewer is not to determine whether the potential employee is the person he wants, but rather to convince the applicant that the job or position is a desirable one for him.

To illustrate that the interview is at best a very difficult device and not a very good device for measuring performance, we describe a study reported by Hollingworth.[8]

Twelve sales managers (A, B, C, D, E, F, G, H, I, J, K, and L) of a rather large company independently interviewed 57 applicants for the job of salesman. Each sales manager ranked the 57 applicants from best to poorest on the scale of 1 to 57, 57 being the poorest. Table 1 shows the lack of agreement among the sales managers in respect to estimating an applicant's potentialities for filling the position. One applicant was ranked 53 by sales

Table 1. Rankings of 4 out of 57 applicants by each of 12 sales managers[a]

| Applicants | Sales Managers | | | | | | | | | | | |
|---|---|---|---|---|---|---|---|---|---|---|---|---|
| | A | B | C | D | E | F | G | H | I | J | K | L |
| I | 53 | 10 | 6 | 21 | 16 | 9 | 20 | 2 | 26 | 28 | 1 | 57 |
| II | 33 | 46 | 6 | 56 | 26 | 32 | 12 | 38 | 9 | 22 | 22 | 23 |
| III | 54 | 41 | 33 | 19 | 28 | 48 | 8 | 10 | 26 | 8 | 19 | 56 |
| IV | 43 | 11 | 13 | 11 | 37 | 40 | 36 | 46 | 1 | 15 | 29 | 25 |

[a]From Hollingworth, 1922.

manager A, 10 by sales manager B, 6 by sales manager C, 21 by sales manager D, 16 by E, 9 by F, 20 by G, 2 by H, 26 by I, 28 by J, 1 by K, and 57 by L. All the sales managers were professionals working in the same company, and supposedly all worked toward the same system goals. The fact that they arrived at data such as this demonstrates that the unsystematic interview has a reliability far lower than that which personnel officers generally attribute to it and, therefore, is not valid. By examining the sources of error in an interview, however, we know that you can improve the interview quite considerably.

**Interview Errors**

There are three principal sources of error in the interview: (1) the applicant, (2) the interviewer, and (3) the interview procedure and setting. Let's look at each of these briefly.

First of all, the applicant is not constant day by day or hour by hour. You are not, why should he be? He changes. You may have gotten him at a bad moment in time. The change in his mood is reflected in the change in his behavior. In other words, he is not a constant reactor. The interview situation itself may introduce variations that result in nonrepresentative performance. The applicant can give faulty or inaccurate information, resulting in inaccurate assessment. One way of eliminating this source of error is to have the applicant interviewed by more than one person. Also information can be gained from other sources. The applicant's arithmetic ability can be obtained from a test. His school grades can be obtained from his high school transcript. One of the keys to securing accurate information is to motivate the applicant to give good answers.

The interviewer is also a source of error. One person may see certain qualities not observed by others. An incomplete picture is attained by one person operating with his own set of biases. The point here is that each interviewer operating with his own set of biases and also using his own set of techniques obtains a very small sample of behavior. The solution to this problem also is multiple interviewing. The errors of interviewee and the interviewer both can be corrected substantially by using multiple interviews. You may feel that it is expensive and time-consuming to have more than one interviewer. Remember, however, that to take an employee into your system and then have him leave that system after a brief stay is also a very expensive operation, costing at least several hundred dollars. It should not be difficult to find another person or perhaps, hopefully, two other people beside yourself to interview a prospective employee. After talking to the applicant you could say, "I would like to have you meet and talk to the nursing supervisor on the floor where you will work if hired." Following this you could arrange an interview with the business manager. Thus, three samples of behavior have been obtained. By combining the three views you can reach a conclusion—a much wiser conclusion than you could reach alone.

We have discussed the interview procedure earlier, but must mention here the setting for the interview. The interview setting should be comfortable, and every attempt should be made to make the interviewee feel welcome and natural. Again the emphasis must be that you want this sample of behavior to be the most realistic sample you can obtain. We have seen amateur interviewers deliberately shine their desk lamp on the interviewees face, as if he were being "questioned" or the venetian blind arranged in a manner to let the sun shine in the interviewee's eyes to determine how he would react. Such nonsense should be avoided along with any other gimmicks. The interview is not a game. It should be a direct straightforward attempt by two people to understand each other and the job in question.

It is important to make sure that you understand several things about interviewing. Interviewing is something we are all going to do; but, without training and pre-planning, and without some systematization, the interview is worthless. You might just as well play pinochle with the job applicant. It is important to systematize your interview, have multiple interviews, and train your interviewers so that the reliability and the validity of the interview procedure can be improved.

### Testing

Interviewing cannot provide all the data needed on everyone to be hired even though some of the tasks in the system require relatively low skills and some of the highly skilled jobs such as nursing are difficult to fill. Formalization of the measurement of certain individual differences and certain skills can be of value.

One means for measurement of various skills and aptitudes of individuals is psychological testing. Of all the instruments devised by psychologists, tests clearly are the most refined. The process has many advantages: it is amenable to objective investigation; we have a lot of knowledge concerning it; it is administratively superior to interviews; and it doesn't require highly trained personnel for its administration. Also, the results of tests usually do not reflect the personal biases of the interview; thus, they are relatively bias free. Although subject to a lot of controversy, the type of bias we are discussing is generally eliminated from most tests. Being objective, they are usually quantitative and therefore can be compared. It is easy to score Sam 100 on a test and Joe 120, but it is much more difficult score Sam 100 on the interview and Joe 120 and assign meaning to these values. Tests can make a significant contribution to the problem of worker selection, placement, and adjustment. They, like interviews, are behavior samples, but are highly controlled behavior samples. Psychologists, in developing the tests, have decided in advance what portion of behavior they wish to sample. They experiment again and again, with arriving at different methods of sampling. As a result, tests have become very sophisticated. They are really samples or short cuts to observing the behavior of the individual in an organization.

Referring to Figure 1, the X axis represents any test scored from 0 to 100. If the X axis is an independent measure of performance, we would like to be able to say that the person who has scored high on the test will score

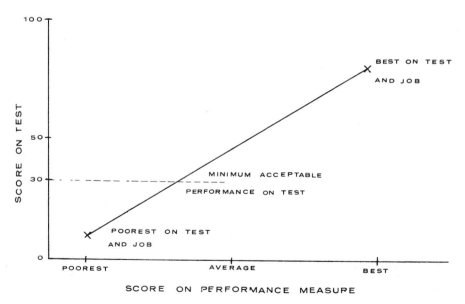

Figure 1. Ideal relationship between test score and measure of job performance.

high on the performance measure, and that the one who scores low on the test will score low on performance. By establishing a cut-off, say at 30 or 40 on the test, we can eliminate all the low performers.

We don't expect all administrators to become test experts; but, we do feel that there are some tests that you can use—and use wisely—even though you may have relatively small organizations. Tests evaluate several different things. As mentioned earlier, there are the typical performance measures to evaluate personality, attitudes, and the like, and there are maximum performance measures to ascertain how much of a particular skill an individual possesses. Let us first discuss measurement of skills.

One of the attributes that you, as a manager, ought to be interested in is intelligence. For a great many jobs, particularly the higher level ones in your organization, you would probably want to hire the most intelligent applicant. As a basic guide to determine intelligence, we recommend the Wonderlic Personnel Test—a fifteen-minute, group intelligence test. You can give it very easily and score it yourself. Tests for many abilities such as clerical aptitude and mechanical aptitude are readily available; these can be easily administered through your own offices, through some arrangement with a personnel organization, or through the state employment agency. Before you hire a clerk there is no reason why you shouldn't have scores from the Minnesota Clerical or the Aurora Clerical Aptitude Tests available to you. If you are hiring someone who is to be a repair or maintenance man, or if you are to train this man yourself, there is no reason why you couldn't use a Bennett Mechanical Aptitude Test administered through the State Employment service or some other suitable agency.

The other large area of testing that you must be concerned with is personality. Personality tests come under the category of typical performance measures discussed earlier. The determination of attitudes or what motivates an individual is perhaps the most difficult area to measure. The results of testing personality traits are less accurate than those of intelligence or aptitude because of problems of defining personality and also because it is possible for the individual taking the test to make erroneous answers to influence the tester. For these and other reasons, personality tests are of less value to you than other types of tests and yet the area that they examine is the very one in which you have tremendous needs for information. One of the tests that you might investigate because it is less subject to the errors described than many of the others is the Strong Vocational Interest Inventory. This is a test that provides an insight into a person's sets of interests and identifies him with others who have similar interests. Quite often you will find that what holds a person in a job is that his interests are like those of everyone else in the organization. And if he identifies closely with the kind of work that is being performed, he will tend to continue in this work and to remain with the organization.

## TRAINING

Now that the new employee has entered into your system through the selection process, it becomes essential to train him in order to obtain from him maximum efficiency in the performance of the various functions required by his job. Training is a necessity. It involves guidance in learning changing techniques as well in improving present methods of performance. The worker must, for example, be trained in the areas of nursing, safety, cost control, or other phases of your operation.

### Tangible Results

What would some of the tangible results of training be? You can experience a reduction of waste and spoilage in your operation. In other words, those spoilages or wastes that could result from carelessness, indifference, or perhaps even improper methods can be corrected through proper training. You may even find that method and system improvement could be a very tangible result of a training program. Well-trained workers will generally volunteer suggestions for improvement.

*Reduction of Absenteeism and Labor Turnover.* Absenteeism and labor turnover usually arise from dissatisfaction of employees. As dissatisfaction is reduced when employees are properly trained so are absenteeism and turnover.

*Reduction of Supervisory Burden.* Adequate training can in one way or other reduce the supervisory time needed for subordinates because once trained these people can perform capably on their own. Employees recognize the direct relationship between the maintenance of quality and job security.

*Reduction of Accident Rate.* When you train in the area of safety there can be a very tangible pay-off in the reduction of the number of accidents sustained by employees.

*Increased Productivity.* Increased productivity is, of course, what we are all seeking in our particular institutions. The employee will give more effort, more of his time, more of his dedication, if he is well-trained.

### Steps to Improve Quality of Training

In the process of training the individual, there are certain steps that can be executed to improve the quality of training.

Step 1: *Prepare the worker.* That is, you should put him at ease and find out what he already knows about the job. It may be that, in the selection process, you may have determined that this individual has a certain level of competency that you may build upon. Explain to him what the function is and what is expected of him.

Step 2: *Present the operation.* Present each step in a logical sequence and stress and explain each key point. Demonstrate slowly one step at a time and allow the worker to ask questions in order that you might check his understanding.

Step 3: *Try out performance.* Have the worker do the job, telling him what he is doing. Observe his performance and correct his errors. Repeat his training if necessary. Question him to check his understanding. Then, continue the performance until you are convinced that he has mastered it.

Step 4: *Follow-up.* In this particular step put the worker on his own. Be specific in what you expect him to do. Be sure to designate to whom he should go for help, and then check frequently. One final word about follow-up: keep in mind that follow-up is not something you perform once and then forget. Follow-up is an essential and continuous part of the training procedure.

## Basic Elements of Program

A suggested pattern for spelling out the basic elements of a training program is as follows.

First: *Objectives.* What are the end results that you expect from training based on the analysis of training needs? The needs may be stated in terms of the number of jobs to be improved or the number of workers to be prepared to fill vacancies in designated positions.

Second: *Scope of the program.* What are the different positions for which training will be given? Give the approximate time in hours, for example, for an average employee to complete the prescribed training for a specific position.

Third: *Administration.* What are the training responsibilities of each person having a part in the direction and conduct of the training? Provide an outline of instruction. What are the work jobs and the lessons or courses of job information that are included in the course of instruction for each position? What factors are you going to consider in selecting employees for training? Who will select them? How do you determine the order in which they shall be trained? How and where will instruction be presented? Who will instruct? During what period of the day will the instruction be given? How will employees be relieved of their work load while in training? What is your policy governing the wages of the employee while in training? How will the progress of the trainees be recorded? Who will maintain the records? What reports will be prepared and who will prepare them? To whom will the training reports be sent? And, finally, what yardstick will you use to determine what performance level the trainee has attained? What procedures and means are available for measuring the degree to which workers are successful in the job? You need standards of accomplishment, some index or yardstick with which the success of workers can be gauged. Standards should be quantitative whenever possible in order to evaluate performance objectively.

## PERFORMANCE EVALUATION

Some means of evaluating worker performance is essential. In reality you are evaluating performance all the time. You discuss certain workers and their jobs with your chief assistant, or, perhaps, you confer with the cook regarding the performance of the kitchen helpers. However, what we are suggesting is that you formalize this evaluation in order that it will be of greater use to you.

There are several different kinds of evaluations of performance or proficiency measures. Some have only limited value while others share a rather wide range of usefulness. Among the latter are the amount and quality of production, and work sample tests. Length of service is a fine but often overlooked means of evaluating proficiency. The amount of training necessary to achieve a certain standard provides a good measure of performance. Ratings by supervisors is perhaps the most common means. Others which you might be interested in, of course, are accidents, the number of complaints by patients or by fellow workers, the accuracy of work that is critical (for example, handling drugs and the like), and neatness, which also is critical in a social-service type of operation.

Let's look at production first. This is perhaps the most common and probably the best single measure of performance. Although it lends itself particularly well to an organization in which "things" are being produced, it might be difficult to assess in some of your operations. In the kitchen, however, it is possible to employ production or output as a means for evaluating performance. The output of dishwashers, food preparers, and other workers could be measured. Wherever there is a set amount of work to be done within a given time, output or actual number of items produced or the time required can be used as a measure of performance. Care must be taken to determine quality as well as quantity of production. In a typing test, for example, it is customary to exact a penalty for errors by deducting the number of errors made from the word-per-minute achievement. With a little ingenuity, it is possible to measure performance in some of the more routine, repeatable kinds of tasks carried out within a nursing home operation. The simple recording of how long it takes a man to mop the floor, for example, is a measure of performance.

Another performance measure is a work sample test. This is relatively simple and yet it is often overlooked. Accurate measurements are made while the worker performs exactly the same tasks as on the job but under a standard set of conditions. Typing provides an example. The typist to be tested is removed from his job, given a work sample to type, and the number of words typed per minute is recorded. In a work sample test the performance of the person tested is compared with a standard that you would like to achieve.

Length of service is another important and valuable performance measurement, although its standards aren't quite as apparent as those of other measurements. The capacity of the individual to continue his work within the system is a very good indication of success on the job, incidently providing a bonus of saving the expense of hiring and training a replacement. Generally, the fact that the person has stayed on the job for some time reflects (1) his ability to adjust to the conditions of work, (2) his ability to get along with his fellow workers, (3) his obvious satisfaction with the job, and (4) his ability to do the job because, if he were incapable, you would have fired him. As time goes on he is certain to continue to develop skills, and thus increase his value to the system and his own satisfaction with the job. Therefore, it is strongly suggested that serious consideration be given to length of service as a measure of job performance or job success.

One of the most commonly used measures is a rating scale. This is a form of personal appraisal. At some time all of us become involved in evaluating the individual. We say, "I don't like Joe's work as well as Steve's," or "Elsie works better than Susan." In a sense this kind of personal estimate is a ranking or a rating of an individual based on some evaluation or observation that you have made of his work performance. Personal estimates such as these are needed in solving many of your personnel problems, but rating methods will enable you to formalize the procedures for obtaining these personal estimates, making them more accurate and thus more valuable. Essentially, personal estimates are expressions of the ideas of the rater. Since ratings are nothing more than opinions, they are subject to all the human errors of judgment—the biases and the inappropriate attitudes that all of us possess. The task for the industrial psychologist is to help in making these expressions of opinion, which are very important and are very real, more valid by reducing some of the sources of error. Let's look at some of these errors. There are two key ones—constant errors and leniency errors.

Before discussing these errors, let us describe the rating scale and the qualities to be rated. Normally, in rating, a series of descriptions is established and then some sort of scale is made for each of these. For example, say that you want to rate a group of individuals on the description "loyalty to organization." The rating scale may be set as numerals 1 through 5, where 1 is high and 5 is low. Or it may be comprised of adjectives, such as superior, above average, average, below average, and inferior. In either case, you have a continuum from high to low. The rating scale need not be confined to five items; it may be extended to seven if you prefer; however, it has been generally agreed that, unless the raters are experts, more than five or seven items will make the rating task more difficult. Also the number of items should always be odd, so that you have a mid-point. Usually individuals are rated on a set of allied traits. In addition to loyalty, you might add promptness, ability to get along with fellow workers, efficiency, and ability to adjust to change. The rating scales (numerals or adjectives) may head columns, placed at the top of a sheet of paper, with the descriptions listed beneath one another at the left; or the descriptions may head the columns with the rating scales listed at the left. The rater places check marks in the columns according to his evaluation of the person being tested.

Now let us return to the subject of key errors. The *leniency* or halo error is made because one overall general impression can control the rating on all the specific items. The halo effect is the tendency to rank an individual high in all items just because he is rated high in a particular one. For example, if the individual is attractive and pleasing visually, then it might be that the person doing the rating will be overly impressed and proceed to rank the individual high in every item. A particular supervisor happens to be concerned about promptness. Tardiness, even if only of a few minutes, really bothers him. It could very easily happen that this supervisor would rate an efficient employee, who occasionally is late in arriving at work, low on all items evaluated. This also is the halo error. The *constant* error is often made because the rater does not want to commit himself, and as a result ranks everyone in the middle range. This avoids having to give any very high or very low ranks. Also, to avoid unpleasantness in discussion with employees about their ratings, the tendency is to give all a high rank. When everybody is ranked high, no one is unhappy, unless, of course, there comes a time when an employee has to be told that his work is unsatisfactory. Then it might be pointed out that not everyone is perfect or average. The employee might be told that, for everyone who is ranked above the middle, someone is ranked below it.

There are means to overcome, at least partially, the key errors. One consists in having ratings made by more than one person. This avoids the individual biases responsible for the halo effect. Another technique is to set up a different series of numbers for each description; for example, for loyalty, 1–2–3–4–5; for promptness, 5–4–3–2–1; and for ability, 1–5–3–4–2. This rearrangement of the scales forces the rater to consider each employee individually in regard to each item on the list.

Another type of rating system consists of comparison of employees—ranking the best employee number one and on down to the poorest employee.

Many descriptive arrangements are available and perhaps the best thing to do is to make certain that, as you go through evaluation of performance, consideration is given to such generalities as loyalty and promptness as well as to specific examples of behavior. If you think that a person is loyal or disloyal, you must have some basis for this and that basis must be the behavior of the individual. If you rank a person high on loyalty, the question to ask is, "What did that person do that makes me feel that he is loyal?" Similarly, if you rank him low on promptness, you ask, "What did he do, or what was the critical incident that led me to the conclusion that he should be ranked low on this item?" In this way, you start collecting samples of behavior as the basis for making appropriate determinations. It is important to remember that it is real behavior that you are concerned with and not just random opinion.

## REFERENCES

1. Charters, W. W., and I. B. Whitley. 1955. Analysis of secretarial duties and traits. As reported in Ghiselli, E. E., and Brown, C. W. Personnel and industrial psychology. McGraw-Hill Book Company, New York.
2. Colby, L. B. As reported in Ghiselli, E. E., and Brown, C. W. 1955. Personnel and industrial psychology. McGraw-Hill Book Company, New York.
3. Cronback, L. J. 1960. Essentials of psychological testing. 2nd Ed. Harper and Row, New York.
4. Dunnette, M. D. 1966. Personnel selection and placement. Wadsworth Publishing Co., Belmont, Calif.
5. Flanagan, J. C. 1949. Critical requirements: a new approach to employee evaluation. Personnel Psych. 2: 419–425.
6. Fleishman, E. A. 1962. The description and prediction of perceptual motor skill learning. *In* Glaser, R. (ed.) Training research and education. University of Pittsburgh, Pittsburgh.
7. Gagne, R. M. 1962. Human functions in systems. In Gagne, R. M. *et al.* Psychological principles in system development. Holt Rinehart and Winston.
8. Hollingworth, H. L. 1955. As reported in Ghiselli, E. E. and Brown, C. W. Personnel and industrial psychology. McGraw-Hill Book Company, New York.
9. Kennedy, J. L. 1962. Psychology and system development. In Gagne, R. M. *et al.* Psychological principles in system development. Holt Rinehart and Winston.
10. Thurstone, L. L. 1966. As cited in Dunette, M. D. Personnel selection and placement. Wadsworth Publishing Co.

# The Management Process

## P. Cayan and S. Davis

3 The management process consists of four fundamental functions. The first is *planning.* Planning is an attempt to determine the objectives and the courses of action to be followed in carrying out the various functions within the nursing home. The second is *organizing.* This particular function concerns the distribution of work within the home and the establishment and recognition of the needed authority in order that the organization may exist as a system; that is, the concern is who is going to do what and with how much authority. The third fundamental function is *actuating.* Here the primary concern is with a true human relations approach to the various problems. You, as an administrator, must somehow cause your employees to carry out their assigned task. *Measuring* is the fourth function. This involves making certain the various objectives that you have established for your nursing home are achieved. You must be sure that your activities are directed in such a way as to gain or achieve particular objectives.

The four managerial functions are performed in relation to the technical functions of the institution such as housekeeping, personnel, accounting, purchasing, and the like. They are also performed in relation to the people who perform these particular technical functions. Each administrator in a sense is a two-headed creature. He must be able to plan, organize, actuate, and control, and he must also be an expert in working with people. To fulfill his obligation the following factors must be given careful consideration. The administrator must first of all have a philosophy—a basic guide that underlies all of his actions in the administrative capacity. What does he believe? For example, what is the justification for the existence of his particular business or institution? What does he think about his subordinates as people, and what ethics and ideals guide him in making the various decisions with which he is going to be confronted? Second, he must have objectives—goals to be obtained by his particular nursing home. His nursing home must provide a worthwhile service to its guests and to its employees. There must be satisfactory monetary and nonfinancial rewards. He is obligated to supply a service to the community. Each part of the institution must contribute in some way to the attainment of the objectives or goals of the institution in its entirety. Third, there are the set of activities engaged in to attain these particular objectives. While many activities are involved, the provision of financial services is of primary importance along with acquiring, developing, maintaining, and utilizing personnel.

There are certain terms with which you should become familiar before pursuing the area of administrative process any further. (1) *Responsibility:* This involves the basic relationships that are pertinent to how well you perform as an administrator. When one says that a person is responsible for some function, what he really means is that the person or subordinate has an obligation to perform a particular function, which has been assigned to him, to the best of his ability. In the nursing home, all segments of the personnel sub-system have responsibilities: the administrator, the employee, the patient, and the owners. (2) *Authority:* Authority is the right to act or to take action of some kind or to require others to act for you. It should be kept in mind that the concept of authority is derived from responsibility defined above. (3) *Accountability:* This is the requirement to answer for or be accountable for a particular performance—that which flows upward from the subordinate to his immediate supervisor or superior.

Responsibility can be thought of as the cement or the glue that holds together the various aspects of a managerial process as we know it. We stated that authority is the right to act or the right to command someone else to act. Authority is really the basis for responsibility and a very essential binding force in the organization structure. Since administrators must work through people to get things done, management theory is necessarily concerned with superior-subordinate relationships. This relationship is based on the concept of authority. The authority invested in a managerial or administrative position is the power to use *discretion,* the power to create and maintain an environment for the performance of the work of the individual and of groups. The true notion of authority is not an autocratic use of power as we know it. Authority can be delegated. This means that you, as an administrator, turn over various aspects of your particular jurisdiction to your subordinates. You let the subordinates do the work for which they were essentially hired.

*The first task of the administrator in delegating his authority is to overcome his reluctance to delegate.* Carrying delegation to an extreme is undesirable; on the other hand, refusing to delegate eventually weakens the administrator as well as his subordinates. Subordinates will never develop to the level of competency that they should unless given responsibility and its accompanying authority. Growth of the individual employee is, after all, one of the primary responsibilities of the administrator. The administrator will often fail to delegate because he doesn't trust his subordinates. He is afraid that they will fail him. This really is an indirect criticism of himself as an administrator. If the administrator spends adequate time in his managerial function of organizing he will have selected and trained a dependable team of subordinates. He will then be able to delegate authority with confidence. Certain administrators may refuse to delegate because it gives them a feeling of superiority to do certain technical jobs themselves, with the result that the subordinates will not have the necessary opportunity or chance to experience growth. Finally, some administrators refuse to delegate because they may fear that their subordinates will become a threat to their security. When administrators, for whatever reason, fail to delegate authority and to share responsibility, everyone suffers.

## ACCEPTANCE OF AUTHORITY

Let us now look at those subordinates to whom you are delegating authority and sharing responsibility. Often subordinates are reluctant to accept authority even though you may be most desirous of delegating and sharing it with them. Unless this particular reluctance is reduced, an administrator will find himself doing the work of others whether he wants to or not. The initial step in removing the reluctance of subordinates is to make certain that they are not avoiding authority because they feel they are incapable of handling it. Perhaps, in such a case, replacement with capable or trainable personnel will be necessary. Assuming, however, that subordinates have the actual potential ability to accept authority, why then are they reluctant to accept it and how may this reluctance be overcome? The key explanation is a lack of confidence accompanied by a fear of failure. A subordinate thinks that he cannot do the job expected of him and may have to pay the penalty of failure. He therefore finds some way of evading or ignoring the authority that is being delegated to him. Subordinates, particularly at lower levels, may refuse authority because they do not wish to lose seniority privileges or the associations of present friends. There is a cohesion between themselves and the people in the various groups within which they work. Finally, subordinates may be unwilling to accept authority because they lack confidence in their superiors. Your subordinates may have seen in the past that the administrator has issued ambiguous orders or played favorites or has even looked for a scapegoat for his own mistakes.

As we continue the discussion of the concept of delegation of authority and sharing of responsibility, there are certain key points to be enumerated that may help. Think of answers to the following: Do you and your subordinates agree in what results are expected of you? And of them? Do you and your subordinates agree on some measures of performance? What type of performance appraisal do you have in your particular institution? Does the subordinate feel that he has sufficient authority to go with the responsibility that you have given him? What more does each of your subordinates think should be delegated to him? How can you best improve your ability to delegate and share responsibility? What really interferes with the effective use of your management time as you relate it to your subordinates? Does it take more time to explain and train than it does to do the job yourself? Honest answers to these questions may put you in a better frame of mind to be willing to delegate responsibility and authority.

## THE PROCESS OF MAKING A DECISION

Everyone makes many decisions during the course of a day; and, yet, most of us do not really understand what actually goes into making a decision. For the administrator the decisions could relate, for example, to a nursing situation, the hiring of a new employee, or relationships with the community. Regardless of the kind of decision, we don't understand the operations that come into play when we make decisions. We should start out (in looking at the decision-making process) with the idea that we have a situation which we will identify by the letter S. Anytime that we are confronted by a particular problem that needs a deciding factor, we will discover that there are before us perhaps several alternatives, any one of which may at the moment seem to be the proper alternative upon which we will base our decision. Identify the alternatives as $S_1$, $S_2$, $S_3$, $S_4$, $S_5$, and $S_6$. Every time we are confronted with a decision to be made, we may not have this number of alternatives. In some instances we may have more and in others less. Whenever we attempt to make a decision, we are really predicting the various outcomes—however many there may be—of the various alternatives with which we are confronted. Alternative number one may have two particular outcomes (i.e., if we were to choose a particular alternative we could conceivably have two situations as a result of choosing that particular route). Alternative number three may conceivably result in four predictable outcomes. The decision-making process really is one of prediction as we estimate various possible outcomes. We will choose the one that we think to be the most favorable and this then becomes our decision. Every time we make a decision, whether it be major or minor, we go through this particular mechanism.

A further exploration of the decision-making process shows that there are certain constraints or restraints placed upon attempts to make decisions. Quite commonly, it is found the financial position of the institution prevents the administrator from making a particular decision. It may be found that a particular decision will establish a precedent that may, in the future, eventuate in a serious situation. Also, the government imposes certain restrictions, through various regulatory agencies, that can be constraining in the administration or management process.

Although making decisions is not always easy, the process does not necessarily involve a tremendous amount of anguish. Here are some guides.

1. Make a distinction between the major and minor problems and attempt to equalize the time spent in resolving both.
2. Delegate or share problems with your subordinates thus making the subordinates part of the decision-making process.
3. Place more reliance on the use of policy guides that can help in relating to the achievement of the objectives or goals of the institution in question. Those problems tending to be routine can certainly be taken care of by the establishment of written policy. Thus the administration is not involved in the constant rehashing of a particular problem week in and week out or month in and month out. Policy can save much work.
4. Make use of consultants and of others through resource material. By this means, the thinking power of other people in other institutions can be employed. One administrator doesn't know all the answers and he should admit this to himself and recognize it early, and make use of the other human resources that he has at his disposal. He should not try to anticipate all eventualities. This just cannot be humanly possible in many cases.
5. Do not expect to be right all the time. This, also, is not humanly possible in many situations. The important thing is to recognize that a decision has to be made and that there is a certain time limit within which it can be made. Don't procrastinate; decide now and free your mind of it.
6. After you have made your decision, don't worry about it. If there is something seriously wrong, you will find out soon enough and can adjust at that time.

### Policy

The need for a written policy was stated in the preceding paragraph. Policies fall into two general categories—broad and specific. In a nursing home, broad policies are established to keep up with the latest developments in the nursing home field so that high-quality care can be provided. Specific policies that specify a certain set of conditions in the performing of the functions within the specific nursing home are needed. The formulation of policies can be shared with subordinates, but the ultimate responsibility for policy formulation rests with the administrator. It is not sufficient to establish policies and then forget about them. From time to time policies must be reviewed and kept up to date. Circumstances may require changes. Constant planning and awareness of the need for change are required.

### Planning

Planning requires a great deal of imagination and is vital to success. What are the values of planning? What can planning do for the administrator? Proper planning will help put things in perspective. It will help to eliminate on-the-spot decisions that are often weak decisions. Proper planning allows the administrator time to iron out many potential wrinkles that he may be experiencing in a particular operation. Well-thought-out plans can be delegated, i.e., can be handed down to subordinates. Planning really provides the basis for control in institutions. The better the planning the better the control. As a manager of a nursing home the administrator must deal with the establishment of many goals and the achievement of many objectives that require planning. The results of good planning are evidenced by orderliness, informed employees, spirit, and adequate productivity.

**Problem-Solving**
One of the key tasks of an administrator is to solve the myriad problems that arise daily. We feel that there is a means for approaching problem-solving that is better than most other methods. Because the approach resembles the means used by scientists in solving the problems of science, it has been dubbed "the scientific method." This does not mean that we are applying any particular scientific knowledge or laboratory techniques to problem-solving. The scientific method is really a process of seeing and approaching problems. Perhaps it should be viewed as an approach, or an attitude, to the development of the inquiring mind.

The successful use of the scientific method requires that one wants his organization to progress. In other words, there must be a constant search to *improve* the operation of a specific institution. It is never possible to attain perfect administration of a nursing home, but we believe that many of the performance errors in the administration of a facility can be discovered and perhaps a much more efficient operation can be achieved if one can learn to solve problems in an efficient, realistic way.

The scientific method uses certain steps that are applied to a particular problem. The first step is *identification of the problem.* The problem must be mentally defined and the entire investigation pointed toward this definition. The second step involves *acquiring some preliminary observations* concerning the problem. At this point the administrator should ask himself: Is there some *pertinent knowledge in existence that I can relate* to this problem at this time? This is somewhat of an exploratory step. The whole question of what has been done in the past and what results were found may very well come into play at this point. You can ask: Has this problem occurred before? If so, how did I or someone else approach it? Is there any knowledge or information in existence that I can bring into play to help me to solve this problem? At this point then, a tentative solution to the problem should be stated, using the knowledge that exists as a result of previous problem solutions. What you are doing is *establishing a hypothesis* or an educated guess about the problem and the solution that you are going to attempt to apply. The next step that must be performed is that of *investigating this hypothesis* thoroughly, using all of the knowledge that you have and any experimentation that you feel that you can bring into play. Ask yourself the question: What is the degree of relationship between the available information and this hypothesis or educated guess? The next step is to *classify the data* obtained. In some cases the quantity of information could be enormous and it is essential at this point that in some way it be pulled together so that you can perceive if there are any patterns in the data. From an examination of the data, you can state *another tentative solution* to your problem, only this time hopefully, your solution is a better one; at least, it is based on a more complete examination of the information available. This last step can be repeated as many times as necessary to achieve confidence in the solution.

## THE ORGANIZATIONAL ENVIRONMENT
The organizational environment in which the employee works is our next concern. Here we take a look at the employees' opinions and attitudes about their company; we will be concerned with employee morale, team spirit, and the like. Instead of thinking about individual differences, we will be thinking about organizational differences. The reason for this is that human beings *interact;* they relate to one another, and, in so doing, they form social structures that have certain psychological and sociological properties. This, in turn, affects the individual's attitudes and performance. There is a social psychology of the work organization that is important and influential in determining the total work output of the organization. Organizations, therefore, not only differ in their physical structure, in their size, and in their methods of management, but they also differ in terms of the attitudes and the behavior they bring about in the individuals who work within them. To state this simply, some people like where they work, *perhaps even for the same reasons* that others dislike it. The reasons given usually have something to do with what's called the *organizational climate*.

Organizational climate, according to one industrial psychologist, is made up of those characteristics that distinguish one organization from another. Certain companies for example are able to retain their employees better than others. In this case the description of the differences between the companies is based on their ability to retain employees rather than on what they produced. This is one way of looking at climate. If employees are easily persuaded to leave an organization to join another, then one wonders what kind of climate exists in the organization that permits people to be attracted from it so readily. Climate is what one reacts to in an organization. "It is the whole context of stimulation and confusion where we work."[3] You might even think of climate as the personality of the company.

There have been numerous attempts to categorize or define the personality of a company. Usually, these involve defining the leadership and the people within the company; for example, if one wants to look at the climate of an organization, it may be necessary to identify the men in the organization whose attitudes count and then determine their goals. Presthus[4] talks about organizations differing in climate based on the number of *upward mobiles, indifferents,* and *ambivalents* in an organization. He uses these terms to characterize the key people within an organization. By looking at what Presthus describes as an upward mobile, an indifferent, and an ambivalent, we might obtain some notion of what he means by climate. Upward mobiles have high job satisfaction, they identify with the organization, and they obtain a disproportionate share of the rewards of the organization in terms of power, income, motivation, and motivational reinforcement. They regard lack of success as a personal failure and not as a failure of the system. They are what have been more typically called "the organization men." The indifferents constitute the great mass of wage and salaried employees. They are withdrawn from system participation. They do not compete strongly for rewards of the system; nor do they share in the ownership and the profits; nor are they even involved in the system itself. They tend to separate their work from their private life. Ambivalents are creative, anxious, and marginal. They cannot reject the organization's promise of success; but they cannot play the roles that are required to compete for these either. The upward mobile is adaptive; the ambivalent is neurotic. The ambivalent resists rules and procedures and is very anxious about change within the organization. Of importance here is the notion that the climate of an organization is generated out of the attitudes of the people who comprise that organization. In other words, the attitude of the people in the system determine the climate of that organization. This brings us face to face with what attitudes are and how we go about measuring them or changing them.

An attitude is a feeling, a readiness to react in one way or another to ideas, to people, to situations. It leads to what we spoke of earlier as "typical performance." An attitude of a person is that which determines how he is going to behave in a particular situation. Attitudes always have a focus, and within the industrial system the focus is on fellow employees and the product, the work place, and the management. The climate of an organization is determined by the attitudes that individuals have about that organization and, in a system, people are bound to have attitudes about where they work and for whom they work. Attitudes, therefore, result in people acting positively, negatively, or neutrally about people, things, or situations, and knowledge of these attitudes is important to the functioning of the system. Thus, a system's managers or administrators have to be involved in measuring attitudes. One way is to analyze attitudes based on what foremen and supervisors report. Often this is unreliable because usually this information is screened on the way up. A foreman or supervisor doesn't usually like to report to management that the attitudes of the people working for him are poor or inappropriate. When asked how things are going in his area, the supervisor will say, "Just fine." Often false ideas are fostered. That is, the foreman will have some idea about what the attitudes of his people should be and will report those rather than what the attitudes really are. Another source of information on attitudes is the grapevine—rumors. Rumors are often distorted also, although they must be listened to because in many instances they do reflect extreme attitudes. Another way of looking at attitudes is through other behavioral manifestations within the organization. Gripes and slow-downs are typical. Unfortunately, these often come too late to be of real value in helping to evaluate employee attitudes.

Perhaps the two best ways of understanding employee attitudes are through interviewing and through the questionnaire. (The questionnaire is really a form of interviewing but differing from an interview by being formalized and written on a piece of paper.) The trained interviewer can talk to an employee, using all of the precautions discussed earlier (page 32). One rather good device that is often overlooked is the exit interview. It is our opinion that every employee who leaves an organization should be interviewed at the time of his departure. Even if the employee is leaving for favorable reasons, such as pregnancy or moving to another town, reasons over which you have no control, a departure interview is important because at this time the employee can afford to be candid. He can really tell you what he feels and knows. As a result, this is perhaps one of the single best sources of information about the climate of the organization as reflected by the attitudes of the individuals within the organization. The questionnaire provides similar information and is more economical and systematic. It is difficult to prepare without expert help, however. Nevertheless, the repeated use of attitude measurements makes it possible for an organization to compare its level of morale with that of other organizations, to observe trends over a long period, and to detect problem areas and situations before they become disruptive.

One key attitude in industry is job dissatisfaction. It has been estimated that approximately 13 percent of all employees are dissatisfied. Other estimators say that the dissatisfaction rate is much higher than this. There are some people who just do not like to work. However, there is evidence that job dissatisfaction is associated with some generalized maladjustment and that as one goes higher up in the occupational levels, one becomes more satisfied. The professional man within the organization is more likely to be satisfied than the hourly worker. Why? Because the professional man's satisfactions generally come from his own efforts. The college, the long-term health facility, or organization where he works is merely the operational setting. He is professionally oriented and he believes that the satisfactions that he achieves come from his own efforts. This is generally not true for the lower-level worker who feels that his satisfactions must come from the organization in which he is employed. This is an important fact for administrators to recognize.

More than any other single factor in the reduction of turnover and the maintenance of a good climate in your organization is ascertaining that all employees share in the system's goals and that those in the low-level jobs in particular somehow derive satisfaction from the work that they do. There is no professional acclaim that can come their way. Their only rewards are good pay, a smile, and acknowledgement of a job well done, even though the job is cleaning the floor or slicing carrots for tonight's supper.

The psychological climate functions in part because people work together and in working together they form two kinds of organizations. The one is the formal organization which you, through your leadership function, provide. The other is the informal organization resulting from friendships, car pools, nearness of work to living quarters, sharing community interests, and the like. These informal organizations within the formal organization can have a very dramatic influence on the climate of the organization and on the general attitude of the workers within the organization. The lazy support one another as do the gripers and the overly ambitious. It would be fascinating to hear a tape recording made while four or five of your employees were riding home together in a car. Groups can be formed on the basis of an issue and can spring up overnight. Friends and relatives also can have a tremendous influence on the organization. And, yet, if you try to do away with informal grouping, you can be in trouble. A prime example of this is provided by a manufacturer who brought a large number of European workers to this country to work in a skilled operation. He thought that these workers were talking too much among themselves. He had partitions erected between each work place to prevent conversation. Production immediately dropped to half of what it had been. The reason, of course, was that the workers whom he had imported had an established friendship; they could relate to each other, and they developed their skills to the point where they could accomplish their work despite the fact that they were engaging in somewhat trivial conversation. As a result, the barriers between their work places didn't enhance their performance but rather interfered with it. When you "get tough" about making rules concerning how much time can be spent at the coffee machine or in idle conversation in the halls, remember that the informal organizations within the total organization are important to you.

Fostering attitudes that lead to a favorable climate, keeping the employee content in his place of work, and the getting together of employees into supportive groups have *motivation* as their basis. People get together in a certain group because each member of the group finds that this group provides a climate that is suitable to his needs. As soon as the individual finds that the group to which he belongs does not meet his needs, he will leave it.

This is true of both formal and informal organizations. That is, the individual must be motivated to stay with you. As soon as he finds that he is no longer motivated to work in your organization, he will leave it. When the needs of an individual in a group are satisfied by the group, then group cohesiveness and high morale flourish. When the needs of the individual are not satisfied within the group, then high morale does not exist and a disrupted organization results. Most of the popular inquiries concerning motives come from trying to answer the questions: Why is a certain individual declining in productivity? What appeal will be productive in improving attitudes of a group of workers? Of all the areas of industrial performance, perhaps the most important and the least understood is the notion of motivation. The real problem of motivation is that it is complex. One of the key problems is in definition, since the word "motivation" refers to so many aspects of human behavior that its meaning is far from clear. We think of motivation as the *process* by which a need or desire is aroused. That is, a motive is not a particular need or desire, but the process by which this need or desire is aroused. Let's examine the following sequence. A man quits his job stating that his pay is low. We conclude from this that his motive is economic gain. We find, however, that he needs money to furnish his home, and therefore conclude that his motive is to achieve gracious living. Then we discover that his wife insisted that he find a job with higher pay, and we conclude that pleasing his wife was his motivation. Further probing reveals that he married his wife because she looked like his beloved mother. From this we conclude that he left his job because he loved his mother. We could, of course, go on with these futile deductions.

We believe that the best one can do is to seek determinants of behavior in terms of three things: the external environment of the individual, his internal or physiological state, and his past experiences. Two of these factors can be controlled in the work place: (1) hire the individual whose past experiences indicate that he is going to work well in the system, and (2) control the environment within the work place so that the individual finds satisfaction for his efforts.

## ORGANIZATIONAL ROLES
We have observed that the organizational climate is created in part by the organizations within the total organization to which various employees belong and in which they participate. As was stated earlier, the organizations may be both formal and informal. One important aspect is the notion that individuals play various roles within the formal and informal organizations. These roles, in turn, are important in achieving the system's goals and a satisfactory climate within the work organization. Roles can be thought of as expectancies— anticipations that the individual will behave in certain ways within a group.

The role that a person plays in an organization, whether the organization is formal or informal, carries with it a commitment to behave in a particular fashion. It also carries a commitment not to behave in certain ways. The appropriate behavior for a particular role is prescribed by several different factors within the organization. One is prescribed by the individual fulfilling the role, another by the members of the formal organization, and a third by the informal group within the organization. The informal group may assign the role of clown and expect this person to be the jester of the group; the formal organization may assign a father role or the role of adviser for the organization, while the individual himself may prescribe a quite different role.

From the possible sources of roles—the individual and both the informal and formal organization—four separate categories of roles emerge.[3] (1) *Self-prescribed roles:* These are the roles that the individual believes that he ought to adopt for himself. As a result of being assigned a particular function within the system, he believes that he ought to adopt a certain set of roles. He has prescribed these for himself. (2) *Roles prescribed by others:* These are the roles the others believe that he should adopt. (3) *Self-perceived roles:* These are the roles that the individual sees himself as fulfilling. He may prescribe for himself one set of roles but feel that he is unsuccessful in this set and actually perceive himself as fulfilling an entirely different one. (4) *Roles perceived by others:* These are the roles that others perceive that the individual is playing. Thus, any individual within the organization has a role that he has prescribed for himself which may or may not agree with the role he actually perceives himself as fulfilling and this role may be entirely different from the role that others assign to him or that others perceive him to be fulfilling. It is the lack of correspondence between the prescribed and the perceived roles that produces friction between the individual and the group. When people behave in ways that are neither desired nor expected, then difficulties are likely to develop. Lack of agreement between the self-prescribed role and the role prescribed by others results from poor definition of the job, poor job specifications, and differences in objectives. Lack of agreement is quite common, particularly in certain kinds of management situations. It has been observed lately in higher education; deans, for example, have perceived or prescribed for themselves a particular role and the students, as we are painfully aware, have prescribed for them an entirely different kind of role. The nursing director may think that she is fair and impartial, whereas actually she may be viewed as strict and biased. Her behavior and the behavior of the people who work for her are a reflection of these perceptions, even to the extent that she may be in difficulty.

To effect correspondence between self-prescribed roles and roles prescribed by others there must be agreement concerning the individual's position in the organization or the informal group. This agreement can be brought about by proper job specification. Whether or not the employee carries his lunch may not be prescribed by an administrator; however, if the employee prescribes for himself the role of being the common, ordinary guy and "brown-bags it" along with the others this action may not be appropriate for the leadership role that has been prescribed. The self-perceived role should correspond to the role perceived by others. The point to determine is the degree to which others understand, comprehend, and have insight into the roles that a particular individual believes himself to be fulfilling. If there is a lack of correspondence, this doesn't result from disagreement concerning the facts of the matter, but disagreement with respect to the interpretation of the facts. This could be largely due to lack of communication, as discussed earlier. The purpose of this discussion is to make certain that you understand that within your organization each individual is playing a role and that, through proper communication, proper motivation, proper training, proper job description, and proper employment and rating techniques, you can attain understanding and agreement between and among the various roles that the individual plays and that are imposed upon him within the organization. Attaining agreement in role perception is one of the key functions of management—one that must be fulfilled if the climate within the organization is such that it will help achieve the system goals discussed earlier (page 45).

## Leadership

A discussion of the management process is incomplete without a review of the concept of leadership. Administrators must exercise sound leadership, evidenced by example; they must be out front leading rather than in back pushing. We believe leadership to be a natural process in that it is something that people want. It must somehow inspire the subordinate, triggering "the will to do" on his part. Leadership that inspires is preferred to one that drives. Driving the employee is termed "non-leadership." Carrying this dichotomy of leadership non-leadership further, we find that a leader accomplishes work and in so doing causes his employees to develop and grow. A non-leader accomplishes work but at the expense of the subordinate. The leader shows his employees how to do the job and provides rewards for successful completion. The non-leader forces the employee to do the job by using fear or coercion and threats to achieve completion. The true leader assumes obligations. The non-leader passes the buck.

The leader and his degree of acceptance by the group certainly have a serious effect on the group. The leader must establish himself, therefore, as a source of authority, yet, at the same time, he must show genuine concern for the group's needs and welfare. The successful leader is usually viewed by the members of the group, that is, his subordinates, as a person who responds to their needs. He must recognize the needs of the group and do something about them. The leader too, will have the ability to determine what actions will best help accomplish the group's goals. It is important to note here that the people working for you also have certain objectives and goals which may or may not be consistent with the objectives of the nursing home. It is essential that you, as an administrator, recognize the difference between goals and objectives of the individuals on the one hand and the goals and objectives of your institution on the other. The real trick of leadership is to merge these two sets of goals or objectives and develop the highest degree of commonality between them so that you can motivate the employee to want to do his job well.

### Leadership Philosophy

A look at leadership philosophy enables one to identify the so-called power styles of leadership. The *autocratic leader* centralizes authority and decision-making within himself. He does not delegate authority. Subordinates do as they are told and do not participate in decision-making. This is not necessarily a poor or bad type of leadership since it has been shown to obtain results in some instances. Its success is dependent upon the type of employees one is dealing with and what these people must do. Autocratic leadership will permit quick decision-making because, after all, the leader is the only person who is making the decision. Less competent employees, including supervisors, can be utilized because they are simply carrying out orders. On the minus side is the risk of poor human relations as a result of the ruthless exercise of power. Autocratic leadership also ignores the potential growth and development of employees.

The opposite of the autocratic leadership style is *participative leadership.* In this, the leader decentralizes his managerial authority. Decisions usually result from consultation with employees. The leader and the group act as a social unit. This leadership gives the employee guidance and support while also providing some freedom for action. Under participative leadership, the leader must still maintain control. Control is an essential point, and its maintenance requires good coordination and communication. Of the two types of power styles discussed, participative leadership provides the best approach to achieving maximum productivity and employee satisfaction.

### SUPERVISION

What is supervision? Supervision is a special position of leadership within organizations. It involves motivating subordinates to do a better job and to do it willingly. Supervision is didactic. This entails the concept of training, measuring, and rating. In this, one is again concerned either with evaluation of the employee or the comparison or measurement of the employee against some pre-established standard believed to be satisfactory or better than satisfactory for institutions. Supervision is correcting, and here one is concerned primarily with the concept of discipline. Supervision is rewarding. This in a sense ties into the points, mentioned previously, of measuring and rating. How do you create desirable atmospheres or climates for work in your institution? How do you recognize the efforts of your employees? Supervision is the attempt to cause things to happen through other people.

The essence of supervision is the generation of change; yet, one knows from many studies that subordinates have a built-in resistance to changes that affect them personally. A supervisor may have this same type of built-in resistance to change. People in an organization develop a particular set of relationships with the various elements within the organization. The typical employee finds a certain security in knowing what is expected to happen. On the other hand, technological and administrative changes are essential elements in any operation if it is to be successful. Technological change includes simplification of manual methods, new materials, new ways of doing things, whereas administrative or organizational change involves the horizontal and vertical grouping of jobs and functions; that is, the changing of their physical location and perhaps even their elimination or addition. Why should technological or organizational change cause feelings of insecurity and therefore be resisted? Fear of unemployment is probably the primary cause. Loss of status is also a threat. Skilled workers feel that their skills may become obsolete thereby reducing the status that they hold in the eyes of their subordinates or of their peers.

Let us look at a few conditions conducive to creating resistance. Resistance can be expected if the nature of the change is not made clear to the people who are going to be influenced by the change. Information concerning a coming change must be complete. Different individuals will see different meanings in a proposed change since each as individuals has a different point of view from which to assess the change. Some workers might see change as an indication that they have not been doing a good job. Others might see the change as doing away with their function. Still others may feel a loss of influence. Resistance may be expected from persons influenced by the change who have had nothing to say about making the change. It will decrease to a degree if these persons are able to have some say in the change. Resistance may also be expected if the change is made on personal grounds rather than impersonal ones. A supervisor posted the following notice: "I have always felt that promptness is an important indicator of an employee's interest in his job. I will feel much better if you are at your job at the proper time." Make the request based on system objectives, not because of personal whim or idiosyncrasy. Resistance may be expected if the change ignores the already established sub-groups in the group. It is important to recognize the informal group structure that exists within the formal structure. Change may threaten the informal group structure.

Management has developed ways to reduce the effects of change and of making change more acceptable. Employers can guarantee employee's protection from economic loss due to change. Offers of retraining at the employer's expense or even guaranteed wages are methods for overcoming fear of economic loss. Change for the sake of change must be avoided. An excellent way to reduce resistance to change is to have those people who will be affected participate in making the changes.

### Discipline

Discipline is perhaps the most difficult job of the administrator. Employees will often tend to keep each other in line. If not, however, the administrator must step in. It is the responsibility of the administrator to develop and maintain discipline in the institution. This can be unpleasant but it is necessary at times. One can rationalize, fortunately, that discipline isn't always a bad thing even for those who are disciplined. An individual can learn from being disciplined. Discipline often involves emotion, particularly pride, and thus easily may arouse fear or even anger. The manner in which a supervisor or an executive applies discipline can make it helpful, or harmful beyond repair. People are disciplined for two reasons: (1) to reform the offender, and (2) to deter others.

A few years ago, a study was made of company rules governing the conduct of factory workers. A number of interesting developments were brought to light. It was found that rules were tending to be fewer in number. Most automatic punishments for the breaking of rules had been dropped. The rule for drunkenness on the job—for a long time this misdemeanor meant discharge—had been changed to read: "May be subject to discharge!" It was found that rules tended more and more to be stated in positive rather than in negative terms, i.e., the rules stated what should be done instead of what should not be done. It was also found that the rules and the reason for the rules were posted around the various areas of the plant. Individuals must be aware that the rules exist if it is expected that they must abide by them. It was also found that many companies were illustrating their rules with cartoons and pictures. Somehow this approach makes rules more acceptable. Cartoons apparently help to put group social pressure on the side of the rule.

There are four methods of punishment available to you as an administrator.

1. *Reprimand:* This can take the form of what is sometimes called a training talk. An individual is brought into the office in private and the infraction discussed with him. This is perhaps the best single method of discipline because it gives the employee a chance to respond. In addition, it retains time within the system, giving an opportunity for learning to occur.
2. *The layoff:* By this is meant time off without pay, not a permanent discharge. This can be very effective, but keep in mind that there is the

risk of having the one reprimanded looked upon as a hero for having "stood up to the boss." The reason, of course, is the visibility achieved by the employee. Keep in mind also that when a person is "laid off" the services of that employee are lost for the specified period.

3. *Demotion:* This is another strong means of disciplining a person. The demoted person suffers from the discipline for a long period, perhaps weeks or months.

4. *Discharge:* Of course this is the ultimate disciplinary measure, and should be used only in extreme cases. Discharge should always be viewed as a failure on the part of management to perform its job adequately. Since the best and most frequently used discipline technique is the reprimand or critical interview, we should discuss it further.

It makes little difference what facet of the man's work or personality is under fire; good management of the interview is vital to success. Criticize in a manner that demonstrates that you are paying direct attention to the person who is being disciplined. Make this person realize that at this moment he is most important to you. Take a counseling approach by trying to help the employee understand his errors so that he will not repeat them. Say the negative first. The positive should be last because this is part of the healing. Talk about real facts, using real examples or "critical incidents." Don't give a critical broadside based on generalities. This is destructive when you want to be constructive. Some experts advise criticizing in the morning early in the first of the week. If the employee is criticized just before he goes home, he goes home unhappy, doesn't eat supper, and doesn't sleep. The same holds for Friday; the individual worries all weekend. Never criticize an employee unless this person is capable of making some improvement. Try to close the interview with a kind word or a word on a positive subject, but don't exaggerate.

## Communication

Communication is the anodyne that facilitates the functioning of the management process. It is the planning, organizing, directing, and controlling. Communication is the process of distributing information and viewpoints from one person to another. Many times one passes all sorts of information to his subordinates but is he instilling a sense of understanding with it? Communication always involves two people—the sender and a receiver. First of all there is a stimulus. The sender of a communication must first experience a stimulus or something that motivates him to want to influence the other person—the receiver. Next the sender must interpret the fact that he wants to send a communication to someone else. When the interpretation is completed, the giver expresses himself in some fashion, as for example, by talking. The sending process thus consists of three parts. From the receiver's point of view, the initial step is that of perception. This, then, includes the hearing or the receiving of the message that is sent. The receiver also experiences an interpretation. And then, of course, some form of behavior is manifested on the receiver's part. The sender-receiver relationship has been called the communication equation.

Effective communication is attained by many means. The sender must be fully informed before he can communicate effectively. He must know completely what he is trying to pass on to others. He should also know what information to share. This begins with what the receiver wants to know: alternation of communication and normal distribution. In an institution, communication is subjected to individual interpretation at every level. Communications must be specific to the extent that each message should deal with a single subject.

The results of a recent study may provide further insight into the problems of communication within a system. It was found that the quickest disseminator of information was the grapevine—amounting to 38 percent of the means by which the employees would most likely get the word first; next was the supervisor—27 percent; then the official memo—17 percent; and, finally, the bulletin board—14 percent. Miscellaneous means accounted for the remaining 4 percent. Results suggest that face-to-face communication carried the message much better than did printed media. The fewer the organizational restraints and restrictions, the faster the communication.

In every institution, whether it be a nursing home or what have you, there are downward communications and upward communications. For example, downward communications are those that flow from the higher to the lower authority—rules, orders, instructions. Upward communications, on the other hand, are those in which the upward flow or the moving up of information is through the organizational structure. These are usually attitudes and feelings that are being transmitted. Unfortunately, there are certain barriers to upward flow of information. The swim upstream is certainly more difficult than the swim downstream. Resistance is strong. The barriers curtailing organization communication, for example, entail the physical distance between the superior and subordinate. You, as an administrator, are isolated and seldom seen. There are also barriers involving superiors. A superior's attitude in listening to the individual must be taken into consideration. Will the superior be discouraging or encouraging? Will the information be passed on upward through the organization structure? One must be very deeply concerned about what his employees are hearing from him and what it is he is hearing from his subordinates. It is of necessity a two-way process and, again, not only of words of messages moving up or down through the structure, but also understanding as well.

One method that can be used in the nursing home to promote communication and at the same time obtain a great deal of participation on the part of employees involves use of the committee. Many things have been said about committees, some of them humorous and some of them not so humorous. A cynic has said that committees are made up of the unfit, appointed by the incompetent, to do the unnecessary. Another has said that the most useful committee size is three, one member of which is out of town and another home sick in bed. It has also been said that a camel is a horse designed by a committee. Much of the criticism of committees is really a criticism of their misuse. A committee is nothing more than a group of people joined together to make a decision, or designated to perform some particular administrative act. It functions only as a group. One of the committee's strengths is the probability of obtaining better decisions than could otherwise be obtained. Sometimes an overburdened administrator or executive doesn't have the time to give every matter the attention that it merits. The administrator needs the advice of people with technical knowledge—the director of nursing, the chief cook, the head of maintenance, and so on. The committee provides the pooled judgment of experienced people representing various viewpoints and thereby helps to enhance the decision-making process. It clarifies thinking and the communication channels. In committee meetings, members have to justify their opinions before the other committee members, and this is good. The committee also has educational value. When people serve on a committee they hear other problems and viewpoints—viewpoints perhaps much different from their own. Newer employees may be placed on committees as an educational process. Exchange of information on committees lets people "in on things." Everyone learns about the problems of other areas and other departments. This lessens the likelihood of anyone passing on conflicting information. It saves time. One doesn't have to explain everything to each person individually. Committees are often the only means of coordinating the various functions of your establishment. Everyone understands each other's problems. As mentioned earlier, new ideas and change win the acceptance of employees when the employees take part in the decision-making process. Committees really are evidence of democracy in the organization.

There are some disadvantages to the committee that one must be aware of. Often there is too much talk and irrelevant discussion. Some members like to be heard more so than others, whether they have something to say or not. In action, committee meetings frequently waste time. For example, if a recommendation is to be approved, often no action is taken because no one wants to stick out his neck for fear of making a mistake. There is the risk also of the dominance of a few. The few who dominate preclude those others who may have some opinion to contribute. One runs the risk also of a low-grade recommendation. A "yes" by some members and a "no" by others comes out in a group as a "maybe," or there is a tendency to compromise. You run the risk of making yourself a weak administrator by leaning too heavily on the committee. It is very easy to use the committee when in actuality you really don't need it. And, finally, keep in mind that committees are expensive. The hourly wages of committee members add up quickly. If you want a committee to develop a proposal or make a forecast of some sort for your institution, give the detailed work to a staff member. If the committee needs to investigate, appoint a subcommittee. Try to appoint to committees only people who express themselves well and are willing to do so. Another failure of the committee is its inability to supervise and get things done, i.e., it can recommend an action, but it cannot carry it out. To accomplish its purpose it must rely on others.

## CONCLUSION

Dr. Mortimer Fineburg, the industrial psychologist and personnel consultant, provides some very good perspectives on the entire area of how to deal with people, to inspire them to participate productively within the organization. [1] He tells us that the best way to motivate a subordinate is to show him that we are conscious of his needs, his ambitions, his fears, and himself as an individual. The goal of a manager or an administrator is not to get people to like him, but if he can keep people from actively disliking him he will have achieved a fundamental objective. An administrator can have every personnel factor in his favor, he can have top wages, top morale, realistic goals, experienced and seasoned employees, and everything else, but if he commits one of the following cardinal mistakes he will critically limit his chance of success in dealing with employees. Fineburg lists the following don'ts.

(1) *Never belittle subordinates.* No man thinks that others regard him as stupid. He may have doubts of his own but he doesn't like others agreeing with him. (2) *Never criticize a subordinate in front of others.* Everyone knows that such criticism is embarrassing and threatening. (3) *Never fail to give subordinates your undivided attention.* You don't have to devote every waking moment to your employees, but it is important to give your undivided attention to every person under your direct control. (4) *Never seem preoccupied with your own interests.* Your own interest might very well be your prime concern, but try not to communicate this to others. (5) *Never play favorites.* This is another cardinal rule of good supervision. When you start to make exceptions because of personal preference, especially when the person you favor is playing up to you, the rest of the staff will soon realize it. (6) *Never fail to help your subordinates grow.* You will recall that this was discussed earlier. Try to be a fighter for your subordinates. (7) *Never be insensitive to small things.* (8) *Never make loose or rash statements.* These you will regret. (9) *Never vacillate in making a decision.* Be affirmative, be decisive, do not procrastinate.

To this point we have been concerned with the pitfalls that should be avoided. Motivating top performance requires positive actions too; therefore, let us look for a few moments at positive ways in which Fineburg suggests that you can motivate your subordinates. (1) *Communicate standards and be consistent.* When an individual knows that he is being evaluated according to a single, fair standard, he has a target to shoot for. (2) *Be aware of your own biases and prejudices.* (3) *Let people know where they stand.* Do this consistently by means of performance review or other methods. (4) *Give praise when it is appropriate.* Properly handled, praise is one of the best motivating factors available. (5) *Keep your employees informed of changes that may affect them.* You don't have to tell them every detail, but keep them aware of what is going on. (6) *Care about your employees.* You must be sufficiently attuned to the fact that each one of your people is individually concerned about his own future and his own self and everyone must feel that you, too, are concerned about him as an individual. (7) *Perceive people as ways and not means.* Avoid the charge that you are using your people for your own selfish purposes. (8) *Go out of your way to help your subordinates.* This relates to the idea that you are concerned with helping your people develop and grow. (9) *Take responsibility for your employees.* This is one of the hallmarks of good leadership. (10) *Be willing to learn from others.* It is assumed that you know a great deal as an administrator about the work of your institution, but be willing to listen to others as well. (11) *Allow freedom of expression.* And, finally, (12) *delegate, delegate, delegate.*

## REFERENCES

1. Feinberg, M. R. 1965. Do you have to inspire people? Business Management. October.
2. Ghiselli, E. E., and C. W. Brown. 1955. Personnel and Industrial Psychology, Chap. 15. McGraw-Hill Book Company, New York.
3. Gilmer, B. von Haller. 1971. Industrial and organizational psychology, Chap. 11. McGraw-Hill Book Company, New York.
4. Presthus, R. 1962. The organizational society. Knopf, New York.

# Legal Aspects of Nursing Home Administration

## Albert C. Neimeth

**4** Before discussing legal problems that face nursing home administrators, it might be well to say that this chapter is not intended to teach administrators to be lawyers. When an administrator has a legal problem he should go to his legal counsel for advice. The purpose of this chapter is to call attention to some situations where legal problems might develop and alert the administrator to these problem areas so that they can be prevented or dealt with before they become needlessly complex or damaging. The areas to be discussed are:

Statutory basis for the existence of nursing homes.

Liability in general, taking an overview of liability problems and the rules pertaining thereto.

Liability as related to the party claimed to have been negligent.

Liability as related to the character of the facility.

Liability as related to the individual cared for in the home.

Malpractice and its prevention.

General problems of labor relations in the nursing home.

Legal problems connected with Medicare and Medicaid.

### STATUTORY BASIS FOR THE EXISTENCE OF NURSING HOMES

Our first area of study is concerned with the statutes that establish and regulate the nursing home industry. In every state, there can be legislation (with rules and regulations promulgated thereunder) that establishes the guidelines that must be followed for licensed nursing homes. As I am a New York lawyer, I will occasionally refer to New York State statutes. While some New York legislation will be similarly applicable in other states, it is the administrator's responsibility to learn specifically about the laws in his own state which may differ.

In New York there are several source statutes providing for establishment and regulation of the private and public health industries: Social Services

Law, Executive Law, and Public Health Law. The Social Services Law pertains to all areas of social welfare for the citizens of the State of New York. The Executive Law, Section 748, has special provisions for private proprietary convalescent homes and homes for adults, and it gives statutory authority and definition for such facilities. The initial paragraph of this section indicates that the legislative purpose of this law is "to assure that the life, health, safety, and comfort of persons cared for in private proprietary facilities will be adequately protected and promoted and that such persons will receive the kind of quality of care, supervision and attention required by reason of their condition."

Article 28-D of the Public Health Law of New York State, entitled "Practice of Nursing Home Administration," covers general provisions and public policy, licensing, registration, violations, and penalties. Section 2895 states, "It is hereby declared and found that the health and safety of the people of the State of New York requires that the administration of medical facilities providing nursing home accommodations be adequate and proper and that the quality of such administrative services is related to the calibre of training and experience of the persons administering such facilities." It is the purpose of this article to establish standards of education, training, and experience and provide for the examination, licensing, and registration of nursing home administrators.

In some states, private nursing homes might be established only by a natural person as opposed to a corporation. New York State allows corporate ownership in certain limited instances. New York State statutes define different types of homes, such as the nursing home, the convalescent home, and the private proprietary home for adults. According to Section 2 of the New York State Social Services Law, "A private proprietary nursing home shall mean a facility providing or operated for the purpose of providing therein lodging, board, and nursing care to sick, invalid, infirm, disabled or convalescent persons for compensation and profit." Look to your own state statute for appropriate legal definition and incorporation guidelines.

With governmental support payments such a major factor in the economic well-being of health facilities, one might first look at distinctly state statutes authorizing and regulating these expenditures. An example of individual state legislation is Section 207 of the New York Social Services Law, Title 6 being entitled, "Old Age Assistance." You should know the rules for state medical assistance to needy persons.

Of greater importance, today states must legislate to be eligible for reimbursement under the federal Medicaid programs provided for under Title 19 of the Social Security Amendments, Public Law 89 to 97. For New York, the appropriate sections of the Social Services Law are 363 to 367. Section 363 is the introductory section of Title 11, Medical Assistance for Needy

Persons. Listed in Section 364 are the standards of responsibility for the Department of Health of New York State. Provision is made for consultive services to hospitals, nursing homes, home health agencies, etc., as is required by the Secretary of the Federal Department of Health, Education and Welfare in order to assist people to qualify for payments under the provisions of this title and Title 19 of the Federal Social Security Act. Other aspects of the law concern care and maintenance under the medical assistance provisions. Again, the federal laws change and you must keep abreast of these changes.

In summary, the state statutes provide the enabling legislation for establishment of nursing homes in each state. Provision for old age assistance had often originally been made under the state welfare laws. Today, to accrue the necessary economic benefits of federal Medicaid statutes, states must also provide covering legislation which indicates the extent the state is going into partnership with the federal government in this area.

## LIABILITY IN GENERAL

In considering the potential liabilities of nursing home operators, we shall look at *negligence,* the doctrine of *respondeat superior, the effect of statute and ordinance violations,* the *doctrine of res ipsa loquitur,* and *workmen's compensation.*

First, what is negligence? How can a nursing home be negligent? How can its employees be negligent? A short definition of negligence is difficult. Negligence has to do with the conduct of the operator and his employees. The question we ask is whether the conduct under consideration is the conduct of a reasonable man. This is usually a jury question. It is a question of fact.

By definition, negligence seems to be that type of conduct, active or passive, that is not the conduct of a reasonable man and results in foreseeable damage to the injured party. It should not be difficult for one to prepare for a possible lawsuit caused by conduct of the nursing home operator or by the home's employees. The facts are in the everyday working situation. In establishing negligence, the question might be whether the act or care by the nursing home employee is reasonable under the customs and mores of the nursing homes in the community. An added aspect of this standard of the reasonable man is the question of injury foreseeability. Is the accident, or is the injury that has occurred, reasonably foreseeable? If it is not reasonably foreseeable, then perhaps there will not be a determination of negligence because a reasonable man would not have foreseen this result from his actions.

In the case of a nursing home administrator or owner, if an employee is guilty of negligence, how does liability for same apply to the owner? The answer to this question lies in the doctrine of *respondeat superior.* Respondeat superior historically is the liability of a master for the acts of his servants. You, as owner or administrator, are in the realm of master-servant with your employees. As a master was liable for the acts of his servants, you, an employer, are liable for the acts of your employees, if they were doing work in the scope of their employment when the negligent act or omission occurred. Whether an employee acted in the scope of employment is determined by the fact situation. Again, a jury will probably make this decision if the case comes to trial.

What type of care is required of the nursing home? Let us consider a typical case decided in 1961.[1] This happened to be an Illinois case, but, basically, the rules apply to all states of the Union. This case discusses what facts need to be established to prove negligence and gives us some degree of care guidelines. The action was for injuries based upon negligence of an employee. A 73-year-old man in a nursing home was supposedly injured when he was struck and knocked down by someone who was drunk and who was likewise a patient in the home. The evidence and the legal procedural aspects will not be considered here. Numerous questions were raised. Was this 73-year-old patient knocked down by another patient who was drunk? Did the staff members know that this man drank? Should they have watched him? The true situation in the case was confusing, as there were no witnesses. The man who claimed he was hurt had a criminal record, and the jury was in doubt as to the veracity of his statements. It was ultimately decided that there was not sufficient proof to establish that the one guest hit the other guest or that the offender was a known drunk, or was drunk at the time of the accident. This case is of interest to us in that it raises the common question: What care does a nursing home owe to its patients? Generally, nursing homes (and similar institutions for the aged) owe their patients ordinary care to protect them from any danger or injury that might be reasonably anticipated; but they cannot be held to be insurers of the safety of their patients. What is required is ordinary care—reasonable care, care that nursing homes in the area hold as the norm.

It might be helpful to discuss a typical respondeat superior case. This case involved a nurse who worked in a nursing home. The question at issue was whether the activity by this nurse was within the scope of employment when she was guilty of negligence. She had burned one of the patients by placing a hot pad on this patient without periodically checking to see if the pad had been left in place too long or if it were too hot. Because this nurse had been hired by the patient and not by the home, the court decided that the nursing home had no relationship with the nurse, did not direct her to do what she had to do, and therefore had no vicarious liability. For the negligent conduct of the nurse, the rule of respondeat superior did not apply, as there was no employer-employee relationship in this case between the nurse and the nursing home.

In another interesting respondeat superior type of case tried in Connecticut,[3] an employee entered his car to drive downtown to cash his paycheck during work hours. On the way out, he hit a patient. Is the home liable for this action of the employee? Was his act within the scope of his employment? The court found that the act was not within the scope of employment, because this was not a work duty even though it occurred during working hours. This was a private chore. Since the employee was not on company business, the home was not liable for his negligence. Respondeat superior did not apply.

Another doctrine of liability is that of *res ipsa loquitur*. *Res ipsa loquitur* is a legal doctrine that applies in a situation where the defendant—nursing home or its employee—is in full control of a facility and the patient—the plaintiff, the person hurt—is in a state in which he has no knowledge of what is happening to him and no control over the activity that brings injury to him. This doctrine might apply, for example, in hospital cases dealing with something that happens to a person while he is under anesthesia. In this situation the patient has the question, "What happened to me when I was under anesthesia?" There is no way for him to know. In such a situation the law provides that the burden of proof is on the home, on the doctor, or on the hospital. Ordinarily, when somebody sues you, the burden of proof is on him to prove that you were negligent. He has to establish the facts to show negligence, and then you, in turn, can defend yourself by showing his contributory negligence, or by disproving that there was negligence on your part. Under the doctrine of *res ipsa loquitur*, the plaintiff—the injured party—does not have any knowledge of the facts because of his condition. As the nursing home or its employee was in control, the burden of proof shifts. If the fact situation is a *res ipsa* situation, the burden is on the defendant to disprove the possibility that his negligence might have caused the injury to the plaintiff.

*Res ipsa loquitur* cases can arise with equipment usage. In the New York case of Davidson *vs.* MacFadden Foundation,[2] there was an action by a patient at a health resort for personal injury received when the examination table upon which she was lying tilted and gave way. The Supreme Court held that the doctrine of *res ipsa loquitur* evidence sustained findings of negligence, on the part of the defendant, as the defendant did not disprove its negligence. A $7500 award was granted. How did the facility, in this case a health resort, become involved in such a situation? The plaintiff came to the resort. As she was being examined on a doctor's table owned by the resort, the table gave way or tilted in such a manner that the plaintiff slid down. Her head became wedged between the table and the wall, and her neck and chest were injured. When the nurse tried to extricate her, the woman's knee was likewise injured. The table was a three-section one that was permanently attached to the floor. Because the plaintiff was on her back when this happened, there was nothing she could do. She had no control over the table and had nothing to do with handling the table. The Appellate Division determined that the facts were sufficient to sustain the verdict. This case suggests that with any equipment owned or provided by the nursing home (such as x-ray equipment, bedrails, or adjustable beds), there is a possibility of liability. If the nursing home is sued, it will have to disprove that the fault lay with its equipment or apparatus (or the operation of same) in a *res ipsa loquitur* situation.

Another area of importance under liabilities in general is the application of *workmen's compensation.* What is the rule in reference to employees suing the nursing home? Basically, in the event of any injury, the employee must proceed under the guidance and procedures of the state's Workmen's Compensation Law. Under these laws, the employee does not have a claim against the nursing home for the job-sustained injuries. The same rule applies when a patient is negligent and injures an employee or a nurse. An employee, a nurse, or a member of the administrative staff can proceed under workmen's compensation laws and be remunerated for his or her injury. On the other hand, the employee may sue an outside third party, for example, another person or an outside independent contractor. In the situation of the injured employee and the nursing home, however, workmen's compensation applies, and the injured employee may not sue the employer for damages.

The last area under liability in general is that of *violation of statutes and regulations.* If the nursing home violates a statute or regulation, does this mean that the home will subject to a damage suit and will automatically be found negligent because of this violation? Is negligence established thereby? The answer is no. To be sued and sustain damages for the actions of employees of the nursing home, negligence must be proved. The mere breaking of a statute or violation of a regulation is not in itself proof of negligence unless statutorily so provided. If it can be shown that negligence was involved and that the damages that resulted were caused by the violation of the statute, then the administrator of the home could be held liable for damages and likewise punished for the violation of the statute. In other words, in proving negligence, a part of the evidence might be that there was violation of an ordinance, a regulation, or a statute. However, it is only together with other facts that negligence can be definitely established in order to impose civil liability and damages. Violating statutes, ordinances, and regulations is a serious matter, even if such action alone might not be sufficient to establish negligence in the civil courts.

## LIABILITY AS RELATED TO THE PARTY CLAIMED TO HAVE BEEN NEGLIGENT

Such parties might be administrators, doctors, nurses, staff, or independent contractors. What liability is an administrator subject to? Consider, as an example, a private proprietary nursing home. Can an administrator *delegate his responsibilities to subordinates* and thereby do away with his liability for them? The answer is no. The administrator cannot delegate to a nurse, an assistant, or to anybody else his ultimate responsibility. Also, an owner has responsibilities that he cannot delegate to an administrator and thereby be relieved of responsibility. As a representative of the home, and of the partners, even if they are inactive partners and the partner administrator is running the home, the owning partners also will be responsible for the administrator's acts, just as he is liable for his own acts. The administrator is generally responsible for the care and treatment of the patients in the home, and he must cooperate with the medical staff and the other staff to see that satisfactory standards of medical and nursing home care are maintained.

A question might arise as to liability when there are two or three owners and only one is sued. In such a case, the rule for joint liability applies. This means that each of the parties is equally liable for damages to the patient or the outside person. They are all jointly and severally responsible. If a suit is brought against one owner, the others must contribute if the one owner who has been sued wishes to be recompensed by them.

Another individual concerned with general obligations and liabilities is *the doctor*. Liability in this area has changed over the years. Questions remain as to the doctor's liability in charitable hospitals and charitable homes as opposed to noncharitable ones. Basically, the current rule is that when a doctor is employed by the nursing home, the home is responsible for his negligent acts. If the nursing home has an arrangement with several doctors and if the administrator asks one of the doctors to take care of a sick patient and the doctor is guilty of malpractice, the nursing home, as well as the doctor, may be sued under the respondeat superior doctrine. A different situation arises with the independent doctor, a doctor who has no connection with the nursing home. In this situation the patient asks his own doctor to visit him, the patient paying the doctor. The home has nothing to do with the doctor other than to allow him to use the premises and perhaps to loan him a nurse or staff member to work with him. The nursing home is not liable for malpractice by an independent doctor. The doctor is in the realm of an independent contractor. He is not an employee.

This brings us to the further question of the *responsibility of a nursing home to supervise a doctor and his orders*. Does not the institution have the responsibility to check to see if the care prescribed by the doctor is correct? If apparently not correct, does not the institution have the further responsibility to follow this up, even though the doctor is acting as an independent practitioner? There may be a trend toward spreading liability a little further than has been done in the past in this situation. Putting a responsibility on institutions to do further supervision of a doctor's work and the work that he is having done by his nurse can create personality problems. Doctors do not like people looking over their shoulders, and there may be disagreement between the hospital or institution and the doctor in reference to the treatment being performed. It might be well for the administrator to consider this a public relations matter to be discussed with doctors. Since the administrator is subject to liability, doctors should be made to understand the possibility that the institution's liability is being expanded. This, hopefully, will help doctors understand the institution's concern in regard to their treatment of patients.

*Individual liability questions also arise in respect to nurses.* Basically, the nursing home is liable for the negligent acts of nurses who work for the home. Like the doctor, if the nurse is brought in from the outside and has been hired by the patient, she is an independent contractor. The nursing home is not liable for the actions of this nurse if she does something negligent to harm the patient who is her client. What might be considered a twist to the situation occurs when a nurse employed by the home is used by an outside doctor who is visiting a patient. We then might apply the borrowed-servant rule. Under this rule, the institution is relieved of liability if one of its nurses is borrowed by an independent doctor and performs all of her actions under his supervision with no regulation by the institution.

*Individual liability questions may arise with regard to staff members* such as kitchen help and clerical workers. Basically, the nursing home is liable for the negligent acts of its staff. Once again, under the respondeat superior doctrine, the master is responsible for the negligent acts of the servant if the act is done within the scope of employment. We previously discussed a case in which an employee of a nursing home drove his car during duty hours to take his paycheck downtown to get it cashed, and, while enroute, hit a patient. In that case, because the employee was not within the scope of his employment the nursing home was not liable for his negligence in injuring the guest. Whatever the facts, the nursing home's liability can be decided by asking: Is the person in the employ of the home? Was the duty performed within the scope of employment? If the answer to both of these questions is yes, then the nursing home may well be liable.

The end result of a negligent action is the award of damages to the injured party. If an individual or institution has been found negligent, there are essentially two kinds of damages that might need to be paid. These are compensatory damages, which might also be called pecuniary damages, and punitive damages. After somebody has been found negligent, the damages awarded for ordinary negligence are compensatory or pecuniary. An individual may be reimbursed for his injury according to the reasonable average settlement or award for this type of bodily injury in the area. In addition, the individual may be paid something for his pain and suffering. He is also reimbursed for wage loss and disbursements. The jury determines this, but the judge reviews the jury's decision. If the judge feels that the amount in damages awarded for pain and suffering and for injuries is far too high or low, he can send the case back for further consideration by the jury because of the inequity of the amount of damages awarded.

*Punitive damages* are damages awarded against an individual who has done something with malice. When an act is performed with malicious purpose, the damages can be quite heavy. Statutes may set the guidelines for applying punitive damages; these can be three or more times the usual compensatory damages. Obviously, in hiring employees, an administrator should be concerned with the employees' malicious tendencies because the knowing administrator can be subject to punitive damages if employees are malicious when they perform negligent acts.

There is one type of situation in which the award for damages can be lowered. If a person is injured, he has an obligation to mitigate the damages. This means that if there is any way for the injured person to save himself from further injury, he has an obligation to do this. If the injured person does not try to save himself from further injury, he will not recover total damages incurred because he will be considered to have been negligent, careless, or purposeful in not mitigating his damages. This point deserves emphasis. When somebody is injured, if there is a question of failure to mitigate, the administrator should note facts to establish this. Thereby, the administrator can help his attorney defend his case. If the injured person has been negligent in failing to mitigate the damages, a considerable saving can result to the administrator in reference to the award against him for his or his employee's negligence.

I want to stress *the importance of care in hiring employees.* The administrator should be thorough in his examination of the credentials and references of the people whom he is hiring, whether they be doctors, nurses, staff, independent contractors, or other workers. If he should have been aware that an employee is an alcoholic, a criminal prone to assault and battery, or subject to fits of malicious mischief, damages can be very high when negligence can be shown. For example, if the administrator did not learn this, he can, on the basis of constructive notice, be liable for negligence of the employee performing negligent acts. Possibly punitive damages could be levied. In any case, compensatory damages would be applicable under respondeat superior.

## LIABILITY AS RELATED TO THE CHARACTER OF THE FACILITY

This liability centers around maintenance of buildings, administrative and medical records, medication and drug facilities, and therapeutic and other equipment. One's liability for building maintenance has similarities to one's liability for maintaining his home, although an institution carries a different and greater obligation. There are various categories of visitors to an institu-

8

76   ALBERT C. NEIMETH

tion, each owed different amounts of care. Among these might be a trespasser—somebody who should not be on the premises and who is illegally on them. Another type of visitor might be a licensee—somebody whose presence is not objected to, but who is not doing a service for the home and who is not being served by the home. A third category is the guest himself—the patient who stays on the premises for care.

*Your obligation to the trespasser* is to warn him of a dangerous condition on the premises when you are aware that he is on the premises and in danger. Examples of this type of dangerous condition would be an unlit elevator shaft or stairways or perhaps excavations on the grounds. If you do not know of the presence of the trespasser, you do not, of course, have the obligation to warn him and are not liable for injury that he might sustain.

*Your obligation to the licensee is greater than for the trespasser for you have invited him to your premises and therefore he is not present illegally.* For him you have the added obligation of maintaining your premises in a safe condition. Using the elevator shaft example again, if a licensee is permitted to walk on the premises, he should be warned of the danger of the unlit shaft and your responsibility is to rope off the area so that a licensee, known or unknown, has reasonable notice of this danger.

*Your obligation to your guests* is even greater because of their condition. The requirement is the use of ordinary care, but because of the usual weakened condition of these guests, ordinary care for them is greater than that for the licensee.

Law suits might revolve around disrepair of stairs, disrepair of sidewalks, objects falling from the roof, failure to clear ice and snow, backyard excavations, and the question of falling on eneven ground or overwaxed floors, or tripping over loose electric cords. There are varied legal problems to be considered in analyzing the question of liability in these instances. For greater amplification of the subject, you should use the services of your attorney. The purpose of this short discourse is to orient administrators to problems that may arise so that these problems can, at an early stage, be turned over to an attorney and thereby not cause unnecessarily heavy damages. Needless to say, the building should be kept in a good state of repair. Basically, this is a matter of common sense and following the statutory rules, regulations, and customs of the trade in your geographical area.

*Questions often arise in the area of administrative and medical records.* All records should be kept in a good state of currency and accuracy, particularly those pertaining to the medical treatment and care given a patient. Questions commonly asked about these records are: How about the individual's right to privacy? Who owns the records of an institution? Is there a confidential relationship established, such as the one between the doctor and the patient? If so, can this privileged information be given out without the approval of the doctor and the patient?

Generally speaking, the institution's general and medical records do not have the same quality of confidential relationship as do communications between the doctor and the patient. There is a physician-patient relationship between the doctor and patient. Even if a physician working for the nursing home comes in at the home's request, the doctor's relationship with the patient is a physician-patient relationship. If the patient so desires and is paying for the physician's services, the patient can request that the medical information be kept private and privileged, and the doctor has this obligation of confidentiality imposed upon him.

As to the home, the administrative and medical records of the home are the property of the home, not the patient. There still remains the possibility of liability in the use of the records by the institution if a question of defamation arises. Defamation, basically, is a written or spoken statement that maligns or hurts an individual about whom it has been written or spoken. As a result, the individual has a cause for action against the institution and may recover damages for his or her injuries. "Libel" is the term for written and "slander" is the term for oral defamation. If the medical records and administrative records are given to an outside person, for example, a writer for a confidential magazine, it might be that the institution is subjecting itself to a defamation action, which could result in a suit for monetary compensation. Thus, for self-preservation, the institution should be very cautious in allowing outside people to see its administrative and medical records without the patient's written approval.

Another important factor in maintaining record security is that an institution cannot maintain a good community image (and it might well discourage future patients) if the public and medical community feel that confidentialities will not be kept by the home or its personnel.

What about the celebrity? Everyone has a right of privacy, but there are distinctions in the degrees of this right based upon who the person is. If Cary Grant or some other well-known celebrity is staying in an institution, general news about him is public and he can expect less privacy than can the average John Doe.

For practical purposes, most homes have tight rules (just as hospitals do) in reference to the issuance of medical records and administrative records. As indicated, a recommended procedure is that these records not be shown unless written authorization is obtained from the patient. You should be alert to the fact that lawyers, investigators, and insurance company representatives are the probable inquisitive persons. They, like all others, should present written authorization before records are opened to them.

*There are many aspects to liability in the area of medication and drugs.* If drugs are stored on the premises, they must be stored in a manner that is reasonable, based upon the standards for similar institutions in the geographical area and in accordance with prescribed governmental rules and regulations. It might be that the general conditions for all similar institutions in the area are sub-par. If this is the case, then your standard should be higher than that of others in an area. Guidance and enforcement of the required standard comes from the state social welfare department that regulates the existence of licensed institutions such as nursing homes. These departments often set guidelines for the degree of security required.

One of the problems that might occur with medication is concerned with who should give medication. The nursing home has to be very careful about this. The doctor establishes the medication dosage, but the nurse generally gives the medication. It is important that the doctor's suggestions and orders for medication are carried out and that the nurse gives the medicine as directed. What is the responsibility of the nurse? In years past, it was a question whether she should have any liability. She was expected to obey the doctor's order and give the patient the medication, and she was not subject to liability if a medication error was made. In recent years, this general rule has been modified. Now the nurse (when she is dealing with medication and drugs) and the home (if the home has been put on notice by its employee nurse) both should check into questions of fact. If the nurse feels that the medication is in error and the institution is notified, but the medication is given anyway, the institution will not be automatically relieved of liability. The administrator should recheck with the doctor when there is any question because, with the large number of people coming under public health care, errors unfortunately will be made. If a nurse with a question in her mind goes ahead and administers the medicine without checking further, she can be subject to liability for the injuries that result from the treatment. The doctor, likewise, would be liable. If the nurse works for the institution, and the institution was informed but did nothing, the institution likewise would be subject to damages for failure to question the treatment.

Most of what has been said about medication and drugs also applies to therapeutic and other equipment. The rule for the *res ipsa loquitur* doctrine, wherein defective equipment is utilized, has already been discussed. If the patient under control of the defendant is injured and has no way of knowing what happened, the burden of proof is upon the defendant, the institution, the doctor, the nurse, and the staff to show that they were not guilty of negligence. The one important point—with application of this doctrine beyond the mere fact that the institution and its employees had complete control of the equipment and provided the treatment—is that it must be shown that the injuries sustained were the direct result of the treatment and of the use of the equipment.

## LIABILITY AS RELATED TO THE INDIVIDUAL CARED FOR IN THE HOME

The obligation of care imposed upon a nursing home varies with the capabilities and weaknesses of its patients. What different kinds of patients are there? How about minors, the insane, the senile? Negligence for each is not measured by the same rule or standard. This applies in establishing both the negligence of the home and the contributory negligence of the patient. In determining whether an individual who suffers injury has been contributorily negligent, such individual is judged by his capabilities, both mental and physical. In many states, a complete defense to a negligence action is contributory negligence on the part of the person injured. In such states, it can well be that an institution, a doctor, a nurse, or a staff member is guilty of negligence and a person is injured thereby; but if the person who was injured was likewise guilty of contributory negligence, that negates any possibility for his recovering of damages. In all cases, it is extremely important to determine what level of performance is demanded from an individual so that it can be determined whether an act is negligent and if there is offsetting contributory negligence.

*This brings the discussion back to the different kinds of patients— children, the insane, and the senile.* A child is not held to the same degree of responsibility as an adult. An insane person is not held to the same degree of capability as a normal person of his age. A senile person is not held to the same degree of responsibility as a younger adult. Each of these individuals, when involved in a liability action, is judged by his own capabilities as limited by his condition whether youth, insanity, or old age. As previously mentioned, in determining negligence, the guide used is the conduct of a reasonable man. However, the reasonable man rule cannot be applied to people who have fewer capabilities than those of a reasonable man. If the child is an 8-year-old, the guideline used is the mental and physical capabilities of a similar eight-year-old child. The same applies to the senile, the insane, and the crippled who are less than whole in the use of their faculties, whether physical or mental.

In nursing home operations, there may be a question of false imprisonment or of assault and battery if someone is held in a room and not released. You ordinarily cannot prevent free ingress and egress of your guests. However, what can be done with a senile person or an insane person? What about the person who temporarily becomes other than normal, but only at rare intervals? What about the person who has an alcoholic propensity, and when he gets drunk has aggressive tendencies against those around him? The institution is charged with the obligation of providing for each individual, depending upon the state of his condition. If the institution lacks the staff to watch over a periodically insane person, for example, or a person with homicidal or aggressive tendencies, this type of patient must be restrained and removed from the premises as soon as possible. Otherwise, the institution is subject to liability if injury occurs due to the acts of its abnormal patients.

As far as the senile are concerned, the institution is under an obligation to note their condition and to provide treatment accordingly. If the facilities and the staff available to the nursing home are not sufficient to provide for the safe care of a senile person, that person should not be taken into the home. The placing, for example, of somebody who is crippled (or who has poor vision) on the second floor, and making him try to come down stairways without aid, might be sufficient to find the home liable for negligence if said person falls down the stairs. The reasoning is that such a person should have been kept on a first-floor area. You cannot lock people up merely because they are senile. Sufficient attendants should be hired to supervise their activities and if this is not possible, these patients should be discharged from your home.

*Suicide is another problem the nursing home may be faced with.* If a person with a suicidal tendency is admitted to the home, the home is responsible for giving him the type of care that will help alleviate the possibility of committing suicide. If this tendency toward suicide is ignored, the home can be subject to a lawsuit and be found negligent. The home may have to pay heavy damages as a result of such a person taking his own life or that of another. If a patient suddenly becomes suicidal, he should be restrained in safekeeping until he can be removed to suitable care. This would not be false imprisonment.

## MALPRACTICE AND ITS PREVENTION

*Malpractice is involved with the acts of a professional,* such as a doctor or a nurse, carrying on his or her profession in a negligent manner that would be subject to liability. This is opposed to a nonprofessional act of negligence as in the case of an administrative error by a nurse or a doctor wherein liability also results from negligence. You might say that malpractice is professional negligence. It is concerned with professional error by a professional in the performance of his licensed duties.

*What are some of the causes of malpractice litigation?* Why has malpractice litigation increased to the degree that it is becoming very expensive for doctors and nurses to obtain malpractice insurance? Why are so many people suing? One reason is that more people than ever before have the opportunity of receiving medical treatment and public health services. With an increase in population and an increase in services, more people are being cared for and therefore more can sue.

In addition, with the greater number of people being cared for as a result of government subsidization of health services, there has been a trend toward less personal relationships between doctors and patients and between institutions and patients. This impersonalization tends to result in people becoming more upset when something seemingly goes wrong. Our population today is more transient than formerly. Fewer people live and die in the same community. A patient is more likely to sue an unknown institutional doctor or nurse than a personal physician or nurse whom they have known well for a long time.

Another factor is the increase in public interest in medicine. Every day the newspapers describe new medical approaches. The government advertises the availability of various medical programs. There are more nursing homes, more hospitals. Television has its doctor programs. The public has been made aware of medicine and of medical facts. People now believe that they are entitled to complete medical service. This awareness makes them more prone to criticize when something seemingly goes wrong. At the same time, medicine is becoming more complex, and the average person is unable to understand this complexity.

Lastly, attorneys have become more proficient and many more of them have gained experiences in trying malpractice cases. As a result, there has been a noticeable increase in the skill and proficiency of the legal profession in handling medical malpractice suits.

*How can malpractice claims be prevented?* Establishing a healthy patient-doctor-home relationship should be the first step. The professional must try to develop a personal relationship with his patient. People need to feel that they are not just numbers, that they are receiving personal care, and that other people are interested in and concerned about them. This will help decrease the bitter feeling of somebody who is injured. There are many ways to keep patients happy, and it is just common sense to use positive psychology in running a nursing home. Practicing good human relations is one of the best ways to avoid possible negligence and malpractice suits against the home and its staff.

Secondly, it must be appreciated that certain patients are suit-prone. If the home knows this in advance, it might be wise not to take such patients into the home. The emotional hypochondriac is certain to be discontented and feel that he is being mistreated. An employer must also beware of the suit-prone doctor or nurse. Some have a history of poor patient relationships and of being involved in malpractice suits. An administrator should analyze closely the references of the people he is hiring in order to be on guard against malpractice claims. As previously indicated under the doctrine of respondeat superior, a home can be liable for the negligence or malpractice of its professional staff.

*Consents are an important safeguard against suit.* When somebody is being treated and there is a question about the person's ability to understand what is being done, the wise course is to obtain a written consent from the patient and, if the patient is senile or incapable, from the person or persons responsible for the patient. In this way, nobody is subject at a later date to a question of whether there was consent to go beyond the minimal scope of treatment. A home should be sure to document, in writing, instructions of doctors concerning patient care to avoid the later charges that care contrary to doctors' orders was given.

## GENERAL PROBLEMS OF LABOR RELATIONS IN THE NURSING HOME

Nursing homes can expect to be increasingly involved with union-management problems. Administrators need to be aware of the right thing to do when they are confronted with questions about labor associations and unionization of their staff. *Why are nursing homes becoming unionized?* Unions desiring to expand have union representatives examining the home, checking with the employees, and trying to generate interest among the employees to become union members. But this alone does not explain why many homes are unionized. There are soft spots in homes that an administrator should look for. These cause problems with his employees and give them the incentive to say, "Sure, why not? Let's have the union in. Our bosses do not care about us anyway. We can do much better with the union." What are some of these soft spots? Wages are always a point of contention. How do the wages in the home compare with the wages of other homes in the area? Also how do the working conditions compare? Are the home's employees being given vacations equal to similarily situated employees? Sick leave, hospitalization, general leave, birthday leave, and grievance procedures are other areas to be considered. Do you as administrator have an open-door policy? Can employees come in and see you? Are you personal with them or are they just numbers? Is there a definite possibility of promotion and wage raises that is known to your staff? Does the home have a well-understood policy with regard to discharge and discipline? Are there avenues for continuous communication between the supervisor and the employee? Are there regular staff meetings? Is there a suggestion box? If the home is large enough to support them, are there employee programs, sporting events, special affairs, and other incentives?

Despite attention to all of these areas in an attempt to maintain a happy and healthy working team, the union still may decide to try to organize your home. What are the rights and obligations of an employer during a union organizational campaign? Under the law, if a union is designated by the majority of the employees of a home in an appropriate unit, that union is entitled to recognition as bargaining representative of the employees. An important point is that the unit must be for an appropriate one, for example, for all the nurses, all custodians, or all kitchen help. It would not be considered appropriate to have the custodians and the doctors in the same unit. Proof of majority employee support of union representation and the appropriateness of the unit must be properly established by the union. The employer has the right to refuse to accept the word of the union representative who comes into his office and says that a majority of the home's employees want to join a particular union. If the employer refuses to recognize the union as the representative of his employees, then the union may insist on an election by secret ballot conducted by the National Labor Relations Board. This is not automatic. If the union decides that it wishes an election, it must file with the Labor Board. The Labor Board will look at the petition. Also the employer can object on the grounds that the unit is inappropriate. This means that a hearing must be held to determine whether the people whom the union claims are its supporters are in an appropriate unit.

It is definitely to the administrator's advantage, if he doubts the union's figures, to sit back and make the union petition for a secret ballot. One reason for this is that people in general, when they are talking in public before union-minded fellow employees, are often afraid to say no. But if a secret ballot is cast, they may vote no.

*From a legal point of view, as soon as the union man comes into the administrator's office, the administrator should immediately retain an attorney.* Labor negotiations are an involved affair, and if the administrator does not start correctly, he can undermine his position. When the union man comes into the office, the administrator should listen politely, tell the man that he has nothing to say, take his name and address, and contact the home's attorney. The union's representative will probably ask for a list of all the home's employees. The administrator is not required to provide this list. In fact, from a practical point of view, the administrator should not give the union the names of his employees. If he does, there will be immediate heavy electioneering to convince the people on the list that they should join the union.

The nursing home's lawyer can arrange for necessary delays in the proceedings before the secret ballot is held. This is important, for the key in union elections, from the union's point of view, is to have the election held as soon as possible. The people who aren't sure become less sure with the passage of time. It is important for the administrator to contact his lawyer at once and say and do nothing before hand; for not only can he innocently prejudice his position by giving out too much information, but he might find himself guilty of an unfair labor practice.

## LEGAL PROBLEMS CONNECTED WITH MEDICARE AND MEDICAID

The final subject to be covered is the application of federal health insurance programs to the health care industry. It seems that everyone involved with an extended care facility has had some problem with Medicare and Medicaid, such as with payment or rates. The issues will vary, but will most likely be continual, as rules change and conflicts sharpen. The following discussion provides only a most cursory review of Medicare and Medicaid.

Both Medicare and Medicaid help pay medical bills. Both are part of the Social Security Act, Medicare being Title 18 and Medicaid being Title 19. They work together, but they are not the same. Medicare is for people 65 years of age or older. Almost every person 65 years old or older, rich or poor, is eligible for Medicare. Some people 65 years old or older are eligible for both Medicare and Medicaid. Whether a person over 65 is eligible for both is determined by the state statutes. Medicaid is for certain kinds of needy and low-income people such as the aged, the blind, the disabled, members of families with dependent children, and other children. Some states, such as New York, include at state expense all needy and low-income people.

Whereas Medicare is a federal insurance program, Medicaid is a federal-state assistance program. The money for Medicare is from trust funds paid by the insured people, but the money for Medicaid comes from federal, state, and local taxes. Medicare is a federal program, while Medicaid is a federal-state partnership. Medicare is the same throughout the United States. Medicaid varies from state to state. With Medicaid, the states design their own Medicaid programs within the federal guidelines.

Medicare hospital insurance provides basic protection against the cost of in-patient hospital care, post-hospital extended care, and post-hospital home health care. Medicare medical insurance, as opposed to the Medicare hospital insurance, provides supplementary protection against the costs of physician's services, medical services and supplies, home health care services, out-patient hospital services, and therapy. Medicaid pays for such things as in-patient hospital care, out-patient hospital services, laboratory and x-ray services, and skilled nursing home services. Medicare pays most hospital and medical costs for those who are insured.

The nursing home that qualifies as an extended care facility might come under both Medicare and Medicaid. Because of periodic changes in rates, I will just briefly note that, under Medicare, there is a deductable fee before hospital insurance applies and there is a monthly charge for Medicare medical insurance. Medicaid can pay what Medicare does not pay for those eligible for both programs. The applicability of Medicare and Medicaid to extended care facilities poses many intricate problems such as the question of rates, the question of lobbying to see that payment schedules are realistic, and the question of regulations. These are matters that an administrator should take up with his attorney. The area is too broad and complex to be covered adequately within the scope of this discussion.

## CONCLUSION

Numerous liability problems face the owners, administrators, and staff of health-care facilities. By being alert to the factual situations from which liability problems arise, nursing home administrators and employees will be able to rectify an aggravated liability situation before injuries and damages become extensive. At the same time, by being alert to legal aspects of nursing home administration, the administrators will have a basis of knowing when they should contact their attorneys for professional advice.

## NOTES

1. Bezark *vs.* Kosner Manor, Inc., 1961. 29 Ill. App 2d 106, 172 N.E. 2d 424.
2. Davidson *vs.* Bernarr MacFadden Foundation, Inc., 1957. 4 App. Div. 2d, 978, 167 N.Y.S. 2d, 684.
3. Libtz *vs.* Jewish Home for the Aged, Inc., 1968. 239A 2d 490.

# Fiscal Administration, Organization, and Techniques

## G. Wheeler

"Every profession does imply a trust
of the service of the public"

Benjamin Whichcote

At the moment the opening quotation may seem a bit obscure or irrelevant. But it is hoped that when you have finished reading this chapter you will see the point and will appreciate the quotation.

You are aware of the impact of the Medicare and Medicaid programs on the nursing home industry. In 1971 some $340 million was raised through stock sales to the public for the purpose of building and operating new nursing homes.

Since 1966, the number of homes has doubled to a total of about 24,000. The number of beds in nursing homes has increased from 875,000 in 1966 to nearly 1 million today. New homes are opening at a rate of about three a day, according to an article in the New York Times. There seems little doubt that the impetus for the rapid growth has been the establishment of the Medicare and Medicaid programs. These programs mean many things to many people, but they do have one thing in common to all—stringent requirements on the nursing home operators to set up and maintain exhaustive amounts of records and paper work. It is unrealistic to expect that this aspect will change much—except to become more and more involved.

Thus, it is necessary to review some of the federal and state requirements for your fiscal administration, and to give you some new ideas and ways and means of coping with the requirements. It will not be possible to go into great depth in any of the areas, but I hope that you will receive a stimulus that will put you on the track of the problems and their solutions.

Initially, we will look at fiscal administration and organization and management controls and then explore the areas of modern methodology for fiscal procedures—cost finding, value analysis, techniques, and profitability.

If we look at management as the *direction of resources to the attainment of objectives,* we see the dire need for sound fiscal administration in any form of business, including nursing homes. In a nursing home the primary objective is that of providing quality services at minimum cost, and, in most cases, there is a secondary objective of earning a reasonable return on the owner's equity in the home. It may be that "reasonable return" is somewhat cramped by regulations, but it is also necessary to have the proper management and administration to have any return at all.

The American Hospital Association's accounting manual for long-term care institutions defines "controlling" as "the process of assuring, insofar as possible, that the objectives of an organization are realized. The main elements of the control process are a comparison of actual and planned performance, an analysis of any significant deviations, and some corrective action."[1]

The effectiveness of the management functions of planning and control depends largely upon (1) the soundness of the organization structure, (2) the adequacy of financial and statistical data relating to each unit within the institution, and (3) the ability of management to make intelligent use of such data.

The accounting process, as a system, is a very vital part of the management process. Organizing for fiscal administration has at least two facets to it in many states at this time. Not only do you have to organize in the most efficient and economical way from the management standpoint, but you may also have to abide by various state codes which have specific requirements to be met in the general areas of fiscal administration.

For example, the New York State Hospital Code,[5] Chapter V, part 713, establishes standards of construction for nursing homes. Among many other standards, Section 713.8 establishes the following requirements for the Administration Department:
1. A business office.
2. A lobby and information center.
3. An administrator's office.
4. An admitting and medical records area.
5. An adequate facility for staff conferences.

Undoubtedly, the interpretations of these codes might be a bit different in different places. My point is that specific requirements of this nature will necessarily affect the organization of your fiscal administration and make it difficult to make the most effective use of your staff.

Organizing your fiscal administration will have to involve many areas, functions, and departments. Typically, your departments might be listed as the following: Dietary, Laundry, Housekeeping, Plant Operation, Plant Maintenance, General Administration, Daily Service, Pharmacy, Laboratory, X-ray, Recreation, and Rehabilitation. Each of these departments is really a cost center and you have to organize so that the true costs of these centers will be evolved. Before you can progress very far in the cost process, you have to decide upon the bases for expense allocations to the centers.

## COMPONENTS OF ORGANIZATIONAL SETUPS

There are five components common to all organizational setups:
1. Definition of objectives.
2. Division of labor.
3. Lines of authority and its delegation.
4. Working relationships of a staff nature.
5. The coordination principle.

### Objectives

For any kind of satisfactory planning, it is essential to form the objectives not only of the whole operation but also for each subgroup as well. The results desired are to be established first; the procedures by which results are measured can be developed later.

### Division of Labor

In all activities, human beings are given jobs or positions according to their skills and thereby their contribution to the activity. Obviously, it is to your advantage to concentrate on placing your employees in the positions in which they will be most efficient, and to hire the best qualified people for the positions.

### Lines of Authority

The lines of authority can be one of the most frustrating, and thereby costly, aspects of an organization. It is not enough simply to put the right person in the right job. The job must be defined for each employee in terms of limits—guides as to what he is supposed to be doing. The employee should know as fully as possible the "what, when, and how" of his job. Otherwise, employees get into one another's way, some functions may be done in a duplicate way, and others not get done at all. In addition, it is just that much more likely that you can develop a smooth-running organization when your staff have clearly defined job outlines.

### Working Relations of a Staff Nature

In any organization there are departments that have no direct lines of authority between them, but to have a smooth and good working relationship all departments have to work together. For example, the bookkeeping department has no authority over most of the other departments of your organization. But to what extent should the nurses and the pharmacist give up some of their time to satisfy the needs of the bookkeeping department? It is self-evident that some time has to be given, but how much and how cheerfully or how grudgingly?

### The Coordination Principle

Coordination of all the departments and functions is the job of management of the administration. This job is comprised of the balancing, timing, and direction of all of the resources of the home in order to realize the optimum contribution of all components to the overall objectives.

The span of control of the administrator is of vital importance. Were he to have a staff of fifty all reporting to him directly, he would never get anything done. The number of people who can report to him will vary with his own strength and capabilities, the capabilities of his subordinates, the degree of complexity in the work, the supervisory control aids available (such as procedure standards, budgetary standards, and possibly work standards), and the number of staff services available.

Generally, approximately six people provide an effective span of control for an administrator, but it is axiomatic that the number should be kept as low as possible in order to free the administrator to use his talents in planning, measuring, and improving the overall operation. If the administrator is deeply involved in the nitty-gritty areas of everyday details, he will gradually become less and less a manager, and more a department head.

Organizing for fiscal administration encompasses far more than the organizational chart for people. It involves budgets, checks and balances, internal controls, cash planning—in fact, almost everything concerned with the fiscal functions of the nursing home.

### MAJOR FUNCTIONS IN ORGANIZING THE FISCAL ADMINISTRATION

### Budgeting

Budgeting is one of the most useful tools of management and is an indispensable device for good fiscal administration. It is not only a forecast of income and expenses, but also, even more important, it should be a comprehensive plan of operations evolved through three functions: planning, coordinating, and control.

Preparation of the budget requires the closest examination of costs, expenses, and sources of income. Budget activities will sometimes reveal duplications, particularly when you rely on cost center managers to prepare their own preliminary forecasts of their needs for the next budget period. Fluctuations in services affect personnel planning and financial requirements. All departments are interrelated in many ways and must be coordinated for efficiencies. And far from the least in importance, expenses must be kept within the forecasts of income—to provide the profit needed to "keep going."

In essence, your budget is your road map. It tells you what direction you are going, where you may have strayed off course, and how far away from the course you have wandered. Your budgetary procedures can be somewhat more flexible than those of governmental variety in which a budget once established cannot be altered and any account cannot be overspent. You do not have that form of restriction, but when you do overspend, you are cutting directly into your profit. Budget time is one of the very best times to review a wide area of possible changes in the organization. Can this job or that job be changed or eliminated? Is this function really necessary?

Although a budget is one of your prime tools, it is also necessary to interpret fully the factors influencing the costs and cost performance as measured by the budget. For example, the budget for the dietary department will have detailed information leading to an overall cost for the number of meals served. It will necessarily rely on some assumptions as to numbers of meals served, labor rates, hours worked, and so on. Your next month's report might show an overall satisfactory situation so far as total cost is concerned. But suppose that you had hired two people in the kitchen at a rate lower than the average budgeted figure. The result could be a satisfactory total labor cost picture, but actually an unsatisfactory picture of efficiency—there were really too many hours worked for the job done.

In-depth analysis and review should be a continuing process.

### Checks and Balances

With respect to checks and balances the following guides should be reviewed:
1. You must have some form of business paper or document to support every transaction. This is the real basis of the *audit trial* for your own benefit, for your external auditors, and for the audits by the intermediaries.
2. For the people in the business office you must establish the working routine that most clearly delegates authority, and that goes as far as possible in separating the various functions of accounting and bookkeeping. For instance, cash receipts might best be handled by someone other than the main bookkeeper.
3. Each employee must initial the documents that he approves with respect to both the responsibility and the work done.

### Internal Controls

Internal controls are part of the measurement devices set up to gauge the budgetary performance. They also function in precluding dishonesty. The following are recommended for internal controls:
1. List all receipts.
2. Make bank deposits daily.

3. Keep complete records of disbursements.
4. File purchase invoices.
5. Establish a receiving routine.
6. Keep patient accounts.
7. Retain payroll records, including time records.
8. Store records.

Regular routines, making certain that the control records are kept, will go a long way toward eliminating the possibility of dishonesty. Yet dishonesty is a factor that has to be recognized and planned for. Some typical kinds of dishonesty that have been encountered are:

1. Forging bills of nonexistent companies, paying the bills, forging signatures, and cashing the checks.
2. Adding figures to checks or vouchers after they have been approved.
3. Collecting overdue, doubtful accounts and listing them as uncollectable.
4. Adding fictitious names to the payroll and cashing checks made out to fictitious individuals. Padding time records comes under this category also.
5. Lapping, a practice in which the cashier diverts payments made by a patient to himself and then juggles other income to that patient's account.
6. Padding expense accounts. This is a fairly common practice.
7. Diverting cash receipts from a patient, entering non-cash allowance credits to the patient's ledger, or even destroying the ledger. (This is why it is essential to have the control of receipts journals so that it is possible to reconstruct a patient's ledger should it have been destroyed.)

Because the business office staff in a nursing home is small, it is difficult to install a high degree of internal control. Usually, internal control is managed by the complete separation of duties among different people. But in a nursing home this method is impractical—the cashier and accounts receivable bookkeeper are apt to be one and the same person. Therefore other means of establishing internal control have to be used; surprise counts, audits, audits by an outside accountant, and one-write accounting systems have all been used effectively. It has been pointed out that thefts by employees may sometimes be regarded as really a "payroll cost" because of poor personnel policies.

One final reminder regarding the question of control of fraud. The American Institute of Certified Public Accountants has an established policy that is worth quoting here, and you may be sure that the Internal Revenue Service takes a similar view of the situation: "Managerial responsibility for the control of fraud is not eliminated by the use of an independent auditor. His liability is clearly limited (the definition is established by the Committee on Auditing Procedures of the A.I.C.P.A.)."[3]

To keep auditing costs from being completely prohibitive, bonding employees who handle money should be combined with sound internal control by management.

## Cash Planning

Cash planning is a primary responsibility of fiscal administration and a definite managerial necessity. Both short-term and long-term planning are required. Usually a daily cash report comprises the short-term situation. A long-term report usually covers a period of six months or a year as outlined in the cash budget, and a review of this is made on a monthly basis. There are definite factors behind, or affecting, your cash position and it is well to keep them in mind at all times:
1. Credit standing.
2. Sound collection policies.
3. Unrealistic rate structure.
4. Haphazard capital expenditures.
5. Unrealistic budgets.

These factors are self-explanatory and simply serve to remind you of the continuing need to review your cash position. The current interest rates alone are sufficient impetus for you to keep abreast of the cash position.

## Follow-up

We have covered the important aspects of organizing for good fiscal administration. It is well to point out here that the efforts (which are quite considerable for nursing homes) directed to producing reliable and pertinent data are wasted in large measure unless the management is ready, able, and willing to use the information. Management must take the follow-up steps of utilizing the information as it becomes available and making sure that any adjustments to the system that have been indicated by the data and information are made.

One very appropriate method of accomplishing this end is *reporting by exception.* This simply means that the routine information showing that all is in order, and is proceeding according to the budget plan, is recapped on a minimum information basis and that the information or data that are clearly out of line or abnormal are highlighted for management's attention. This is where management can most profitably spend its time—in finding out the reasons for the unusual situations brought to its attention. Reporting by exception can readily be done by use of any of the usual current methods of accounting. It will be absolutely essential for the management of a nursing home when it does reach the point of computerized accounting.

The Systems and Procedures Association[2] warns that industry's experience with electronic data processing (EDP) to date indicates that:

1. Clerical cost savings rarely materialize from EDP equipment applications.
2. Any significant savings realized can largely be identified with improved systems work preceding or in conjunction with mechanization.
3. Faster report production (more paper) has not provided more valuable management information. Instead it increased the problem of management scanning more data to determine significant information.

Although the above would seem to indicate that it might not be advisable to concern yourself with computer accounting, I do not believe this to be the case. You should at least be aware of its possible application in a nursing home.

## OFFICE LAYOUT AND FORMS ADMINISTRATION
It may seem a bit unusual to refer even briefly to office layout and forms administration when you are concerned primarily with fiscal administration. Yet, in the nursing home these two aspects have practical application to efficient operation.

### Office Layout
Even in a small office, time spent in developing the optimum layout will prove worthwhile. A well-planned office will minimize the time consumed by nonproductive motion, eliminate space as a communications barrier, reduce confusion, conserve costly space, and possibly eliminate some inter-office friction. An analysis of the layout can be done without a tremendous outlay of time and money. The usual procedure is to use grid paper and block out the overall space available. Then a systematic procedure can be implicated in developing the following information:
1. A floor plan showing utility and structural details.
2. A flow chart showing the flow lines of the paper work in the office (and outside if applicable). The flow lines should go between major functions, not section to section.
3. Volume of paper work and its urgency.
4. The relative priority of each function.

After this information has been gathered, a flow chart showing the existing procedures can be made. Very likely this will show a complexity of crossing lines.

The next step is to study the possible alternatives. Templates of the office furniture which can be moved around on the grid paper are made. You may find out that your office supply house can be of direct assistance to you in this project, at least by providing layout paper and templates. It will be less likely to be helpful with the charts showing work flow. It should be of assistance in the minimum space requirements for employees (between 50 and 75 square feet for each person, depending on furniture and equipment), aisles, and so on. The main point to remember is that you must present the facts on paper and make a logical analysis of the situation. It will soon become obvious what improvements are possible.

## Forms Administration

As has been pointed out previously, the paper work requirements of a nursing home are tremendous and it is very easy to almost lose control of the situation. In Webster's Dictionary a form is defined as "a printed or typed document with blank spaces for insertion of information." According to this definition, almost every piece of paper used in your business is a "form." It follows that regular attention to forms in your nursing home should pay off handsomely in terms of more efficient operation, reduced space requirements, and reduced costs. The usual practice is to consider forms costs solely in terms of their purchase price. A good program of forms administration would go well beyond the initial cost factor. It would consider such factors as: copy requirements, design, types of paper, method of reproduction, type of binding (if necessary), cost of using the form, and time and money involved. You would do well to "pick the brains" of your forms suppliers and to talk to several of them about the help that they can give you. It is customary in the forms industry for the representatives to give considerable service in the way of design work at no cost to the prospective buyer. The forms business is one of the most competitive in the country and this knowledge may be of real help to you when you will need to determine what forms you will need to operate your nursing home.

## COST FINDING

It is not my purpose to detail the information readily available in guides and manuals put out by the Federal Government and the various intermediaries. These agencies are quite explicit for the most part, and in large measure spell out what records they require you to keep. It seems to me, however, that very little about how to accomplish the record requirements that they set up is stated in the manuals. There is a lot of unanimity among nursing home operators in regard to the paper work requirements established by the Social Security Administration, their intermediaries, and, in addition, by many states.

However, you must also look at the other aspects of the costs situation. You are in the business of performing essential services for ever-increasing numbers of people, and you want to give these people the best possible care, and, in addition, make a profit. Recent articles make it clear that sizable numbers of nursing homes have not found it possible to break even with their overall costs of operation and are withdrawing from Medicare and Medicaid programs. Others are remaining with these programs and seem to be able to provide excellent services and to make a profit at the same time.

Cost finding is not only necessary to meet federal and state requirements but also is an essential management tool for use over a wide area. You must have an accurate knowledge of the costs of each function and each department of your organization. You must know in which departments the costs are in line, and in which they are out of line. Accurate and complete cost records will be your basis for numerous immediate actions, long-range planning, and ultimately will determine the profitability of your nursing home.

Some of the objectives of cost finding are:
1. To provide the basis for establishing the rates for services, and to check the profitability of existing rates.
2. To provide a negotiating basis and to determine the totals of reimbursable costs.
3. To provide the necessary information for the multitude of reports.
4. To provide management information for decision-making in other areas.

It is a good idea at this point to review some of the principles involved in setting up the methods of cost finding. It is essential to have the basic requirements in mind, because you need them both in satisfying governmental requirements and for your own management requirements. The Social Security Administration principles in brief recap are:
1. Only the proper costs for that type of patient are to be borne by that patient.
2. The costs must be reasonable (it is intended to cover all "proper" costs, both direct and indirect), and the costs must be determined in accord with regulations. "Proper" costs are defined as the:
   A. Common and accepted occurrences in the field of the provider's activity.
   B. Appropriate and helpful in maintaining the operation of patient care facilities and activities.
3. Adequate records and cost data:
   A. The nursing home must provide adequate cost data for reimbursement.
   B. Cost data must be based on records which can be audited.
   C. Cost data must be on accrual basis.
4. Financial and statistical records must be kept in a constant manner (that is, not jumping from one basis to another), but desirable changes in procedures will likely be allowed.

The question of "adequacy" of records is certainly open to discussion, as is the question of what is needed to audit records. For instance, there is already substantial debate as to what is sufficient checking for a reliable audit in the cases of businesses using complete computer accounting. There are no simple answers to that question and doubtless will be none for some time. Keeping of records on the accrual basis causes little disagreement as it is generally recognized that to know one's cost picture accurately, the cost data have to be kept on the up-to-the-minute basis, including all costs incurred but possibly not yet paid.

The general reimbursement principles as established by the Social Security Administration can be summarized:

1. Determine expenses by departments.
2. Reclassify expenses by cost centers.
3. Distribute overhead cost centers to revenue-producing centers (cost finding).
4. Allocate costs between types of patient activities and programs.

As most of you know only too well, the major part of the "cost finding" work is in the area of coming up with the final costs of revenue-producing centers and program costs. This involves the most detailed kind of what used to be called "Cost Accounting." Only a few methods of cost allocation are approved by the Social Security Administration or recommended by AHA manuals as well, and they are complicated, to say the least. Naturally, if your nursing home is not involved in the Medicare or Medicaid programs, you need not adhere to all of their required procedures. However, in our opinion, you can do little less than is required by these programs and still come up with meaningful cost data for your own management decisions. The kinds of records that the Social Security Administration manual suggests and recommends are:

### Journals
1. Cash receipts
2. Cash disbursements
3. General
4. Voucher or accounts payable
5. Payroll
6. Charges

### Supporting Documents
1. Vendor invoices
2. Check vouchers and requests
3. Bank statements and cancelled checks
4. Charge slips

### Supporting Records
1. Payroll
2. Daily census reports and monthly summaries
3. Inventories (perpetual records or physical inventories)
4. Patient medical records

### Ledgers
1. General
2. Fixed assets
3. Accounts receivable

### Other Documents and Records
1. Auditor reports
2. Service department cost-finding statistics
3. Schedules of charges
4. Appraisal reports
5. Agreements with outside parties
6. Personnel files
7. Chart of accounts
8. Standard operating procedure manuals
9. Articles of incorporation or founding papers
10. Minutes of director's meetings, shareholder meetings, and committee meetings.

The paper work seems endless. The requirements are there, and the next aspects to be explored are the ways and means of setting up the records as easily and economically as possible. It is well to mention here that the current clamor on the part of politicians regarding all Medicare and Medicaid program costs will only tend to require you to keep even more records.

## VALUE ANALYSIS

An activity of vital importance to any business, and perhaps even more essential to nursing homes where income is somewhat restricted and, as a consequence, everything possible must be done to keep costs under control, is called Value Analysis. This term means exactly what it implies—analyzing everything possible to see whether you are getting the best value in total for the money expended. The General Electric Company is credited with having initiated the formalized procedures of Value Analysis, or Value Engineering, as designated by General Electric. After some months of experimentation, General Electric adopted the procedures on a company-wide basis. The annual savings rapidly rose to the level of hundreds of thousands of dollars. The procedures were adopted rapidly by some branches of the Federal Government, but mainly by profit-minded businesses. There is no reason whatsoever that Value Analysis can't be applied to nursing homes and become a regular part of the routine. What is it? Simply a systematic analysis of *procedures* and *purchases* to obtain maximum performance at minimum cost.

Every product purchased, every activity, and every service should be examined in the light of its performance and its utility as well as its cost. Value Analysis involves more than the usual cost-reduction procedures. In cost-reduction procedures, for example, in order to reduce your administrative overhead and office costs, which you feel to be too high, you may make studies showing that some reduction is possible in office supplies and perhaps work loads can be increased. These measures could result in some temporary savings. But if you think about it, behind that kind of study was the basic thought, "We'll keep our same old procedures, accounting systems, and office equipment, and just rearrange things so fewer people can do the work." Well, that is NOT Value Analysis. Value Analysis would make a complete analysis of the functions to see how they could be performed better, faster, more accurately, and more economically. In Value Analysis, questions like these are asked:

1. Does the function contribute value? (Of what real value are some of the data, information, and reports that are accumulated?)
2. Is the cost in line with usefulness? (How much does it cost to gather and maintain some accounting records in relation to their actual use to the business?)

3. Does the function really need all the features it possesses? (Are all parts of the various procedures essential to the end product or service?)
4. Is there any equipment that would enable the function to be performed more efficiently?
5. Can a usable product be purchased at a lower cost than the one employed?
6. Instead of using customized products and/or procedures, can a standard product be found that will do the job as well, or better?
7. Can some supplier provide the end product (reports, for instance) for less? Can some routine data processing work be farmed out?

Before we proceed any further into the discussion of Value Analysis possibilities, I believe it would be a good idea to consider some of the road blocks that General Electric Value Engineers encountered over the years as they were applying the Value Analysis techniques to areas of investigation.[8]
1. I agree but—.
2. We've tried that too.
3. We did it this way.
4. Procedures won't permit.
5. It won't work.
6. There is no money budgeted for this.
7. Don't move too fast.
8. You can't do that.
9. It's never been done that way before, etc.

Such "road blocks" are probably familiar to you. It is too easy to maintain the status quo.

How can Value Analysis help you? If you have someone on the staff who has a genuinely inquiring type of mind, it is highly advisable to make some of his time available for Value Analysis work. A simple Job Plan involves the use of a six-step or phase procedure:
1. Information phase.
2. Speculation phase.
3. Analytical phase.
4. Program planning phase.
5. Program execution phase.
6. Presentation and follow-up phase.

Obviously, all functions being analyzed would not need a great amount of time involved in all six steps of the plan. The check list should be used simply to remind you of the ground to be covered.

Basically, Value Analysis is the application of logical reasoning and common sense to as many functions of your operations as possible. For many a company, the savings resulting from its use improved the profit picture considerably.

## Payroll Preparation

As a specific example of one area of Value Analysis we will use payroll preparation. Let's assume that your employees are paid weekly, by check, and that they are fifty in number. Thus far in the field of technology, the preliminary work of time cards, rates, and so on, is pretty much the same for any of the methods of payroll preparation. There has to be some way of determining the number of hours worked, the hourly (or weekly) rate of pay for each employee, and allied information before the actual process of payroll preparation is begun.

We will discuss three methods of completing the payroll and compare their costs. The three methods are:

1. Regular hand method whereby a payroll summary for the week is usually made first, the data are then posted to individual earnings ledgers, and finally the checks are prepared.
2. The one-write method, wherein the three steps of Method 1 are performed simultaneously.
3. A computer payroll system as carried out by a service bureau. In this direct comparison, we begin with an elapsed time card for the employee, so that the comparison of the three methods is on an equal base.

*Method 1.* Time studies have shown that it takes an average of ten minutes per employee to make up the payroll by the step-by-step procedure. In this method, three sets of records have to be proven out separately because, being made separately, there is always the chance of copying errors. Who among you has not experienced hunting for errors due to transpositions, and taken a lot of time not only in finding them, but also in rectifying errors due to them?

The annual cost of forms would average about $65. But the bookkeeper's time involved would be considerable, taking a minimum of eight plus hours weekly for an average cost of $25 weekly, using an hourly rate of $3.00. Thus, the total annual cost of this system for fifty employees would approximate $1365.

| Materials | $    65 |
| Labor | 1300 |
| Total annual cost | $1365 |

*Method 2.* The standard "one-write" system eliminates about two-thirds of the time involved in the regular hand method (Method 1) for preparation of the payroll. Time studies have shown that it takes an average of three

minutes per employee for the processing of his records and preparation of his check by the "one-write" method.

In the "one-write" method the stub of the check is the employee's statement. The employee's earning record card and the payroll summary are placed under the check, and the earning information is typed on the top stub of the check. This information is automatically posted on the earnings ledger and on the weekly payroll summary at the same time. Not only is two thirds of the mechanical time saved, but the accuracy is improved considerably. The forms for a fifty-person weekly payroll would run about $100 per year. On starting the system, there would be a one-time cost of about $25 for equipment. The labor costs would run about $390 annually, with the book-keeper's rate of $3.00 per hour. Therefore, the total annual cost of this system would be $515 for the first year, and under $500 for each subsequent year.

*Method 3.* The computer service bureau has gained considerable popularity in the last two or three years. In checking several bureaus I find that each has a slightly different method of computing the costs of payroll services. The costs quoted by a national bank that has been offering the service for several years will be used. This bank has a running charge of $15.00 per pay period and, in addition, a charge of $0.32 per check, making the weekly cost of a 50-person payroll of $31.00—an annual cost of $1612. This would be less than the true cost because there are added expenses in starting a new employee into the system, a start-up cost for all employees at the outset, and a cost anytime a change in pay rate, deductions, or in any other existing memory data in the computer is made. A low estimated cost for the computer payroll service would be $1600 per year. And to this you must add the cost of picking up the checks from the bank.

One unique feature of the computer payroll service is the preparation of the quarterly payroll reports and the year-end W-2 forms for each employee. Although this is an excellent feature, on a strictly economic basis it does not compensate for the added costs of the EDP system.

*Cost Comparison of the Three Methods.* The following table summarizes the costs of the three methods of payroll preparation.

On a purely economic basis the one-write system would easily be the winner. But this system may, or may not, be the final answer. Perhaps your office staff is at a level where you know that you must add another person to the payroll, and this person would be the one who processes the payroll. If you could avoid adding this person to your staff by farming out the payroll to a service bureau, that would probably be the most economical thing to do. Labor is almost always the single highest cost of your operation. However, in the majority of cases, Method 2 will be the most feasible and economical to install. A good rule of thumb to use in estimating overall costs of a computer

Annual Costs for 50-Person Payroll

|  | Regular P/R | One-Write P/R | Computer P/R |
|---|---|---|---|
| Forms cost | $    65.00 | $125.00 | (included) |
| Labor | 1300.00 | 390.00 | negligible |
| Service charge | – | – | $1600.00 |
| Total cost | $1365.00 | $515.00 | $1600.00 |

payroll system at this time is 60 cents per check. Usually there is also a minimum charge of $20 to $30 per week, regardless of number of employees.

I have given you a quick look at a simple and typical cost comparison. Most comparisons will be far more involved, but if the systematic approaches are used, you will be able to end up with the most economical and logical solutions to your problem. Use the Value Analysis approach wherever you can, and you will select the procedure that will give you the most benefit for your money.

## One-Write Accounting

A recent article by Harold Steinberg, CPA, published in *The Journal of Accountancy* in the "Management Controls and Information" section is of interest.[7] It states:

> Pegboard (one-write) accounting is a simple and very low cost system for eliminating time-consuming and repetitive office procedures. Unfortunately, however, its use among even the small businesses is relatively limited. One major reason for this limited use—the lack of understanding of how the system works—can easily be overcome by just a brief exploration of the system's capabilities.
>
> The accounting result of a business transaction is the entry of data in various records. However, once the original determination of the data is completed and entered in the initial record, all the entries in subsequent records are no more than copying tasks. Only the format is different. One-write accounting takes advantage of this situation in that the entries in the many records are made all at once.

In one one-write system which handles the disbursement side of the records, four steps are carried out with one writing. And, of course, one-write systems are available on a full accrual basis, incorporating purchase journals and vendor ledgers.

Many other one-write systems are available to cut down the paper work load. Among them are accounts receivable systems, counter receipts systems, and some non-accounting ones such as prescription records, and narcotics record system.

### Work Measurement and Setting of Standards

I would be remiss if I didn't point out that, as I have stressed previously, your labor force is your biggest single cost of operation. Measuring its efficiency is a requisite for keeping costs under control. *Business Week* reported that more and more businesses have turned to borrowing some tools from the factory production line. Work measurement programs for all forms of clerical jobs are catching on. The Chase Manhattan Bank assessed its personnel by means of the scientific measurement yardstick. In three years, more than 800 jobs were eliminated. Payroll savings were "about $4.5 million per year." Utica Mutual Insurance Company crossed off 23 jobs from the organization chart in just 6 months. Its executives expect a 30 percent payroll savings when analysis is completed. It would appear that Chase Manhattan and Utica Mutual had been operating with excessive costs.

The techniques of work measurement and setting of standards have been available for more than fifty years and have been continually refined since the early days of "scientific management" under Frederick W. Taylor and Frank and Lillian Gilbreth. You will find that some exploration in this area will be well worth your while. Here are some suggestions about how you might obtain the data and information you need:

1. Your accounting firm is a most logical place to start, especially if it has a Management Services Division.
2. Numerous industrial engineering firms are able to assist you in Value Analysis work, work measurement, and similar fields.
3. Don't forget the services offered by systems and procedures firms. Often there are no consulting fees if the firms are interested in supplying systems for you.
4. Don't hesitate to pick the brains of the technical salesmen who stop by regularly. They can be a font of information if they know that you are interested.

### COMPUTERS AND THE NURSING HOME

To date I know of no true computer systems which are at a cost level affordable by a nursing home. There are several bookkeeping machine systems that fill the bill quite well, but they cannot handle all your cost accounting work. Again, a very close cost analysis is indicated to see whether one of these systems is the right one for your operation. In my opinion, there is a strong probability that in the not-too-distant future some one of the computer services will develop an accounting package expressly designed for nursing homes. Because of the particular accounting problems of a nursing home, such as the involved methods for allocation of overhead and indirect costs, the computer programming will necessarily be much more sophisticated than the usual general ledger programs now offered by computer service bureaus. The current state of technology makes your kind of programming entirely feasible, but, to the best of my knowledge, this service is not yet available from service bureaus.

## FUTURE POSSIBILITIES

One other possibility which is logical and seems to me to be a step that could be taken at almost any time would be to form regional groups of nursing homes. These groups could form a central buying organization to reduce costs of supplies and perhaps to eventually utilize a central computer service.

Many, many innovations are just around the corner. Some are already available, as I have already pointed out, and others will follow. It will pay you to keep abreast of technology and to plan reviews of almost all of your procedures regularly.

"Businesses planned for service are apt to succeed; businesses planned for profit are apt to fall."

Nicholas Murray Butler

## REFERENCES

1. Accounting manual for long term care institutions. 1968. American Hospital Association.
2. Business systems. 1966. Systems and Procedures Association.
3. Hechert and Kerrigan. 1967. Accounting systems. Ronald Press.
4. Martin, Thomas L. 1958. Hospital accounting principles and practice. 3rd Ed. Physician's Record Co., Chicago.
5. New York State Hospital Code. 1969.
6. Seawell, L. V. 1964. Hospital accounting and financial management. Physician's Record Company, Berwyn, Illinois.
7. Steinberg, H. I. 1965. Exploring peg board accounting. The Journal of Accounting. Cost finding and rate setting for hospitals. American Hospital Association, Chicago, Illinois.
8. Value analysis. 1961. Technocopy, Inc.

# Physical Therapy
# in a Nursing Home

*J. Alexander*

6 During the past decade, physicians and the public have come to expect that physical therapy will be one of the services provided by a nursing home. Conditions of participation in federally financed programs underscore the need for inclusion of "restorative services" to the total medical care offered. In response to this pressure for inclusion of physical therapy, criteria for referral have sometimes been misinterpreted and have sometimes led to inappropriate use of physical therapy services. Retroactive denial of payment is less likely to occur if motivation for referral is based on a rational analysis of the patient's need in keeping with his total medical management, and not merely on the desire of the nursing home to meet the "code," obtain added reimbursement, or to keep physicians and/or families satisfied that something is being done. It is essential that the physician and the therapist evaluate each patient's needs, identify his problems, and develop an appropriate treatment plan based on a physiological approach.

A large percentage of nursing home residents tend to be confined to bed[2] or are physically inactive. Frequently they have experienced hospitalization or prolonged illness at their homes prior to being transferred to the nursing home. Their general health is usually impaired. Unfortunately, many people see nursing homes as a custodial residence for patients with a terminal illness. Thus, the patient tends to assume a passive role, and the staff may have a tendency to project the expectation that patients should conform to such behavior. Physical inactivity combined with passive behavior may result in a general depressed and depressing attitude; this need not occur. Keeping patients active results in an improved level of health, better morale of patients and staff, and less need for nursing intervention. For a physical therapy program to be able to succeed, it is essential that the management and nursing staff give the program its wholehearted support and carefully evaluate the needs of the residents to determine how extensive a program, how large a staff, and how much space and equipment are needed to meet the objectives.[4]

## OBJECTIVES OF PHYSICAL THERAPY
## IN A NURSING HOME

Physical therapy can be employed to:

1. Minimize or prevent deleterious effects of inactivity.
2. Maintain or increase the patient's capacity for independent function.
3. Permit the patient to maintain his dignity and self-esteem.
4. Motivate the staff to participate in keeping patients self-reliant and demonstrate methods of accomplishing this objective.

## DELETERIOUS EFFECT OF INACTIVITY

Caillet[1] outlines the effects of a prolonged period of inactivity. Muscle atrophy or loss of muscle bulk can result from loss of nerve supply and/or disease. Muscle bulk constitutes a major portion of the body's protein. It serves as a covering over bony prominences and permits the body to tolerate the pressures of sitting or lying in bed. As atrophy progresses, metabolic changes occur, resulting in a negative nitrogen balance. One of the manifestations of negative nitrogen balance is reduced viability of skin. Prolonged pressure on capillaries unprotected by muscle bulk results in "squeezing out of blood" or ischemia of the skin and underlying tissue. If this process is permitted to continue for any length of time, the skin breaks down. Patients who are paralyzed also may have impairment of sensation and thus the usual discomfort signals may not remind them to turn. Incontinence has a tendency to macerate tissue and increase the danger of skin breakdown (decubitus ulcer formation). Decubitus ulcers can easily become infected and thus lead to chronic sepsis.

Reduced level of activity increases the likelihood of decrease in vital capacity and pulmonary reserves and increase in residual air. Respiratory infection is frequently concomitant with inactivity. Many patients may also have decreased cardiac reserves or a history of illness involving the cardiac or pulmonary systems. It is essential to institute activities that will balance the demand made on the patient with his capacity for function. Overprotection and inactivity tend to produce cardiac deterioration and reduced vital capacity and, in the "cardiopulmonary cripple," sudden excessive activity can lead to additional insults to already precariously functioning vital organs.

As a result of decreased muscular activity, bone tends to lose its ability to retain calcium. Osteoporosis presents a constant danger of fracture induced by minimal trauma. If a patient is on a prolonged course of steroid therapy this threat is increased. Calcium washed out of bone may be deposited in kidneys, bladder, or soft tissue.

Patients with neurological disorders may be unable to empty their bladders completely and thus develop increasing urinary retention. The ambiance of moisture, darkness, and warmth in the bladder constitutes a perfect breeding place for bacteria. Attempts at emptying the bladder by catheriza- tion can also result in introduction of infectious organisms due to carelessness while changing catheters.

Contractures and joint deformities are frequent byproducts of loss of elasticity of tendons, shortening of muscles, and tightening of joint struc- tures. Loss of joint mobility may seriously interfere with the patient's ability to move about and to perform activities of daily living, thus resulting in greater need for nursing care.

It may be easier for a staff member to perform an activity for a patient than to assist him in performing it himself. Eventually, the patient "gets the message" and doesn't even try, and thus, instead of maintaining some inde- pendence, becomes even more dependent. As his physical dependence in- creases, he also becomes more passive intellectually. He must go to bed when it is convenient for the staff; he can only participate in activities when there is someone willing to take him to the site where they are taking place. If he requests special consideration, he is labeled as a trouble-maker; or, even worse, he is deliberately ignored. Patients who have left rehabilitation centers with a fair degree of independence frequently lose much of the gain they have achieved during their course of treatment when they are sent to their homes, nursing homes, or convalescent centers, since the organism tends to respond on the level at which it is challenged. Thus, if little is demanded, functions tend to decrease.

Prevention of most of the problems resulting from inactivity is possible through intelligent management. Appropriate mobilization of patients within their physical limits may initially be more time-consuming, but will be a sound therapeutic investment.

## FUNCTIONS OF THE PHYSICAL THERAPIST

The physical therapist assumes many distinct roles. He is an evaluator, a provider of services, a teacher, a consultant, a director of group therapy, and a supervisor.

### Role as Evaluator

As an evaluator, the therapist is responsible for establishing base lines regard- ing a patient's strength, range of motion, functional status, integrity of skin, sensory modalities, and communication skill. He must perform manual mus- cle tests, or modifications thereof, to determine where muscle weakness can be identified and to what degree. He employs range of motion tests to determine the degree of movement(s) which can be performed passively at any given joint. He uses activities of daily living (ADL) tests to ascertain the areas in which the patient can function independently, in which he requires some assistance (by means of either a person or equipment), and in which he requires maximal assistance. From a realistic point of view, the length of time required to perform a given activity may be important and hence should be one of the parameters measured. Skin breakdown, if present or threatening, must be noted and considered in respect to the way in which the patient is to be treated. A simplified sensory examination is essential to determine whether there is loss of position sense, two-point discrimination, or loss of pressure, pain, temperature, visual, or tactile perception. Lack of information regarding deficits in the perceptual modalities can lead to serious accidents and open the way to a malpractice and/or negligence suit.

All findings must be recorded in a manner that is understandable to all who come in contact with the patient and must be available in the regular patient chart.

### Role as Provider of Services

The physical therapist serves as a provider of services. Based on his evaluation and in concord with the referring physician, the therapist develops a treatment program, carries it out, or delegates certain aspects to supportive personnel. Initially, *all therapy* should be performed by the therapist himself to permit direct observation of the patient's reaction to treatment and to facilitate modification as dictated by the patient's response to the therapy. Once a program is well-established and when the objective of therapy is to increase endurance, to practice skills previously taught by a therapist, or to maintain activity at a specific level, it may be permissible to delegate particular aspects of the treatment to well-supervised and carefully instructed supportive personnel. It must be pointed out, however, that many patients have multiple disabilities requiring careful and continuous monitoring to permit changes in the rate or intensity of therapy. Furthermore, fiscal intermediaries generally take a dim view of paying for physical therapy unless it is performed by a qualified physical therapist.

To accomplish treatment objectives, the therapist may devise exercise to increase strength, endurance, movement, agility, and balance as well as cardiopulmonary function. He may use *heat* or *cold*, in many different forms, to reduce pain or edema or to facilitate movement. Massage, hydrotherapy, and electrical stimulation are used according to the patient's needs. The therapist will teach the patient how to move from his bed to a chair, to a tub or shower, or to equipment. He will instruct the patient in ambulation with the use of canes, crutches, braces, or prostheses and in self-care activities. It is essential that when these activities are taught, re-enforcement by all people coming into contact with the patient be provided in a consistent, continuous, and patient manner. This can be hoped for only when all personnel are agreed on the treatment goal and are informed how the patient has been instructed. A consistent approach is especially important when dealing with brain-damaged patients, such as those with hemiplegias, who frequently have learning difficulty and low frustration tolerance, and, therefore, require a very structured setting in order to function.

### Role as a Teacher

The physical therapist in the nursing home should also be prepared to serve as a teacher. In-service training of nursing personnel in body mechanics, proper method of lifting and assisting patients, protecting patients from falling when they are ambulatory, and ways to minimize or prevent the development of contractures or the loss of muscle strength are the responsibility of the therapist. While the demand for therapists to work in nursing homes has increased, few physical therapy students are exposed to this aspect of physical therapy during their education. Attention should be given to creating an atmosphere that is conducive to learning. Admittedly, it takes time to teach and supervise students. Students may not be allowed to perform treatments or evaluations unless they are physically supervised by a licensed physical therapist. In a one-man department, it is difficult to ensure that this condition is always fulfilled. In addition, it is customary to provide some remuneration to full-time students in the form of meals, housing, and/or stipends. Students should only be accepted if there is adequate supervision and a sufficient variety of patients and patient problems to permit meaningful learning experiences. Students should never be considered as "cheap help."

### Role as Consultant

As a consultant, the therapist assists the nursing staff in developing means of coping with the problems presented by individual patients. He demonstrates how activities should be carried out and ascertains that they are carried out correctly. He monitors the patient's progress from time to time and alters the program in keeping with the changes in the patient's condition.

Again it must be emphasized that delegation of given tasks carries with it the responsibility for making sure that the person who is asked to assume these tasks is properly prepared to accept them. Responsibility can never be given away—only tasks may be shared.

### Role as Director of Group Therapy

In selected instances the therapist may work with a group of patients. In addition to increasing his ability to serve more patients, this technique also permits socialization and re-motivation. It reduces the patient's tendency to see his problems as unique and facilitates the development of a more realistic outlook. It may be necessary to have the aid of supportive personnel in order to safeguard patients and to guarantee their full participation. If therapy is a chargeable item, group therapy should be treated distinctly from therapy performed on a one-to-one basis. Group therapy cannot take the place of individual treatment, but it can supplement it. Specific objectives that can be accomplished by group therapy, provided the patients have similar problems and similar levels of performance, may include general conditioning exercise to maintain general body strength and modified ball games and rhythm activities to increase balance or socialization.

### Role as Supervisor

If there is more than one therapist or if supportive personnel assist the therapist, the therapist must also function as a supervisor. He must develop appropriate standard operating procedures and methods of record keeping and budgeting, and must requisition supplies and equipment. He must assure an equitable distribution of workloads and develop his staff to meet the objectives of the institution. He may be responsible to interpret the physician's request to his staff and ensure that the patients receive the appropriate treatment. Just as any other supervisor, he must evaluate his staff and take corrective action when this may be indicated.

### RECORD KEEPING

One of the immediate results of increased public participation in the health field is the growing demand for accountability. Nursing homes have been identified as one of the areas where prevailing medical practices, as well as therapist's actions, have been questioned. Utilization review, if not already an established fact, will no doubt become a prerequisite for continuous accreditation of the institution, as well as a condition for reimbursability.

Weed[5] introduced a system of record keeping that is designed to facilitate auditing the appropriateness of patient management. A systematic review of objective and subjective findings is used to develop a complete patient profile. Based on the initial data, a list of problems—not diagnoses—is established together with a suggested plan for solving each specific problem. As a problem is solved, it is marked closed, and new problems can be added to the list as they are discovered. Subsequent progress notes are always oriented to the numbered list, and only those problems in which change can be reported or which require further attention (because none of the hoped-for-change has occurred) are cited. At time of discharge, the complete list is reviewed with an appropriate statement regarding what has occurred during the course of treatment, and recommendations are made for home program of further therapy and follow-up.

A chart organized in this manner ensures that all of the patient's difficulties are kept in mind and minimizes the likelihood of forgetting an important aspect of the patient's management.

Problem-oriented charts can be used to teach all personnel, to serve as a checklist during evaluation conferences, and to permit ready examination by utilization review committees or third-party payers.

Care must be taken that management problems, rather than diagnoses, are listed. For instance, a patient with a diagnosis of diabetes might be admitted to the nursing home with a number of specific problems, each of which can be managed:

1. Blood sugar—elevated.
2. Peripheral neuropathy—sensory deficit.
3. Decubitus ulcer—over right heel.
4. High blood pressure.
5. Decreased arterial supply—right leg.
6. Decreased visual acuity.
7. Depression.
8. Disorientation.

After an examination of the patient the physical therapist might add:

9. Weakness (right) upper and lower extremities.
10. Difficulty in ambulation.
11. Difficulty in transfer.
12. Lack of initiative or motivation.

Based on this problem list, a treatment program becomes self-evident and permits more complete interchange of information between the active treatment team. It is recommended that the problem list become the top sheet of the chart and that everyone involved in the patient's management be instructed to add to the list as the information becomes available.

If physical therapy is a separate billable service, all treatments must be itemized. In some instances, identifiable notes written into the chart at the conclusion of every visit are required for reimbursability. Unfortunately, this demand leads to voluminous, repetitious, and meaningless charts. On the other hand, third-party payers, as well as physicians, want to be assured that the patient has received a specific treatment and what was done. Simple charge forms can be devised to include this type of information without cluttering up the history record. Charge forms also facilitate preparation of a monthly activity report, which may be necessary for institutional accreditation.

Medicare has made a most unfortunate distinction between "restorative" and "maintenance" services. The latter service has been defined by the Social Security Administration as a skilled nursing function and as such is not reimbursable. This short-sighted decision is detrimental to the welfare of the patient who comes to the nursing home with a multiplicity of problems which are constantly changing and which require the use of immediate and critical judgments to avoid adding to the patient's difficulty. It is, therefore, essential that restorative *versus* maintainance services be considered when establishing criteria for referral. In addition, records must document this medical decision and problem-oriented initial and follow-up notes permit ready auditing of the appropriateness of therapy.

## SPACE, EQUIPMENT AND STAFF NEEDS

Schlossman[3] suggests that equipment and space requirement depends largely on:

1. Anticipated caseload.
2. Actual space available.
3. Budget.
4. The preference of the therapist.
5. The number of people working in the department.

Therapists can work with minimal equipment. They frequently do so when treating patients at home. However, some basic equipment will increase the efficiency of the therapist and the safety of the patients.

Minimally, a treatment table (30 inches in width and, if possible, of adjustable height), 12-foot adjustable-height parallel bars (weights, pulleys), adjustable canes (four-legged canes, crutches, walkerettes), some form of heat equipment (such as a hydrocollator unit and/or infrared lamp), ice machine, filing and storage cabinets, chairs, screens, expendable supplies, and pillows and linen should be available. A sphygmomanometer, stethoscope, and reflex hammer are needed to monitor patients' responses. Whirlpools and ultraviolet lamps are most useful in maintaining healthy skin. A tilt table may facilitate getting a patient who had been on prolonged bedrest accustomed to the upright position.

Additional equipment, such as diathermy and ultrasound apparatus, paraffin baths, and cold pack units, is desirable but may not be used frequently. A therapeutic pool may be extremely impressive but will usually not be utilized to any extent unless there are sufficient staff members to warrant the extra time and effort entailed.

Ideally, a spacious, well-ventilated, cheerful area should be provided. Plants and decorations which can be changed from time to time will add to the setting. A generous area permits group programs combining physical, therapeutic, and psychosocial objectives. Suitable music provided by FM radio, record player, or a background music system will be enjoyed by the patients. If a whirlpool is considered, it is helpful if this equipment is in a separate room where floor and wall covering are of moisture-resistant material and where there is a drain in the floor. A Hoyer Lift or a similar mechanical device for lifting patients is highly recommended.

The therapist's capacity to treat patients can be materially increased by a supportive staff. These assistants can be responsible for housekeeping, simple record keeping such as attendance forms, getting patients from the domiciliary area to the treatment area on time and returning them at the completion of the therapy session, preparing whirlpool baths and getting the patients in and out of these baths. They can prepare patients for treatment by assisting them with dressing and undressing as necessary. They can help patients in putting on braces, artificial limbs, or other adaptive equipment. If indicated by the therapist, aides or assistants may apply hot packs or infrared lamps and assist patients in performing activities initiated by the therapist. The aides should be well-instructed, and oriented to their part in the program. It is highly recommended that they not be permitted to provide services which could be described as physical therapy and which carry with them a certain degree of risk unless a physical therapist is physically present.

Initially, a therapist may need to see a patient for 30 minutes to an hour at a time to permit him to perform the necessary evaluations, develop the treatment program, and observe the patient's response to therapy. As the patient improves and as he becomes more familiar with the routine of therapy, actual time per patient spent by the therapist can be decreased.

It is most helpful that time be planned for nursing staff, physical therapist, the physician, and other staff members to periodically share their experiences and to exchange suggestions for continuing patients' activities beyond therapy time. At times, it may be beneficial for the patient to skip the planned therapy and in its stead permit the patient to talk about how he feels about his problems. An astute therapist can utilize this opportunity for helping the patient to accept realistic treatment goals. Variation of methods for accomplishing treatment objectives may help to prevent ennui and keep interest and participation at a high level.

## LEGAL IMPLICATIONS

Physical therapy practice is regulated by law. A physical therapist must meet the requirement of the licensure of the state in which he expects to practice. Reciprocity or endorsement of licensure is possible in specific instances. The law requires that a physical therapist accept patients only on referral from a duly licensed physician.

Physical therapists may work as salaried employees, as independent practioners, on a fee-for-service basis, or on a contractual basis.

Increased third-party payment has resulted in the development of guidelines to determine who is eligible for physical therapy reimbursement. These guidelines are constantly changing and must be carefully monitored. State medical aid programs and Medicare regulations have been accepted in many instances as models for decisions by other insurance carriers. It is recommended that, in all instances, authorization and conditions for treatment be obtained in advance to avoid "retroactive denial" or a post facto refusal by the intermediary to pay for services rendered.

## DEFINITIONS

Some confusion arises as to who is a physical therapist, a physical therapy assistant, and a physical therapy aide.

*A physical therapist* is a professional member of the medical team. His education is minimally on a baccalaureate level. In addition to subjects of a broad liberal nature, he is prepared in basic sciences, gross and functional anatomy, physiology, pathology, and psychology. He is made aware of the problems encountered by medical, surgical, and neurologically impaired patients of all ages and he is atuned to the psychosocial implications of illness or disability. He is skilled in evaluation of a patient's functional status and in developing and executing appropriate treatment programs based on the patient's needs. He is knowledgeable in the use of supportive equipment to increase the patient's functional ability and to minimize deleterious effects of inactivity.

*A physical therapy assistant* is a recent addition to the allied health manpower. He (or she) is a graduate from a community college program which meets the basic guidelines set forth by the American Physical Therapy Association. He must work under the supervision of a licensed, professional physical therapist. Some disagreement exists about how close this supervision must be. One can be guided by Hippocrates who warned that we should do no harm to those under our care. Therefore, the amount and directness of supervision would depend on the types of patients treated, the degree of judgment necessary, the caliber of the assistant, the specific stipulations of the law, and the terms of malpractice insurance covering the operations of the physical therapy department.

*A physical therapy aide* is a person who has received on-the-job training and assists the therapist and physical therapy assistant by assuming responsibility for general housekeeping, giving messenger service, preparing patients for therapy, and helping in "handling" difficult patients. Selected treatment procedures may be delegated to the aide if, in the judgment of the therapist, this will not be injurious to the patient.

It is necessary to reiterate that mobilizing patients through physical therapy carries some degree of risk to patients. It is essential, therefore, that adequate insurance be maintained. If the institution provides this coverage, the physical therapist and his supportive personnel should be designated and the therapist should be apprised of this coverage. If the therapist, under the terms of his contract, is held responsible to provide his own coverage, he should also supply the institution with proof of the adequacy of the insurance and indicate whether his helpers are included.

## REFERENCES

1. Caillet, R. 1961. Exercise in multiple sclerosis. *In* S. Licht Therapeutic exercise, 2nd ed., E. Licht, Publisher, New Haven.
2. Damato, T. F. 1967. Trained physical therapy aides extend professional skills. Hospitals, JAHA, 41:77–82.

3. Schlossman, S. M. 1968. Physical therapy in a small nursing home. Nursing Homes. 17: 7–12.
4. Utt, W. H. 1968. Physical therapy planning. Nursing Homes. 17: 16–17.
5. Weed, L. L. 1970. Medical records, medical education, and patient care. Yearbook Medical Publishers, Inc., Chicago.

# The Roles of Occupational Therapy within the Nursing Home Setting

## V. N. Ferrante

7 The continuously increasing population within the setting of the nursing homes has had marked effects and made dramatic changes within the profession of occupational therapy. Until recently, the profession was not attracted to the care of the elderly as a field of endeavor but we must now meet the ever growing challenge and responsibility to improve the care and understanding of older individuals. It is evident that the needs of these residents to live life in its entirety has given to occupational therapists a "new face" and a multi-faceted role. The acceptance of this new role is evident in the changing trends of programs in homes and extended care facilities for the aging which must have characteristics of flexibility, diversity, and ingenuity.

### DEFINING OCCUPATIONAL THERAPY

There are no strict delineations of needs; in fact an overriding and inter-mingling of the general areas of physical, emotional, social, and intellectual needs have necessitated the formulation of programs closely inter-related and one relevant to the other so that by the very definition of *occupational therapy* accepted by the American Occupational Therapy Association as *the art and science of directing man's response to selected activities to promote and maintain health, to prevent disability, to evaluate behavior, and to treat or train patients with physical or psychosocial dysfunction,* the goals within the facility for the care of this age category may be brought to fruition. They are a reflection and implementation of the facility's philosophy and objectives pertaining to total overall care of its residents, which hopefully should emphasize maximum utilization of assessed capabilities and involve residents in decision-making group situations as well as individual relationships.

## STAFF PATTERNS AND PROCEDURES

Considering health service needs and related programs in a nursing home or extended care facility, staffing patterns ideally would include an occupational therapist on a regularly scheduled part-time or consultant basis, at least. In what ways can the therapist best serve the nursing home—its administrators, staff, and residents? The therapist, by training and experience, provides skills and contributes to the optimum quality and quantity care essential in these facilities. The direct service care on the part of a regularly employed therapist has specific methods and procedures.

First, and foremost, direct service care requires referral from a physician who requests specific goals to be achieved or worked toward based upon his diagnosis. Nursing staff and other professionals, such as social workers, may also be sources of referrals since they frequently, by the very nature of their close relationship with the resident, discover problems which may evolve during the course of their stay in the facility. Upon referral, the therapist evaluates the individual, in order to plan an appropriate and realistic treatment program dependent upon the data accumulated.

The procedures for data collecting involves evaluation of physical status, covering capabilities, degree of limitations, and possible potential levels. This determination is based upon testing via the use of standardized methods, to evaluate:

1. Range of motion.
2. Muscle strength.
3. Coordination level.
4. Activities of daily living such as dressing, feeding, toileting, transfer, and the numerous other related self-care components and every day activities.
5. Psychological assessment by observation of behavioral reaction within structured or non-structured situations.

In addition to the above procedures, to develop a composite picture of the resident, every effort must be made to acquire pertinent information—physical, emotional, social, intellectual, vocational, from all available sources, such as other professionals, physicians, nurses, social workers, physical and speech therapists. The occupational therapist is in a unique position to identify problems—observing reactions to his or her environment—and alerting other team members on her findings in order to provide a supportive program. It is only in this sharing of pertinent information that the "whole" individual may be understood thoroughly and thus realistic physical objectives and goals of adjustment be proposed and developed to meet his or her needs.

## THE TREATMENT PLAN

The treatment plan now to be outlined must also take into consideration the attitudes of the resident toward his physical status—acceptance or rejection—and the degree of motivation for self-improvement. What does the individual consider his primary need? It might be wise, in order to achieve a higher degree of cooperation, to plan a program attaining that need first, if not medically inadvisable, so that by demonstrating success in one phase, other goals, considered by the therapist to be equally, if not more important, may be worked upon with fewer objections. To a great degree, people's feelings, about themselves and others influence goal setting as much as strictly physical factors. Thus, establishing a mutually acceptable treatment goal, the therapist by skillful interpersonal relationship can direct or guide a resident in the selection of carefully analyzed activities or work-related projects, providing the opportunity to have some degree of personal choice and challenging mental capacities. Whether emphasis is upon increased range of motion, muscle strengthening, hand-eye coordination, or increased tolerance, the option of selection should be presented to the patient, thereby stimulating participation and interest on a graded level. Visual evidence of accomplishment or progress sustains interest and promotes a good mental attitude toward increased activity and environmental involvement. Any degree of improvement—no matter how small, particularly with the aged—helps to achieve a more satisfactory attitude and adjustment in coping with the process of living. Maintaining this sustained interest and motivation by the use of properly analyzed, devised projects to provide required motions to be transferred at a later time into normal activities on the basis of range, strength, and coordination, is the responsibility of the therapist or any occupational therapy staff personnel, implementing the program plan under her supervision or guidance. It is the encounter between giver and receiver in a well-balanced setting of environment and services that is stressed as a means of reactivation improving the inherent capabilities of an individual. Active participation in the treatment plan is the most essential facet of any program. The implications are that in all planning, the factors most important and basic to the elimination of unsatisfactory adjustment are: (1) maintaining good physical function, (2) a useful and productive role, and (3) satisfying social interaction and positive attitudes with vital programs working to overcome dependency fostered by the sheltered environment so prevalent in care of the elderly.

These goal-related projects or activities, providing proof of abilities and productiveness, have a real psychological impact, resulting in increased self-confidence and a willingness to explore new avenues of activities and improved interaction with his object and interpersonal world.

## MINIMAL ASSISTANCE AS A GOAL

To this point, the therapist has evaluated and formulated a program plan providing the resident with the opportunity to participate in goal-directed projects, not only physically and reality-oriented, but creative and social as well, fostering alertness, alleviation of depression, and the building of attitudes of well-being. The knowledge of capability to function instills *self-confidence* and *self-respect*. Higher levels of *self-esteem* and *broadened horizons, an awareness of the things around him, greatly diminishes feelings of uselessness and rejection.*

*Security, self-confidence,* and *ability to function independently* are the cornerstones in program planning in activities of daily living. Any deficits in the component factors of daily living noted in the initial evaluation are eliminated by teaching techniques within the abilities of the individual to function with minimal supervision or assistance. Basically, individuals are much more comfortable in a situation requiring this minimal help; if a device for completely independent functioning is the only answer, then it is fabricated by the therapist. Every attempt is made to train without special or extra equipment. However, such devices, if wisely selected, frequently increase ability and may make it possible to start training earlier than would ordinarily be possible. Perhaps just an elastic palmar band with pocket to hold eating utensils is the solution to inability to feed oneself; it is most logical to encourage the resident to utilize this piece of equipment, thus releasing some member of nursing staff for other duties. Whatever progress is achieved in any area of self-care should be reported to the nursing staff in order to have it followed through and re-enforced on the nursing units.

## THE TEACHING FUNCTION OF THE OCCUPATIONAL THERAPIST

It is also the responsibility of the therapist to teach the appropriate and safe techniques of transfer and other self-care activities to provide a continuum of care. This may take place at the time of initial activities of daily living evaluation or at the scheduled times for training as required or determined by the evaluation. Such an arrangement is mutually beneficial to the staff and resident. The resident learns by continuous, correct re-enforcement to do things safely and more independently and eventually nursing staff is released to provide more pressing nursing care to others.

Demonstration of proper applications of splints, slings, or other special devices is also essential on the part of the therapist so that their use will be encouraged. The impact of a good activities-of-daily-living program effects not only the resident, but also the nursing staff; as self-care abilities increase, the demands upon staff decrease. Additionally, now being able to function on a higher level of independence, the individual is more inclined to move about more freely, thereby increasing his or her sphere of social and intellectual interaction.

## RECORD KEEPING

Any program, whether restorative, psychological, or maintenance, must be recorded in resident charts for implementation and coordination with other therapeutic goals. Periodic reviews and re-evaluations are likewise essential to re-adjust or adapt activities to either progress or regression as noted. Changes in program reflect not only the observations of the resident by the therapist during this process of treatment but also any information acquired in team conferences with other personnel involved therapeutically in the care of the individual.

## STAFF PARTICIPATION

Staff working with the person must be made aware of any goal or treatment technique changes, either on a verbal or written basis in the matter of goals, and verbally or by demonstration in the use of techniques.

To carry out programs effectively, the therapist should be provided with sufficient staff—if the facility is fairly large—the physical space to work comfortably in a pleasant atmosphere with wheelchair as well as ambulatory people, and materials and equipment adequate for carrying out planned programs. Number and types of staff personnel would reflect the needs of the residents as indicated by planned programs. The certified occupational therapy assistant (COTA) who is a graduate of a curriculum meeting the standards of and approved by the American Occupational Therapy Association and properly certified through examination, can follow through the program therapeutically planned by the therapist. However, the COTA does need guidance, supervision, instruction, and evaluation of her performance. In addition to functioning in the treatment process, under the registered occupational therapist, activity, maintenance, and supportive programs could also be included in her sphere of position requirements. The occupational therapy aide, in addition to the assistant, contributes to the effective implementation of any program. She can assist in routine treatment duties such as re-enforcing and continuing training in areas of activities of daily living, exercise, preparation of and assistance with projects, group work, and observation of reaction and behavior which are to be recorded and reported to the therapist. Assistance in record keeping, routine office work, supply and equipment maintenance, as well as general housekeeping responsibilities frees the therapist or assistant from routine chores and increases time allocated to function in direct resident care for which each in her own position is technically trained.

## ROLE OF THERAPIST

The therapist, in a direct service situation, therefore functions to:
1. Evaluate.
2. Plan.
3. Treat.
4. Supervise.
5. Instruct both resident and staff.
6. Coordinate her program with all other disciplines for the effective total care of the resident.

In situations where full-time or regularly scheduled part-time services of an occupational therapist are not available, a consultant occupational therapist very frequently, through her experience and knowledge in health care of the elderly, is the source for pertinent and vital information. The repertoire of occupational therapy consulting service covers a variety of areas and levels. On the administrative level, interpretation of the principles and scope of occupational therapy as related to the fulfillment of the health needs of the facility's residents is of primary importance. The development of a philosophy of care can assist the staff substantially in planning programs for patient participation; recommendation for types of activities and expansion or changes required to meet particular resident needs all fall within her province as a consultant.

In this role, the therapist incorporates rehabilitation concepts into the activities program in the initial planning stage in order to encourage higher caliber of physical and mental participation of the resident. Periodic consultation allows for re-evaluation of the programs as to effectiveness in relation to the total facility population. Guidance can also be given to assist individual patient needs and incorporating some of the skills learned through occupational therapy into the media of purely diversional activities. Program formulation, planning, and coordination is based on the premise that no matter what the discipline, the focus is on the physical, psychosocial, and intellectual needs of residents.

## FACILITY PLANNING

The occupational therapy consultant may be utilized in the initial structural planning of a facility to provide the requisites for adequate space for all programs. This may involve assisting in the initial planning of the department on a physical basis: space requirements to allow freedom of movement by wheelchair and ambulatory residents, proper height working surfaces, adequate light, heat and ventilation, and amount of storage needed. Items such as grab bars, toilet seat heights, width of doorways, and other architectural considerations would all fall into this area of facility requirements. To stimulate favorable response to goals established in planning for the individual, it is essential that the physical facilities for carrying out treatment have the following provisions:

1. Large enough to allow freedom of movement of wheelchair and ambulatory residents.
2. Adequate lighting and ventilation.
3. Working surfaces adjusted to comfortable heights—for both wheelchair and ambulatory residents.
4. Easily maintained work surfaces.
5. Clean-up and toilet facilities close to, or more ideally within, the working area.
6. Storage facilities for supplies and current projects under way by the residents.
7. An area free from or with minimal distracting stimuli for work in perceptual-motor skills.
8. A small kitchen area which provides an opportunity for male as well as female residents to attempt once again those homemaking skills which comprised such a large part of their lives.
9. Assist in planning for general elimination of architectural barriers such as narrow doorways, lack of grab bars, commodes of incorrect heights, etc.

All the above factors are essential for an environment fostering successful achievement of program and treatment goals resulting in gratification and fulfillment of needs.

## OCCUPATIONAL THERAPIST AS TEAM MEMBER

The consultant should also be available to nursing staff in any occupational therapy-related problems. These mainly involve demonstration of techniques of activities of daily living, range of motion exercises, to prevent contractures, proper use of wheelchairs and adapted equipment for encouraging optimum functional level of self-care.

Consultation with the occupational therapy department may pertain to identifying resident-care problems, formulation of policies and procedures, organizational structure, program planning, job description, recruitment of qualified personnel, resolving staff relationships either within the department, to other departments, or residents.

The consultant should be available to attend staff meetings and conferences where some of the problems may surface for discussion. Recommendations for their solution may be made orally, at this time, to be followed by a written summary. In-service education and development of educational materials also fall into the scope of consultant services.

All consultations should be summarized in writing and cover such facts as time and place, persons seen, what took place during the visit, the topics covered, and recommendations for a course of action based on information collected.

These are all made on an advisory basis as they pertain specifically to the field of occupational therapy but contingent upon the recognition of the fact that interpersonal relationships exist between all disciplines in the care of nursing home residents.

## CONCLUSION
To serve in these capacities, the occupational therapist must have a broad field of experience, an ability to accept challenge, satisfaction in and ability relating to people on a service level and within the framework of a team. An ability to teach, patience, flexibility, understanding, powers of observation, maturity, creativity, and imagination are as important to the success of an occupational therapy program as are the medical and technical skills acquired through the process of education.

## REFERENCES
1. Hagen, P. M. 1967. Nursing home residents: a challenge to the occupational therapist. Am. J. Occup. Therapy. 21: 151–155.
2. Judd, M. W. 1971. Why bother, he's old and confused. Winnipeg Municipal Hospitals, Winnipeg 13, Manitoba, Canada.
3. Kaplan, J. 1957. The social care of older persons in nursing homes. Am. J. Occup. Therapy. 11: 240–243.
4. Moore, B. M. 1954. Interpersonal relations. Am. J. Occup. Therapy. 8: 100–103.
5. Mosey, A. C. 1968. Occupational therapy: Theory and practice, training grant from RSA to the Medical Foundation, Inc., Boston, Mass. Pothier Broitus, Printers, Inc., Medford, Mass.
6. Mosey, A. C. 1973. Meeting health needs. Am. J. Occup. Therapy. 27: 14–17.
7. Weidman, L. 1970. The sunset years. Nursing Homes. Nov: 14–15.

### Special Brochures
1. Occupational Therapy Reference Manual for Physicians. 1960. American Occup. Therapy Assoc. Wm. C. Brown Book Co., Dubuque, Iowa.
2. The Consulting Process for Occupational Therapists: Committee on Continuing Education, Council on Standards. American Occup. Therapy Assoc.
3. Manual on Occupational Therapy in Nursing Homes. 1969. Missouri Occupational Therapy Assoc.
4. Guideline for interpretation of Occupational Therapy in general practice

and rehabilitation. 1970. Michigan Occupational Therapy Assoc., Ann Arbor, Mich., Comm. on Practice.

5. Occupational therapy job descriptions. Special Grant #5 DO2 AH00964-01, 2 Dept. H.E.W., Public Health Service. 1972. The Ohio State Univ., Columbus, Ohio, School of Allied Medical Professions.

6. Restorative occupational therapy in the extended care facility. 1971. California Occup. Therapy Assoc.

7. The O.T. as consultant: workshop excerpts. 1969. University of Puget Sound, Tacoma, Wash., School of O.T.

8. Guidelines on occupational therapy in nursing homes and related facilities. 1970. Wisconsin Occup. Therapy Assoc.

# Communication Problems of the Client in a Nursing Home or Rehabilitation Center

*Ralph W. Jones*

" . . . I was in a furious state . . . the consultant saved my life, but at the time he addressed me as though I were deaf, a foreigner, or mentally deficient. He used to pitch his voice up and ask me how I was doing and then he would lower his tone and say to my wife, 'I think he understood that.' I lay helplessly silent—and above all, angry."

Patient, Mr. A.

8 The above passage from the writing of a stroke patient shows just one of the problems that a nursing home administrator will encounter with perhaps a half-dozen of the clients in his facility. The people who are having such thoughts are most likely those with aphasia. A person suffering from aphasia usually finds himself suddenly flung into a difficult world that leaves him frustrated and with a feeling of helplessness.

## WHAT IS APHASIA?

Aphasia is a medical term meaning inability to deal with the symbols of communication. In recent years, it has been used to designate both total and partial loss of communication ability, although literally "dysphasia" means partial and "aphasia" means total loss of ability to communicate.

Aphasia can take various forms. A client (I prefer the use of this word rather than "patient" as I feel it to be a more appropriate designation for an active participant in communications therapy) may be able to understand words, but not be able to write or utter them. He may not be able to use numbers or to read. This does not necessarily mean, however, that he has lost the power to think clearly. Usually he can think reasonably well.

## WHAT CAUSES APHASIA?

Aphasia is caused by brain damage. From birth to old age there are several disorders that can affect the blood vessels of the brain, impairing the functions of the brain itself. The five main ones, all of which are familiar, are hemorrhage (bleeding), thrombosis (clot formation), embolism (blocking of a blood vessel by a clot), compression (pressure), and spasm (tightening and closing down of the walls of an artery). In young children, aphasia is usually the result of brain damage suffered prior to birth, during birth, or in infancy. In teenagers it is usually the result of a serious automobile accident.

One possible result of cerebral vascular disease is the "stroke"—referred to by most physicians as a cerebral vascular accident (CVA). A stroke usually occurs suddenly when an artery supplying blood to a portion of the brain ruptures or is closed by thrombosis, an embolism, or by any of the other conditions mentioned above, thus resulting in loss of oxygen to a portion of the brain. A patient who has had a stroke may have paralysis of an arm and leg and, often, difficulty in speaking and using language—aphasia.

I often liken aphasia resulting from a stroke to what happens when a telephone wire is cut. The two telephone instruments (perhaps the brain center and the speech organs) work well but somewhere in between is the cut wire (neurological damage) that prohibits communication. Because the aphasic cannot always say what his brain tells him to, a specific therapy needs to be designed. Failure to provide this can lead to increased depression.

Not all communications problems represented in your facility will be due to strokes. Although stroke will probably be the most prevalent cause, some patients will suffer from other neurological problems such as cerebral palsy, epilepsy, multiple sclerosis, muscular dystrophy, brain tumors, and Parkinson's disease. You may also have a few patients with cancerous growths at sites that interfere with the speech organs.

## INCIDENCE OF COMMUNICATIONS PROBLEMS
## IN NURSING HOMES AND REHABILITATION UNITS

The most accurate estimates that I am able to obtain from the federal government, and from my own 25-year experience, leads me to estimate that, in a 72-bed rehabilitation facility, there would probably be six to eight clients with a communications problem due to stroke, with a maximum of twelve having this problem due to all causes. The "hard of hearing," who are not included in this chapter, might add considerably to this number. There would probably be little, if any, outpatient services, although these may expand in the coming years. In a nursing home, 72-bed facility, for example, there would likely be fewer at any one time—perhaps five to six (of all types)—than in a rehabilitation center.

Of an estimated 2 million persons who suffer from cerebrovascular accidents, one-third are wage earners, under the age of 65, who have been made unemployable by the residuals of these "accidents." It is especially important that these comparatively young people have every opportunity to regain as much of their communications ability as possible. One-third or at *least* 200,000 of these people have acute communications problems. Moreover, in the American Heart Association's publication, "Seven Helpful Facts about Strokes," printed in 1969, appears the statement: "Since 1950 the stroke death rate has dropped 32% among middle-aged men (45–64 years of age)." Medical skills are keeping these people alive; we must help to rehabilitate them.

In a rehabilitation unit, there may also be two or more victims of brain damage resulting from an automobile or other type of accident. Since these people are usually in the lower age group, their prognosis for at least a partial recovery and return to the stream of life is far better than for the individual who is 65 or older.

## WHO SHOULD DIRECT THERAPY FOR APHASIA?

The need for a speech pathologist who specializes in aphasia—for administering therapy to an aphasic client cannot be overemphasized. The New York State Hospital Code, Section 731.13 on speech and rehabilitation services, begins, "The operator shall employ or otherwise arrange for a qualified speech pathologist to provide speech and language rehabilitation services for patients when such services are ordered by a physician." Note especially that the code specifies speech *pathologist*. Codes of other states should be checked and up-to-date information kept on file, since changes may be made frequently.

Occasionally, experts from some other fields or within other areas of speech pathology have a sincere desire to help the aphasic. It is almost inevitable that these people will use techniques and materials employed in their usual type of work. The results are often worse than those of no therapy at all. The efforts can be likened to trying to fit a tractor tire to a passenger car.

Depending on the resources available in your community, you quite naturally may feel the need to turn to the person who provides speech therapy and services to the "hard of hearing" in your public schools. However, this individual is usually not qualified to provide training to the aphasic client.

There may be a nearby college in which speech pathology is taught and in which a professor skilled in aphasia is available to give some consultative services. The professor may choose to use some student help. Some exceptional students are able to handle specifically assigned segments of the work with the aphasic and other similar clients if the evaluations are complete and clear, and if they have constant supervision by skilled aphasiologists who not only observe but actually demonstrate the types of techniques essential for the program.

The worker whom the administrator secures should be someone with a flexible time schedule and a deep dedication to the cause. He should expect to be available occasionally to see relatives or others on a Saturday morning, a Sunday, or in the evening. He can, or course, avoid off-hour commitments, but not in the best interests of his clients. Hopefully, a qualified individual will be available to your clients for from 6 to 20 hours a week.

A communications therapist working with clients having acute CVA problems should have, or have had, at least the following:

1. The usual courses in speech science, speech pathology, audiology, voice, linguistics, and allied subjects.
2. Certification from the American Speech and Hearing Association.
3. Further education in the related fields of perception, learning disabilities, neurology, public relations, behavior modification, and especially study in the problems of the aged.
4. A dedicated desire to be of real service, and the intelligence and integrity to continue to learn.
5. The insight and ability to really reach the apparently "unreachable."
6. At least, a specific 3-hour course in aphasia.

## FEES

For reimbursement for communications services (aphasia, the "hard of hearing," etc.) fee schedules are usually available. It is essential, of course, that your aphasiologist meets your state's qualifications as to experience, training, and the like, if he is to be eligible for reimbursements. Although New York State's requirements may be somewhat higher than those of most states, it is hoped that the aphasiologist whom you employ will measure up to the qualifications listed and described in the preceding paragraphs.

## WHEN DOES THERAPY FOR APHASIA BEGIN?

No matter what the cause of a client's communication problems, the sooner he starts to be retrained to communicate, the better off he will be. Formal therapy should be initiated as soon as the attending physician considers it expedient.

## PREPARATION FOR FORMAL THERAPY

The aphasiologist will want to discuss with the administrator of the nursing home the lines of communication and details of other aspects that need to be followed in the facility. Perhaps there are professional staff sessions or special times when he may be best able to secure additional data from the physicians or others. The aphasiologist will need to know the policy regarding initial evaluations. If he is a regular (albeit part-time) staff member, then it is likely that he makes his first evaluation in a routine manner, but policy must be set up and followed.

### Evaluation of the Client

It should be kept in mind that even the half-dozen or more excellent evaluation sets of materials for true aphasics will likely have to be revised by the therapist to meet the particular needs of the client. This is why I recommend a complete case history and evaluation before therapy begins. Even in this technological age, allowance must be made for the individual characteristics.

Of what will a speech pathologist's evaluation consist? Just as an architect will not think of beginning his drawings for a new home until he knows the size of the land, its topography, the size of the family, the number of cars needing to be garaged, and other relevant matters, so a therapist cannot make a therapy plan until he has knowledge of all the related material.

I believe that everyone who has a communications problem ought to have, as soon as he is reasonably able, an evaluation of all aspects of his communication deficits, including reading, writing, hearing, and seeing. A determination of the parameters of the client's abilities must be made first. Since hearing problems are discussed in another chapter of this book I will merely mention that they also need a careful evaluation. The aphasiologist will require close contact with the audiologist, since many of his clients will have multiple problems.

Regular evaluations of a client's progress are important for everyone's benefit. If they are not being made, it is the administrator's responsibility to determine, with the help of the clinician, how often they should be made and who should receive copies.

Be sure that the diagnosis is complete. Several years ago I evaluated a 90-year-old client considered to have aphasia. In reality this man was also profoundly hard of hearing. My therapy to fit his needs brought about quite remarkable results in this gentleman whose other faculties proved to be quite capable. As a result of the correct treatment he enjoyed several years of a "better life."

### Records

The nursing home administrator should facilitate the preparation of records by the specialist who is evaluating the client. It can be assumed that items pertaining to the case history have already been recorded on the chart—names of relatives, addresses, telephone numbers, whom to notify in case of emergency, and so forth, as well as an adequate medical history including onset of the cerebrovascular accident or other cause of aphasia, and records on previous care. These items needed by the communications specialist will not duplicate standard items in the case history.

In addition to the usual data already secured, the aphasiologist is most interested in further information concerning such items as:

1. Onset of the CVA, previous episodes, any closely related factors such as dizziness, blurred vision, weakness in either hand or foot.
2. Recent hospital stays and reasons for admission.
3. Related conditions, including lessening of visual acuity; hearing loss; use of hearing aid (how effective, how often used); if dentures are worn, their fit and comfort.
4. Other physical problems present before stroke.
5. Education, job, hobbies, etc.
6. Family, children, other important associates.
7. Reading habits and the extent of his reading.
8. The degree of spontaneous recovery in hand and leg movement, speech comprehension, as well as ability to speak.
9. Capability in respect to activities of daily living, including dressing himself, going to the bathroom and other personal care, and reading and writing letters.
10. The report of the attending physician concerning the diagnosis, prognosis, and general condition.
11. If any other specialists have examined the client, who they were and of what their special recommendations consisted.

The client's relatives will usually give quite a bit of data without much prodding and, in fact, this probably provides a good catharsis for them. Unhurried, skilled, and early conferences with relatives are essential for all who are involved. Quite often the relatives have unrealistic, vague ideas of what the client can do. I try gently and tactfully to bring them to a closer realization of the actual abilities of the client.

## FORMAL THERAPY

### Initial Sessions

The first sessions (while the client is "stabilizing") may be short and informal; possibly, the therapist will begin by holding conferences with attendants and relatives.

The therapist's initial visit to the client will probably be a short, casual, "chatty" one, and should follow an introduction to the client. (The start should be gentle and tactful!)

The therapist may talk about the weather, the room, the client's attractive pajamas, and so on, but in reality he will be gaining a great deal of pre-evaluation knowledge. He will be able to observe how much comprehension the client has, which arm, if either, is involved in paralysis, if facial paralysis is evident, and if the client can make sounds, is friendly, vague, or perhaps belligerent.

It seems as though anyone who knows a little about an aphasic says, "He can always swear." Swearing, however, is not usual. It is true that most aphasics will use some expletives which have become a sort of automatic speech pattern for them. Must CVA subjects can sing, count, or utter a casual and quite appropriate "Hello," "Nice day," or "Thank you." But if you ask what comes after three or what kind of day it is, they may not be able to answer. Their speech usually reflects an over-learned type of expression that is emitted automatically. Therapists use this sometimes to give the client some confidence and to get him to vocalize. This type of speech, however, will not really provide an insight into a client's ability.

The therapist, while first visiting with the client, will also be able to determine to some degree the state of his hearing and vision. Much can be accomplished during the casual visit if one knows where to look and what to look for.

The therapist will need to consult with the physical therapist, occupational therapist, social worker, and charge nurse as well as others concerned with the care of the client. He will also consult with these people during regular visits after the therapy has started.

The buyer of a house may be misled by having his attention diverted by such relatively unimportant things as a lovely view from the window, but the builder will see the less obvious things such as ancient plumbing, evidence of leaks in the cellar, and a crumbling foundation. So the aphasiologist is trained to "perceive."

## Continued Therapy

The administrator should not question the amount of time that the aphasiologist spends with a client at one sitting. The competent aphasiologist does not try to complete a hard-and-fast 30 minutes of drill. He will pace each session to the needs and abilities of the client on any particular day. One should try to put himself in the place of a client who has the inability to make even one sound. The one who can almost be understood but lacks a few key words may even suffer greater distress. The therapist must always start treatment at the stage of recovery that the client has reached.

The therapy schedule will be flexible and the administrator should make it possible for it to fit easily into the nursing home routine. Some clients must be seen every day. At the beginning of therapy, some can accept only a casual, unstructured 10-minute session, while others may be able to accept 60 minutes easily and want still more. After therapy is under way, 20- to 30-minute sessions about three times a week will usually be reasonably effective. However, many clients will require much more time.

All work that the therapist does should be practical. The client needs to know the word "toilet," and phrases such as "light off" or "it's too cold" and perhaps fifty other life-sustaining and ego-retaining expressions. He does not need to learn the terms so often recommended in booklets. An aged client, who is confined to a bed or chair and is having difficulty making known his basic needs, does not need to know how to say "horse" or "airplane."

The basic number of words that are important for adult aphasics to learn in order to communicate with a sense of dignity is about sixty. I usually give the staff this basic list so that they can help the client to use these words whenever possible. But again I urge, one must not insist or even ask for a correct oral response.

From the following list one can readily choose the most important words that a specific client might learn to use.

| | | | | |
|---|---|---|---|---|
| no | yes | hi | hello | fine |
| good | good-bye | goodnight | good morning | water |
| coffee | tea | want | eat | drink |
| bed | warm | cold | move | over |
| I | you | me | my | your |
| doctor | nurse | wife | husband | book |
| paper | match | cigarette | go | come |
| walk | give | cards | watch | wash |
| bath | bathroom | chair | table | car |
| radio | T.V. or | belt | coat | dress |
| hat | television | pants | shirt | shoes |
| socks | pajamas | tie | underwear | apple |
| banana | suit | bread | cup | dish |
| egg | fork | juice | knife | milk |
| meat | salt | sandwich | cake | hungry |

In some instances the following may be added:

| | | | | |
|---|---|---|---|---|
| nurse | blanket | pillow | light | dishes |
| cane | crutches | wheelchair | clock | too cold |
| too hot | telephone | money | pocketbook | write |
| mail | comb | pencil | toothbrush | glasses |
| Bible | newspaper | stockings | slippers | |

For various individuals, days of the week, months of the year, special addresses, counting from one to twenty, primary colors, plus any special interest items may be included.

## The Team Approach

The "team approach" is strongly endorsed for each and every brain-damaged client. More and more physicians are beginning to subscribe to this total approach and this is good since they are, of course, key figures in its implementation.

The administrator's role is not over when he has helped the communications clinician with the preparation of a case history and an evaluation. It is the administrator's responsibility to make certain that the schedule runs smoothly, that the orders of the attending physician are carried out, and that the rest of the staff is involved in the therapy so that it continues at all times—not just while an actual session is in progress. The effect of the staff's cooperation in the therapy for a client cannot be overemphasized.

The client and the therapist can probably be helped the most if the staff is encouraged to follow the suggestions, given below, for dealing with the client.

1. Keep your conversation simple and practical.
2. Speak directly to the client after making certain that you have his attention.
3. Take into consideration any weaknesses of vision or hearing that the client may have.
4. Obtain some idea of the prognosis for the rehabilitation of the client's affected side.
5. Consider that the client may have some difficulty in seeing well either to the right or the left. The usual CVA subject whose right side is the affected one will experience some difficulty in seeing to the right. When the involvement is on the left, the visual problem, if any exists, will be to the left.
6. Avoid talking about the client over his bed. He may understand quite fully.
7. Avoid talking "down" to the client as if he were a child. Be fundamental but adult.
8. Encourage any and all efforts at rehabilitation.
9. Try to realize that one's usual speech consists of several concepts spoken quite rapidly and in an offhand manner. The aphasic needs fewer concepts and should be spoken to directly. Do not "mouth" your words or raise your voice. If the client is hard of hearing, get to know which ear is his "good" one and whether the loss is in high- or low-pitched sounds.
10. Keep the room and its equipment in a manner that will make the client most comfortable. If he cannot speak or even gesture efficiently, he cannot tell you that there is a glare in his eyes, that he would like the television or radio on or off or louder or softer, or that his leg aches, or

that he might like any one of a number of things that might add to his comfort.

An aphasic who originally learned a language other than English is likely to revert to his mother tongue. In such an instance an interpreter, perhaps the spouse, should be available for part of the time to help the staff and the therapist.

It is important for the administrator and staff to know that there sometimes appears to be a curious relationship between educational ability and ability to improve—the less education, the greater the improvement. This may be because the less educated client will more readily accept the fundamental work or because he does not have a need for a high-level vocabulary or, possibly, speech had not been essential in his work. If he has been a mechanic or a maintenance man, his communications needs are served with only a few hundred words, whereas, if he has been a minister or a professor, he most likely will not be content with a minimal vocabulary.

I frequently post standing suggestions in the room of the client with whom I am working after checking with the administrator of the nursing home. I then ask the staff to carry on direct and fundamental conversation whenever they come into the room, whether to help the client in eating, to make the bed, give medicine, or perform other necessary chores. The staff member can casually and naturally ask the client such questions as "How many *pillows*?" or "Shall we pull up the *curtain*?" However, the client should *never* be held to saying a word before he gets something, or in any way be made overconscious of his deficits. This neither helps the therapist nor the client.

I like to allow the staff to observe me at work, but I do not recommend observation of an inexperienced aphasiologist, since the staff may fail to properly interpret the objectives.

I encourage staff members to report to me changes in the client's behavior. Frequently, a nurse may tell me, "Joe said, 'I want to get up,'" or some such phrase. I try to find out the circumstances under which Joe said this and the motivation. It can help me and the staff in motivating the client toward further rehabilitation. (Caution: A staff member in her eagerness to help often exaggerates what she actually hears the client say.)

In speaking to the client the staff should not use the suggested words, listed on page 134, in isolation; they should be put into a phrase or sentence; for example, "I am your *nurse*," "I will make your *bed*." Do not even ask for a response; that is the work of the aphasiologist.

## Cooperation of Relatives
As soon as possible it is a good idea to have the relatives of the aphasic attend some therapy sessions, since ultimately they may be the ones who will be

responsible for the continuance of any work that the therapist can do. The therapist must help relatives and others to face the fact that obtaining communication adequacy usually takes far longer than relearning the fundamentals of walking and caring for oneself.

## EQUIPMENT

If you are going to have a successful communication program in your nursing home or rehabilitation center, you will need to have certain equipment available. Obviously, no aphasiologist can say just what another aphasiologist would find essential for his program. However, there are certain items that I have found especially useful in the development of a program and from my experience I recommend the following:

1. A small office suitable for at least four or five people. This can be used for group therapy or conferences with relatives.
2. A Language Master (a special type of tape recorder put out by Bell and Howell) with sets of cards.
3. A regular tape recorder with a supply of tapes.
4. A supply of pamphlets and at least some of the reference books and autobiographies listed in the bibliography at the end of this chapter.
5. A lockable filing cabinet, a lockable desk, and a typewriter. A portable electric typewriter may also be needed for some clients.
6. An audiometer.
7. Some evaluation tests for aphasia with protocol booklets, plus other tests within the scope and interpretation of the layman.
8. Various sets of cards and toys (to simulate regular objects such as cars, sewing kits, carpenter's tools).

The collection of useful items can be added as they are needed. The word cards, for instance, can be matched to fundamental pictures. There is no limit to what can be useful. There are also some workbooks available which your aphasiologist may request.

In some situations, if a facility is close to a college clinic which handles similar work, it may be possible to borrow equipment, such as an audiometer, that will be used infrequently. You should also consider the possibility that a service club might be willing to purchase a Language Master or other electronic equipment for your use.

## VALUE OF THERAPY

How valuable is communications therapy for the brain-damaged client? Its value cannot be overestimated, not only for the reduction of frustration on the part of the client and relatives as they learn to "understand" the problem, but also in helping the client to make the most of his intact or less-injured channels and modalities of communication, and to do this before he becomes increasingly depressed or develops wrong habits and efforts at communications.

Just as you would give even the least likely-to-live patient in your care all the comfort and the most skilled help possible, so the aphasic deserves the best possible help for his very essential need. The therapy starts with a skilled evaluation, and lucky is the rehabilitation unit if a capable aphasiologist is a part of the regular staff! My experience indicates that the skilled aphasiologist is able to be of some service to every brain-damaged aphasic no matter how hopeless the prognosis. He can help to guide the development of new pathways for clients to communicate in various modalities. He can interpret abilities and deficits to those who take care of the client, and he can be a bulwark to the family in this their hour of need. When constructive activities show their value, then frustration and strain are generally lessened.

Even the most skilled clinician cannot accomplish a miracle, but, perhaps with a complete evaluation, he can unlock a new pathway or emphasize the use of an unexpected one. If communication ability has been severely damaged, for instance, in lieu of the "impossible" or very difficult and limited speech the therapist may be able to teach the individual a manner of writing, the use of gestures or pointing to a meaningful picture, or employment of word lists. But this is considered a stopgap; all reasonable possibilities to work toward oral communication should be continued.

Two things must be constantly uppermost in one's mind in dealing with the individual with aphasia: first, a "little progress" may mean a lot; and, second, sometimes an erratic, tedious, and discouraging start may lead to far more accomplishment than one would ever dare to hope for!

## GLOSSARY OF APHASIOLOGY (FOR ADMINISTRATORS OF NURSING HOMES)

The following is *NOT* intended to be a scientific glossary; you will find such glossaries in several of the references listed in the bibliography. It will give you some insight into the problems of the dysphasic as he tries to make his adjustments to the "unfamiliar" world into which he has suddenly been thrust with no preparation and little, if any, understanding of the causes.

APHASIA:    Inability to deal with the symbols of communication. (The diagnosis is preferably made by both medical and psychological personnel.) In comprehending aphasia it helps if one thinks of all the avenues of communication for the *normal* individual who feels, comprehends, sees, hears, tastes, writes, spells, uses arithmetic, tells time, and is well-oriented and emotionally stable. However, with *Aphasia* many of these "avenues" are more or less impaired, and quite often in what appears to be an illogical and erratic manner. You will note that I use the term "aphasia." It has become entrenched in the literature and is easy to recall and to use. However, it means "complete loss;" hence, "*dysphasia*" or a partial loss is what is really meant. A true "aphasic" would be pretty close to being a "vegetable."

## Sub-classifications of Aphasia

AGNOSIA:    The client having agnosia suffers various degrees of inabilities to recognize what various things are *for*. He may not be able to tell what a fork or an apple is for, or to understand the difference between the word "hello" and "good-bye," or to view the landscape as it really is. He may be unable to read, and to perform various tasks, yet he may readily eat the apple, use the fork correctly, and wave "good-bye." He may also fool you by holding his magazine in the usual fashion and even turn pages, apparently normally. Such phenomena may occur in all areas: verbal, visual, tactile, auditory, etc.

APRAXIA:    The client with apraxia cannot with normal efficiency and accuracy imitate a sound or an arm action, or tie shoes, etc. These inabilities may be quite inconsistent and are *NOT* the result of impaired neuromuscular facility.

There are, of course, many other "inabilities," also quite irregular and erratic in degree and in various situations such as:

ANOMIA:    Inability to recall nouns. Usually this is one of the most upsetting of the language problems for the aphasic, who sometimes gets into all sorts of oral, syntactical, and grammatical difficulties trying to express orally what we may think of as a simple concept such as "book" or "car." (This is sometimes called "word finding;" it's usually the key word that cannot be spoken.)

ALEXIA:    Complete or partial inability to read (dyslexia).

AGRAPHIA:    Inability to write, complicated by the fact that the subject may have to relearn writing with his "noninvolved" hand (usually the left).

DYSARTHRIA:    Partial inability to produce accurately articulated speech. This is what sometimes used to be called "baby talk." Caution: A superficial evaluation of the client's speech may lead one to believe that he has articulation problems when in reality these might to a great extent "clear up" once he overcomes some of the fundamentals of his aphasic condition. So be sure that you do not waste therapy time as well as discourage the client, who will quite likely realize that this type of treatment does *not* meet his basic need, although he may not so indicate to the therapist.

HEMIANOPSIA:    Involvement usually of the right quadrant of both eyes, with resultant vague or poor vision to the right.

JARGON:    A phenomenon in some aphasics wherein they use a jumble of words and phrases that may be meaningful, in part, to them.

LABILITY:    Excessive emotional outbursts, usually crying but sometimes laughter, in most instances due to the subject's weaknesses rather than to any situation.

PERSEVERATION:    The continuance of the same oral response even after one has switched to different verbal materials. For example, perhaps you have been talking about "telephone" and used the term in many ways, then you switch (with pictures, sentences, etc.) to the concept "house" and ask the client to use the word "house" and he replies "telephone."

SPONTANEOUS RECOVERY:    Usually some degree of spontaneous recovery takes place after almost every CVA, during a period of six months or so following the episode. It is helpful if all therapeutic modalities can be working to improve on this usual asset. The sooner the formalized work is begun the better.

## Terms Which May Help in the Approach to Aphasic Therapy

ASSOCIATION:    In association, the therapist tries to bring in many aspects of a concept; i.e., he does not merely say "chair" but "we sit in a chair" or "there are three chairs in the room," etc.

ESTABLISHMENT:    In establishment it is made reasonably certain that the client knows what the therapist is talking about. For example, if "cup" is the subject a cup is displayed and its use is explained and demonstrated.

FRAGMENTATION:    Fragmentation is *eliminated* as much as possible. Seldom should a word be spelled out, used in isolation, or taught without giving it as complete meaning and as practical usage as possible.

FRUSTRATION:    Try to avoid frustrating the client (or eliminate it before it occurs)! I believe that a person learns better with the inner satisfaction of accomplishing something of value to him, especially if he has made an honest effort to do all that he can. Thus, do not pressure! But rather assume that the client is reasonably eager to accomplish and that it's up to you to set the situation that fits his irregular and erratic abilities.

FUNDAMENTAL:    This term is preferred instead of "easy," "simple," "primary," and the like. It helps to preserve the adult integrity of the client.

Correct and exact terminology is, of course, important; otherwise chaos results. However, sometimes it is essential to supplement the specific terminology with a description of what the client can and cannot do at certain times and in certain situations. I may not even use the "term" itself and thus I avoid too specific a label on this complicated and ever-changing individual, the stroke patient.

In "Conference on Research Needs in Rehabilitation of Patients with Stroke," a Vocational Rehabilitation Administration study, January 19–20, 1966, p. 127, Dr. Joseph Wepman states:

> In conceptualizing the role of the central nervous system in language, a somewhat arbitrary distinction has been drawn between the input problems of reception (the agnosias), the output problems of expression (the apraxias), and the central integrative problems (the aphasias). We consider the input and output problems as being transmissive in nature and affecting specific modalities. By transmissive, we mean that they are disturbances that affect the capacity of the individual to transmit specific stimuli to the central process or to transmit a specific motor act from the central process.

## REFERENCES

It has been a most difficult task to select the following from literally hundreds of publications. However, I have been guided by thinking of the busy administrator of a nursing home who has a relatively small amount of funds with which to purchase materials. Some may believe that I have omitted some of the better materials. My aim is to provide the basics without appearing too "scholarly." I estimate that all of the nineteen publications listed can be purchased for about $75.00.

### General Information Books on Aphasia

1. Buck, McK. 1968. *Dysphasia*: Dysphasia, professional guidance for the family and patient. Prentice-Hall, Inc., Englewood Cliffs, N.J. The book is a well-written account of the author's CVA that occurred when he was Professor of Speech Pathology and how he and his family dealt with the trauma. It's full of insight. (I could have placed this with autobiographies except that it contains much additional material.)
2. Griffith, V. 1970. *A stroke in the family*. Dell Publishing Co., New York. This author acted as a companion-teacher for Patricia Neal; the book is full of suggestions that worked *for those involved*. (Note: Not all of the therapy methods described would be indicated for every client.)
3. Page, I. H. 1963. *Strokes*. Collier Books, New York. A compilation, by seven experts, on the various aspects of strokes. A well-written paperback.
4. Sarno and Sarno. 1969. *Stroke, the Condition and Patient*. McGraw-Hill, New York. One of the most practical books ever written on the topic of strokes; most highly recommended.
5. Schuell, H. *et al.* 1964. *Aphasia in adults*. Harper and Row, Hoeber Medical Division, New York. A "standard" in the field.
6. Schuell, H. 1974. *Aphasia theory and therapy: selected papers and lectures of Hildred Schuell*. Edited by Luther F. Sies. University Park Press,

Baltimore. A complete textbook on aphasia, and a practical clinical guide to its diagnosis, therapy, and management.

## Autobiographies of Those Who Made Remarkable Recovery from Strokes

These works, in part, help the client to understand his plight, but, since each has a few paragraphs on frequent thoughts of committing suicide, *I DO NOT* recommend that they be given freely to the client. Some judgment needs to be used. Selected parts, however, *could* be read *with* the client and could prove to be inspirational.

1. Farrell, B. 1969. *Pat and Roald.* Kingsport Press, Kingsport, Tenn. This book will be of special interest not only because it's exceedingly well-written but also because it is the story of the recovery from a stroke and aphasia experienced by the Oscar winner, Patricia Neal.
2. Hodgins, E. 1964. *Episode.* Antheneum Press (Wolfe Co.), New York. This book is quite humorous; and displays great insight. (The author calls it "the report on the accident inside my skull.")
3. Ritchie, D. 1960. *Stroke, a diary of recovery.* Faber and Faber, Ltd., London.
4. Wint, G. 1967. *The third killer, meditations on a stroke.* Abelard-Schuman, Ltd., New York.

## Pamphlets

For all American Heart Association pamphlets, contact your local or regional heart Association office.

1. A handbook of rehabilitative nursing techniques. 1968. Kenny Rehabilitative Foundation, Minneapolis, Minn. Several authors, excellent illustrations.
2. An open letter to the family of an adult patient with aphasia. National Easter Seals Society, 2023 W. Ogden Avenue, Chicago, Ill. Ten cents a copy.
3. Boone, D. R. 1965. An adult has aphasia. 3rd ed. The Interstate Printers and Publishers, Danville, Ill. Price $1.00. Very fine presentation.
4. Cerebral vascular disease and strokes. U.S. Government Printing Office, Washington, D.C.
5. Strike back at stroke. U.S. Government Printing Office, Washington, D.C.
6. Strokes, a guide for the family. American Heart Association, New York. No author noted.
7. Taylor (Sarno), M. Understanding aphasia, a guide for family and friends. New York University Medical Center, 400 E. 34 St., New York. First published in 1958; 6th printing in six languages in 1970. Seventy-five cents a copy, most attractive, understandable, and complete. Highly recommended.

8. Up and around. U.S. Government Printing Office, Washington, D.C. A booklet to aid the stroke patient in activities of daily living.
9. Wepman, J. Aphasia and family. American Heart Association, 44 E. 23rd St., New York. The author is one of the outstanding authorities in the field.

NOTE: In both "Strike Back at Stroke" and "Up and Around" it is stated that the exercises described should be carried out *ONLY WITH THE SPECIFIC DIRECTION AND APPROVAL OF THE PHYSICIAN ATTENDING THE PATIENT.*

# Psychological Aspects of Recreation: Socialization Programs for Nursing Home Administrators

*Thomas Kavazajian*

9   When we think of the word "play," we almost automatically think about children. This is as it should be, since play comes as naturally to children as swimming does to fish. Although my real purpose is to emphasize the value of play for older people, I believe that the best approach is to discuss children's play, first, bearing in mind that what applies to children applies equally to adults.

For purposes of this discussion, I will define *"play"* as any activity that is pursued by an individual purely for the sake of enjoyment, fun, or pleasure, as opposed to those activities called "work" that must be done for some purpose other than personal enjoyment or expression.

Since play activities seem to be natural to most higher-order animals, it is not surprising that play comes naturally to children—the offspring of the highest-order animal. Not only does play come naturally to children, but it is necessary for both human growth and development, and a natural consequence of the maturational process. According to analysis, children's play provides the following:

1. *Physical stimulation and activity which are necessary for physical growth and well-being.* Here fine muscle movement as well as large muscle involvement is important. Through physical interaction with others, the child learns to get along with others by developing competitiveness and aggressiveness, cooperation and sharing, tolerance for defeat, tolerance for winning, mutual physical respect, and tolerance for physical discomfort or hurt and frustration.

2. *Play provides intellectual stimulation and activity which foster mental development.* The child learns to use intelligence for planning and organ-

izing in play. He further learns to invent and discover and characteristically reacts spontaneously and naturally. Imagination and fantasy life, which are the forerunners of productivity and creativity, are often put to use and therefore developed. Communication skills are also enhanced through practice and improvement.

3. *Play fosters emotional stimulation, activity, and reactivity which contribute to the development of emotional maturity.* The gamut of emotions is experienced in play activities. Children learn to laugh, cry, be happy, be sad, and so on. They learn how to interrelate or get along with one another by developing consideration for others, how to share and do things together, and how to acquire mutual respect.

Another significant factor, which falls under the category of emotional development, is that play gives the child a chance to act out and often work out his problems, concerns, and conflicts in a harmless and acceptable fashion. This is the basic principle behind the type of child psychotherapy called "play therapy" which is very relevant to our topic since a capable, well-trained, recreation-socialization worker is essentially a therapist in his approach to motivating, handling, and helping those in his care.

It should also be mentioned that children do not necessarily need complicated toys for their play activities. In fact, these often detract from play, since complicated toys and contraptions detract from enjoyment by stifling imagination and creativity. Sophisticated toys leave little to the child's ingenuity.

In the final analysis, it can be said that children grow, learn, and mature through play. Their learning is physical, intellectual, and emotional. When growth, learning, and maturation are arrested, life and living halt. What applies to children applies to nursing home residents as well. These people require activities that will continue to stimulate them physically, intellectually, and emotionally. The physical aspects may become far less important to the older than to the younger person, but the emotional and intellectual aspects remain essential. It is because of this that every nursing home should have a well-endowed, well-organized, well-developed recreation-socialization program.

## ROLE OF THE ADMINISTRATOR

In spite of the fact that most nursing home administrators are usually directly or indirectly answerable to some type of governing board, in most instances it is the administrator rather than the governing body who is most influential with regard to the policies and procedures that are operative within the home. Most importantly, it is the administrator who sets the general tone of the home. Many administrators are not sufficiently aware of this fact. Those who are aware often don't realize to what extent this is true. The nursing home is certainly not unique in this way, since the same principle applies generally to practically all institutions such as public schools, colleges, prisons, municipal governments, and even our nation.

The administrator's role in establishing the general tone of the home may be a very direct, easily apparent one if he exercises very strict authoritarian control over the various institutional operations, programs, and procedures. Direct control often takes the form of explicit verbal requests or orders, and of strong memos of approval or disapproval to various department heads or employees. The views, opinions, and attitudes of the administrator are evident by his recommendations for or against certain procedures and by what he supports or discourages. Then, too, there is the matter of direct financial control over which the administrator has a great deal of responsibility. His recommendations as to how funds are to be budgeted and then spent undoubtedly reveal the type of institution that he is interested in developing.

In addition to direct control, the administrator exercises a great deal of indirect influence, which, though more subtle, may be equally instrumental in determining the nature of the institution. A few examples of this type of influence include casual remarks or comments to employees about the programs and operations of the agency, attendance or non-attendance at certain functions within the home, and expressed interest in certain phases of functioning and obvious disinterest in others.

## THE TRICKLE DOWN EFFECT

The most usual way in which the administrator will influence the home consists in a combination of the aforementioned direct and indirect modes. However, regardless of the manner of influence, it is felt that there is what we might call a *"trickle down effect"* which eventually operates in all institutions when the top administrator, regardless of title, sets the priorities and tenor of the institution. Most, if not all, of the other employees or subordinates on down the ladder of hierarchy, importance, influence, or function tend to fall in line with the direct dictates or indirect expectations of the "top person."

When the subordinate personnel disagree with top administrative wishes, they will sometimes protest or fight for what they believe is right. This occurs especially when personnel feel very strongly that the attitudes, policies, and procedures are detrimental to their area of concern or to the agency. Then, too, if they feel that their own professional functioning or personal philosophies are being seriously violated, they may object strenuously. As a result, they may be dismissed, or they may resign. On the other hand, sometimes they may be able to convince the administrator and influence others to accept their point of view. This is, of course, especially important if there is merit in their ideas. Hopefully, a good administrator will be aware of, and in some way be responsive to, this kind of professional dissent, rather than stubbornly adhere to his own ideas regardless of the possible merits of the views of others.

It is my contention that the nursing home administrator must be aware of the fact that his ideas and attitudes (biases, if you will) have a profound influence upon every aspect of the nursing home, including all of its programs. I especially call your attention to this fact since my area of interest, namely, recreation-socialization programs, is one of those programs that can be so influenced.

Let me analyze some possible sources of the administrators' attitudes without going into an esoteric discussion of individual personality dynamics. My analysis or explanations may appear to some to be a gross oversimplification, but I feel that, from a practical point of view, there are two key questions to be considered. These are:

1. *How does the administrator perceive his institution?*
2. *Why does he perceive it as he does?*

## MODELS

As far as I can determine, there is no one prototype or model for a nursing home. The nature of the resident population may, to a large extent, determine the nature of the home. For example, a very infirm population will necessitate extensive medical services while a relatively *well* population might demand extensive activities programs. In spite of this factor, it is my contention that the way in which each administrator perceives his institution may well determine not only the nature of the home, but also, more importantly for this discussion, the nature of the recreation-socialization services within the home.

I believe that there are a number of distinct perceptual models that can be described and that will assist each administrator in evaluating how he views his institution. The various models, as we see them, might be:

1. *The Medical Model.* This nursing home is viewed primarily in terms of providing for the health needs of the elderly patients. The emphasis would most probably be on medicine, diet, exercise, and the like. This institution is thought of first and foremost as a hospital. Consistent with this orientation, the recreation-socialization program would be geared toward therapy of one sort or another.

2. *The Custodial Model.* Here the agency is seen as primarily custodial in the sense that it provides shelter or a roof over the heads of the elderly tenants. Emphasis would be on protection, safety, and comfort. This nursing home might best be characterized as a protective sanctuary. If recreation-socialization programs are developed they would probably be of a safe, passive type.

3. *The Hotel Model.* In this view the nursing home is responsible for providing food, relaxation, and entertainment for the elderly guests. In it the recreation-socialization program might well be geared toward the entertainment of the guests.
4. *The Social Club Model.* Social companionship is the key word to be provided for the elderly club members. The emphasis within the nursing home would be on establishing friendships, forming social groups, and similar services. The recreation-socialization program would be geared toward developing and encouraging the socialization process.
5. *The Activities Center Model.* In this model the members of the center must always be doing something; they must be involved, participating, whether alone or in groups. Here, the aged are considered as participants. All sorts of individual and group activities would be featured in the recreation-socialization program offered in such a model.
6. *The Religious Retreat Model.* Here the nursing home is considered to be a religious retreat where the parishioners or the congregation members are being prepared spiritually for death or, possibly, life after death. Naturally, the recreation-socialization program would pertain to religion and religious activities.
7. *The Jail Model.* Although difficult to conceive of in this day and age, it is possible that the orientation of a particular nursing home might actually be dedicated to isolating and segregating the older people from society as though they were inmates of a prison. In this model there might not be any recreation-socialization program or, if there were, it might be geared toward providing a limited degree of exercise.

I don't doubt that many of this book's readers can describe other models. For example, both a family model and a military model have been suggested.

Naturally, all of the different prototypes are, in a sense, ludicrous, but I believe that they help in making my point, which is that any administrator may lean more toward one or another view without being aware of it. He won't realize his point of view if he hasn't thought about it in some way or examined the programs and activities to which he gives priorities in terms of money, time, space, personnel, and equipment.

Ideally and hopefully, each administrator will perceive of his agency as a combination of many of the models indicated, with the exception of the jail approach which hardly seems appropriate to any nursing home. And yet, interestingly enough, the feeling of being "in a jail" is probably experienced by a good many aged nursing home residents. It is our task to change this perception if possible, and, frankly, good recreation-socialization programs do a great deal to achieve this objective.

Naturally, it is impossible to have a perfect combination or balance in one's viewpoint. Therefore, virtually every administrator will emphasize certain approaches while possibly minimizing or neglecting others. It is of paramount importance that each administrator try to determine his perceptions and biases objectively.

## FORMING ATTITUDES

A valid question at this point might be *where do nursing home administrators' viewpoints come from?* A list of some determinants might include the following factors:
1. The field or occupation that the administrator was trained in or worked in prior to entering the profession of nursing home administrator.
2. The nature of the administrator's educational background.
3. The administrator's personal philosophy of life.

Naturally, one and two often, but not always, are combined.

*The most usual fields from which nursing home administrators arise seem to me to be:*
1. The medicinal or the paramedical field, such as nursing.
2. Business, management, or accounting.
3. Health, recreation, and physical education.

In addition to these broad occupational fields, there are a number of other fields from which the majority of nursing home administrators come from. These are:
4. Teaching.
5. The social sciences such as social work and psychology.
6. Administrative-military.
7. The clergy.

It is rather obvious that, having been trained and having worked in one of these fields, a nursing home administrator might quite naturally lean toward perceiving his agency in a way that reflects his background. For example, the administrator who was a nurse may inadvertantly be overly concerned with medical care while neglecting recreation-socialization. On the other hand, a person from a business background might be more concerned with balancing the budget than with any particular program.

*The type of education to which an administrator has been exposed may have a strong influence upon his views.* For the sake of discussion we have categorized arbitrarily the types of education as:
1. Technical-scientific.
2. Liberal arts tradition.
3. Business-finance.
4. Philosophical-religious.

Of course, these types are not mutually exclusive and one person might have been exposed to any combination. To illustrate how these different educational backgrounds might influence thinking, consider the fictitious case of the administrator who allows the nursing home residents to take trips to a distant museum because he has a fine-arts background, yet will not authorize a trip to the local hydroelectric power plant, since he is not particularly interested in science. The same type of prejudice could be imagined in reverse as well. Actually, the way in which various biases operate is extremely subtle and often difficult to detect clearly.

Lastly, I believe that one's own personal philosophy and human value system play a decisive role in occupational decisions. With regard to personal philosophies there are countless possibilities. Again, for discussion purposes only, I offer a few broad types of *philosophical outlooks* against which your own philosophical outlook might be gauged.

1. The view that man is a working, active being with no time for play or recreation.
2. The view that man is essentially a social being.
3. The conviction that man is, first and foremost, a religious or spiritual being.
4. The belief that man lives only for pleasure.
5. The idea that man is merely a biological entity.
6. The viewpoint that man has no purpose but merely exists as best he can until death.

To illustrate the influence of philosophical outlook, I will cite the make-believe case of the nursing home administrator who, because he feels that religious belief is the only human value worth cultivating, does not allow his recreation-socialization personnel to organize any activity unless it pertains directly to religion in some way. This example is farfetched, but I hope it makes the point.

*To summarize,* it seems to me that each nursing home administrator must be aware of his own value system and how it relates to his personal, educational, and occupational background. He must also cultivate some insight into his attitudes toward life and living and especially toward aging and the aged.

Sometimes posing questions such as the following is helpful in learning about ourselves. Try this self-test of your attitudes.

1. What is more important to you—a good meal or an enjoyable companion for an afternoon?
2. Which is more important—physical well-being or emotional well-being?
3. Which would you rather have—a beautiful room or a pleasant roommate?
4. Would you prefer to spend an afternoon reading, in church, watching T.V., or playing a game with others?
5. Do you regard senility as reversible or irreversible—totally, partially, or to what degree?

6. If you had to cut something out of your budget, would you lower the quality of food and keep recreation activities on the highest level, or would you keep food quality as high as possible and lessen expenditures on recreation-socialization?

These questions may seem old; however, I believe that they will help you to evaluate your thinking on the subject. Many of you in the field have had to consider those types of questions time and time again. One fact never changes, namely, that life is full of choices and the choices one makes reflect how he really thinks and feels.

Also you might ask yourself: When the budget gets tight, how and where do I look to cut back and save dollars?

Finally, consider your answers with respect to how they relate to your personal values and outlook on life.

## SOCIALIZATION AND PSYCHOLOGICAL
## NEEDS IN RECREATION—SOCIALIZATION PROGRAMS

Any residential setting responsible for the care of human beings of any kind must be equipped to fulfill man's basic human needs. In addition, specialized institutions (such as a nursing home or extended care facility) must be able to provide for the fulfillment of other specific needs as well.

Most of us are familiar with the *basic inborn physiological needs.* These are the needs for food, water, elimination, rest, sexuality, activity, and stimulation. The last two are relative newcomers to the scene, but are extremely important and very basic.

As an interesting aside, recent experimentation suggests that the socially acquired need for affection may actually be directly related to the need for stimulation. It appears that it isn't that infants require affection or love as such, but, rather, that they require stimulation to which they can react. There appears to be a definite physiological need for the organism to react both internally and externally to stimulation. Many different types of stimulation seem to answer the need. However, in our culture it is the parents or parent substitutes who do most of the stimulating, usually in the culturally dictated and approved form of affectionate play.

*In addition to the aforementioned basic physiological needs, there are numerous social or acquired psychological needs.* A list of these would depend upon two factors: (1) *the culture with which we are dealing;* (2) *the subjective views of the person drawing up the list.* With this in mind, it might be appropriate to outline some needs that come to mind which you might also find acceptable as being essential to people in our society.

1. The need to receive affection from others (to be loved, accepted, wanted, preferred, etc.).

2. The need to be affectionate toward others (to love, accept, care for others).
3. The need to be with others, or companionship (being physically and emotionally near others).
4. The need to be alone, to have solitude (to have time to think, meditate, and recuperate).
5. The need to communicate with others (through verbal or gestural language, to interrelate).
6. The need to share experience (to participate with and therefore experience the same thing as someone else).
7. The need to excel (to do something well or better than another, to experience one's capabilities, strengths, or powers).
8. The need for intellectual activity (to think, reason, and imagine).
9. The need to feel (to experience one's emotions, be they positive or negative, loving or hateful).
10. The need to belong (to be part of something higher, stronger, or more powerful than ourselves).
11. The need to mature (to continue to grow and develop as human beings).
12. The need to create (to make, to do, to accomplish, and to produce).

I'm certain that many of you might disagree with items on this list, feeling that some needs were left out or too many have been included. However, the specific differences should not detract from the importance of recognizing that all human beings have, in addition to their inborn biological needs, acquired social needs that must be met if life is to be worth living.

It is interesting to note that, although socially acquired needs are not considered to be biological necessities for the sustenance of physical life, many people die for no apparent physical reason, for example, in prisoner of war camps where only basic biological needs were fulfilled. Apparently, the fulfillment of physiological needs is not enough for civilized man.

With more specific reference to the social needs of older people, Clark Tibbits[1] has developed a list that might be of interest to you, and that illustrates the subjective nature of what are considered acquired needs.

1. To render some socially useful service.
2. To be considered part of the community.
3. To occupy increased leisure time in satisfying ways.
4. To enjoy normal companionship.
5. For recognition as an individual.
6. For the opportunity for self-expression.
7. For health protection and care.
8. For suitable mental stimulation.
9. For living arrangements and family relationships.
10. For spiritual satisfactions.

At this point it should be emphasized that it is the recreation-socialization program of the nursing home which addresses itself to the fulfillment of most of the socially acquired needs. This alone is the justification for developing the best program possible in each institution, especially when one accepts the fact that the fulfillment of socially acquired needs is as important to man as is the fulfillment of the biological needs.

To describe specifically how various recreation-socialization programs fulfill the various needs is not within the scope of this presentation. However, you can be assured that this could be developed by an experienced nursing home recreation worker or director.

## MINIMIZING ADMISSION TRAUMA

*The importance of an effective recreation-socialization program* as it focuses upon the psychological problems of the new resident as he first enters the nursing home cannot be minimized.

To begin, it should be pointed out that, in a sense, any given nursing home is a family. Hopefully, most, if not all, of the residents feel like part of the family. This is especially true where a good recreation-socialization program has been in operation. At any rate, there is the situation in which the old-time residents feel relatively secure in their family and therefore do not wish to have the status quo disturbed.

On the other hand, the new resident feels like the unwelcomed stranger. In addition, and as a backdrop to this feeling, let us look first at how the older person about to enter a nursing home for the first time feels with respect to society. It goes without saying that he has gradually become more and more isolated and painfully alone. Not only has he lost his social identity in terms of work, there has been a complete identity reversal in terms of family roles. Whereas others had been dependent upon him, he is now dependent upon them. He has usually experienced physical and mental loss which further affect his personal identity and he is usually fearful of death and feels that there is no future for him. It is with these feelings and the additional feeling of being unwanted or rejected by his family, friends, and society in general, that he comes to the nursing home which he is just as sure doesn't want him either. It is no wonder then, that he feels unhappy, depressed, and angry as he reacts to another drastic change in his life with so many unknowns before him. He feels like a stranger and, in a sense, he is a stranger. The long-time residents see him as an outsider or intruder. They resent the new person, an unknown, who is usually looked upon as a threat.

Very often the newcomer is shy and tries to rely on himself. He is very guarded and is afraid to extend himself to others for fear of rebuff. He wishes to remain unnoticed and anonymous. In addition, he may be very embarrassed or self-conscious about physical disabilities or his appearance. The fact that others have disabilities offers him no solace. He is often suspicious of others. Here it should be noted that many physical illnesses have certain emotional side effects. For example, hearing loss is often accompanied by suspicious paranoid reactions. The newcomer feels useless and, in a way, feels that he has nothing to look forward to but death.

This, then, is the composite picture of the new nursing home resident. It seems to be very negative and it usually is. The only positive feature is that sometimes, deep down, the older person feels relieved that finally someone is really going to look after him and provide the care and attention that he needs. Along these lines, perhaps, we should do more in terms of educating an older population to accept eventual institutional care.

In spite of all of the negative aspects ascribed to the situation of the new resident, an effective recreation-socialization program can aid the newcomer in a number of interesting ways:

1. The professional personnel gently encourage the newcomer to join in some activity, helping him to take the risk while supporting his efforts in joining.
2. The newcomer is protected from the others who can be cruel, especially since some older people tend to be very outspoken and opinionated.
3. He is given an opportunity to enjoy the company of others.
4. He can utilize his knowledge for some activities.
5. He can draw upon his past experiences.
6. He might have an opportunity to teach others.
7. He can experience physical and mental activity and stimulation.
8. His feelings of self-worth can be redeveloped.
9. He may begin to have something to look forward to.
10. He can be helped to feel important and needed again.
11. The program can provide continuous opportunity for making friendships.
12. The program can help to keep the newcomer physically dexterous in terms of small and large muscles.
13. It can help him to take his mind off himself.

The last point is an important one, since very often persons who become immersed in recreation-socialization activities often forget their illnesses. They enjoy doing what they want to do in spite of their infirmities. In fact, when busy, they often forget to take their medication!

*To summarize,* the important results of an effective recreation-socialization program lie in the fact that the program helps the new resident in becoming part of the family. In addition, it continues his feeling of belonging and continuity to the overall family. As an additional bonus, it can also be one of the strongest factors in creating and continuing good morale within the institution. In this respect an effective recreation-socialization program may be more important than good food.

Physical disabilities should be no barrier to participation in recreation-socialization activities. Workers in the field can devise programs for everyone. There is practically no physical barrier that can prevent a motivated, interested older person from participating in some type of personally rewarding and meaningful recreation-socialization endeavor.

Whether you measure the worth of programs by individual human happiness or group institutional morale, it pays to have effective, well-endowed recreation-socialization programs operating in your nursing home.

Last, but not by any means least, hire a professional (when possible), experienced recreation therapist. Colleges and universities in America now have educational programs for this profession. In addition, some states now have specific standards for accrediting therapeutic recreation workers.

## REFERENCES
1. Tibbits, C. 1960. Handbook of social gerontology: societal aspects of aging. University of Chicago Press, Chicago.

# Recreation and Socialization: Preparation and Pre-planning

*Florence Olsson*

**10** The question of progress in recreation, socialization, and activities in nursing homes usually stirs some controversy. As an administrator, your own thinking regarding this may be influenced by your past experiences, your attitudes toward the aged, the size of your nursing home, geographical location, and, most important, the degree of patient illness and incapacity.

It is generally recognized that strides have been made in the past decade. This is evidenced by an increase in training programs, special courses offered for activities leaders and others in the field, the increase in the number of published articles on the aging, and radio and television programs on related topics. Also, there has been an increase in communications among geriatric agencies.

There is no denying that we still have a long way to go before we surmount obstacles such as lack of funds and shortage of well-trained personnel, but we have begun to roll up our sleeves.

## OBJECTIVES

After World War I, therapeutic recreation came into being, but it was not until World War II that it became a profession. In the years to follow, it held a rather dubious place in the institutionalized setting before it was established as a necessity. It thrived mostly on donated funds and was often conducted by well-meaning volunteers, ladies' auxiliaries, nursing staff, and social workers.

In recent years, colleges and universities have been offering graduate programs in therapeutic recreation with credits toward master and doctoral degrees. The graduates are called "Therapeutic Recreation Specialists," but because there are by no means enough of these people to fill the demand they function primarily in the area of administration, education, supervision, and consultation.

The New York State Code for Nursing Homes, in the chapter on the activities program, provides the following general definitions:

*An activities program* means a planned schedule of recreational, social and other purposeful activities for nursing home patients designed to make their lives more meaningful, to stimulate and support the desire to use their physical and mental capabilities to the fullest extent to enable them to maintain a sense of usefulness and self-respect but not specifically to correct or remedy any disability.

*Occupational Therapy* shall mean the evaluation and treatment of physical and psychological dysfunction through the use of such activities as creative, manual, industrial, educational, recreational, social and self-help activities to enable the patient to achieve his optimal level of self-care and productivity.

State codes frequently define the minimum qualifications for employment in these types of programs. In the absence of qualified activities personnel, the codes require that there be as a program consultant, a therapeutic recreationist or an occupational therapist in at least a consultive capacity. Consult your state's code for exact rules.

Personnel in activities and occupational therapy must realize that they are equally important in the total picture and must leave lines of communication open with one another as well as with all related departments within the facility. Occupational therapy, physical therapy, and nursing all work with the sick portions of the body. Normally, recreation treats the whole person but must be guided by other departments as to limitations in referred cases.

In the same vein, a physician's approval for a patient to participate in an activities program is not considered a prescription from the physician for occupational therapy treatment.

It is the responsibility of each administrator to see that clarification in these areas is stressed in the orientation and in-service training of involved personnel. Only with such understanding can administrators effectively direct their efforts toward the primary objective, that is, service to the patient.

## PREPARATION AND PRE-PLANNING

Before one can begin to set up a program, careful consideration should be given to choice of staff. It must be recognized that even well-planned programs will only be successful when high-ability activities personnel are available to carry them out.

The activities leader should be versatile and should understand all phases of activities in order to supervise the staff and relate to the aged and their needs. In addition, he or she has the responsibility of thoroughly explaining job descriptions, policies, and procedures.

Whether your facilities are large or small, proprietary or voluntary, or have a particular religious or ethnic population, much of the content of this chapter can be modified to suit your needs. Whether there is a full- or part-time staff employed, its members will need proper training in order to apply the necessary skills. Since the majority of activities personnel are women, serious consideration should be given to drawing more men into the field. Men tend to give a good balance to the program, especially in the area of drama and discussion groups.

Initial training and supervision are most important, since the inexperienced activities worker is prey to becoming personally involved with the patient. It takes time to acquire a professional attitude, but the warm, friendly approach with a good balance of objectivity is best for everyone. More than once I have witnessed a very close relationship develop between a patient and a worker only to have the relationship end with the patient in a state of depression after the worker has departed. Although it is important to look for skills when recruiting activities personnel, a good balance of emotional stability, intelligence, and common sense is equally necessary.

Sometimes, an activities worker who does not function well may have a fear of working with the aged. If this is deep-seated, it would be a disservice not to advise this person to pursue another occupation.

Inexperienced persons with good potential often make excellent workers, but, of course, time must be spent in good training and close supervision. It has been my experience that this time is well spent.

Once the members of the activities staff have proven their ability to conduct a well-balanced program, you, as administrator, should give them the necessary freedom to work. Seriously consider their suggestions and requests for the tools that they need to keep the program in operation. If the request for additional staff is not financially feasible, extra effort might be put into recruiting volunteers. If working space is a problem, think in terms of converting likely areas or turning dining or other areas into dual-purpose rooms. Several sources can be explored to obtain equipment for arts and crafts, games, and other activities to avoid a strain on the budget. A well-worded letter to likely donors can sometimes work wonders.

Board members and women's auxiliaries may have some influence. One very good source of help is the relatives of patients, especially those of patients who respond to activities. To cite one case: The daughter of a patient was constantly trying to convince her mother that she should become involved in some form of activity. After each visit to the home the daughter left in utter frustration. With the special approach of the activities worker, the patient began to take an interest in mosaic tile work. The daughter was so pleased that she asked that a supply of tile be purchased at her expense. The enthusiasm that is the earmark of a successful program is contagious, and interested observers will want to help.

Before any program can be launched there are several important considerations:

*The activities staff must acquaint themselves with the people whom they are to serve.* This can be done by visiting with them and talking with them to determine their interests.

*A patient-interest questionnaire can also be helpful* but that which appears on paper and that which can be put into actual practice often differ.

*Personal contact with the patient also serves to give them a voice in program planning.* This is important since too often programs are geared to the interests and talents of the activities workers. These visits will also serve to determine limitations and attention span, and, as stated previously, there should be good communications with medical and paramedical personnel for additional information, if needed.

*The social service department routinely should share that part of the social summary that would be of concern to activities.* This is most valuable in gaining an insight into the cultural and religious backgrounds along with other information that can aid in the proper approach to an individual.

Getting to know the patient is only half the picture. The activities worker has to withstand scrutiny by the patient. This provides good reason to pause and reflect, for only too often are we guilty of assuming that apparent senility renders the patient incapable of making judgment. A worker who is not accepted favorably can expect difficulty in gaining participation.

It is true that patients often take part in activities to escape boredom, but, more often, it is because they are lonely and welcome the presence of the friendly worker. Usually, after continued association, the activity itself becomes the important factor.

## SETTING UP THE PROGRAM

A schedule of events is most commonly recognized as a piece of paper showing the days of the week and the time of day for each activity. It will contain the usual assortment of attractions such as arts and crafts, games, music, current events, parties, and so on. It looks fine tacked up there on the bulletin board, but let us recognize this schedule for what it really is. It is an outline—a plan—that, hopefully, will be followed fairly closely. But the best-laid plans can go awry. This should be no surprise to the well-trained worker, since sudden changes in programming may be necessary for as many reasons as there are patients. The worker should be capable of dealing with this situation by drawing from her skills to fill the gap. There must be flexibility. There have been instances in which the worker became indignant over the cancellation of her planned performance while the patients calmly accepted the interruption in routine.

## SELLING THE PROGRAM

Once the program is set up, the biggest challenge to the activities personnel is selling it. Most importantly, it must be sold to the patient to give him a feeling of adequacy. It must be sold to the administrator to justify the activities program and to substantiate its needs for supplies and staff. It must be sold to other departments within the agency for their cooperation in carrying out the program. It must be sold to groups such as board members and women's auxiliaries to gain their approval and support. It must be sold to the community; to local banks and merchants to obtain contributions and places to have exhibits; to local schools and churches for volunteers and entertainment; to chambers of commerce and political organizations for public interest and community participation. It must be sold to the people of the community, not just the aged, but the younger adults for better understanding of its purpose. This is a large order; however, in this ever-expanding field, we need all the help we can get.

## COMMUNICATING WITH THE PATIENT

A schedule of planned activities should be posted one month in advance for all to refer to. This should be done not only because it is recommended or demanded by a state code, but also because it is an efficient manner in which to operate. Posting a monthly calendar is fine for staff and volunteers, but I have found individual weekly programs for patient distribution to be a better means of communication. Other media for helping the patient to know what is going on are bulletin boards or blackboards, special invitations or notices at each patient's place at meal time, and reminders by word of mouth during grand rounds. On one occasion, when I had scheduled a very unusual vaudeville performance and wanted to call special attention to it, I had sandwich signs made by craft workers. Two residents volunteered to wear them and circulate in the dining room on the eve of the show. This caused much amusement and was well received because it was in keeping with the event.

With such information coming to the patient regularly, you will find that eventually, whether or not he participates, he will begin to notice changes, make suggestions, and even point out errors. Being a good listener takes practice, but here is an area where it becomes necessary. To illustrate: A patient came to me once with the suggestion that a certain area in front of the building would be much more attractive if flowers were planted in it. I agreed with the suggestion and, after making the proper contacts, gained approval and the flowers were planted. It would be difficult to describe the pleasure that was enjoyed by so many during the course of the summer.

Another patient suggested placing large numbers on a wall opposite the elevators for easier identification of floors. All this proves that, if you listen, you just might hear something worthwhile!

## AREA
Activities workers will be the first to know whether or not an area is right for their purposes. Frequently, there are complaints of too much heat, too much noise, and uncomfortable furniture. These problems are sometimes difficult to solve, but they have a great bearing on the quality of service to the patient. Ingenuity on the part of the activities workers could come to the rescue here.

## APPROACH TO PATIENT PARTICIPATION
There is a kind of "numbers syndrome" among persons conducting activities. Concern about the number of persons participating in a session sometimes overrules interest in the activity being conducted. It is difficult to determine at just what level this anxiety has its origin, but when it exists there should be a serious review of agency philosophy. Admittedly, there is no better morale booster for the worker than to have a large group in attendance. But whether a group is large or small the important question is: Why are the participants attending? Is it because they want to; because the activities leader insisted; or because they were too timid to refuse? If a given activity continually shows poor participation, the cause must be determined and a change made. If the average attendance is good, the fluctuation should be accepted by the conscientious worker as routine.

The nature of the approach when inviting patients to participate is dependent upon many things, all having to do with their physical, mental, and emotional conditions. The sensitive worker will soon learn what works best with each individual. I recall a report from the activities staff about a patient upon whom the staff had spent a good deal of time for a number of days in an effort to involve her with the group. Finally they gave up. The patient apparently had enjoyed the attention she was getting, and when it ended she felt neglected and decided, on her own, to join the group.

Empirical studies in gerontology, some done in sociology at Louisiana State University,[1] confirm the assumptions that must underlie any really beneficial programs for the aged:
1. Older people wish to remain self-directing. They are not 'just like children.'
2. Older people can learn, though the process may take longer.
3. Being old does not imply inadequacy. Dependability, if affected by age, is increased.
4. Age and illness are not coincidental.
5. Older people do not look alike, think alike, or act alike.

6. Each person takes through the threshold of old age the attitude, personality, character, and life organization which are the products of earlier years.

## RECORD KEEPING

It is recognized that making reports and keeping statistical records is time-consuming and presents difficulty, especially when there is limited clerical personnel, but these chores are necessary. Each activities staff member should keep his own daily log. This could be a simple chart with columns for listing the date, kind of activity, where the activity was conducted, the number attending, and, most importantly, a space for recording notable changes in behavior patterns of patients. This information can be correlated at the end of each month to supply base information for the administrator's monthly report. I have found the use of a role book helpful. The patients' names are listed alphabetically on lines with small boxes representing each day of the month. Each activity is represented by a letter of the alphabet and each phase of programming in which the patient becomes involved is recorded in the box under the proper date. In this way, it is possible to follow the total pattern of participation of each person. A patient whose participation has been regular and then suddenly drops off would be identified. Keeping such a role book can be time-consuming, but could be a good assignment for a capable volunteer.

Activities persons are notorious for not putting their experiences on paper. This is unfortunate, since many good ideas or observations which could have been shared or set aside for future reference have been lost. Keeping notes on special events for reference the following year is useful in making changes or improvements. Also, it will help a new staff person to pick up where another leaves off.

## ACTIVITIES

### Arts

Participants in the arts are usually those who have some talent or are adventurous enough to try their skill. Others can be drawn into the group if the worker is capable of demonstrating ideas that will lead to fun rather than possible failure.

The more capable individuals may work with water colors, pastels, charcoal, acrylic paints, or poster paints, which are less expensive. They may enjoy painting original pictures or copying favorite subjects. This is fine, but what about the others? Here are ideas that can serve as ice-breakers for the timid would-be-artist and that are also failure-proof.

*Blow Painting.* The only equipment needed is: colored inks, drawing paper, and straws. The method is to place several drops of ink on the paper, then blow at them through a straw while turning the paper, causing the ink to form interesting designs. Nurses, visitors, and just about everyone can get into the act.

*Leaf Painting.* The materials: drawing paper, poster paints, and assorted fall leaves. Patients enjoy searching among the leaves brought in from outside. One side of the chosen leaf is placed on the paint (paint can be poured into a dish or painted on with a brush). The leaf is then gently pressed on the drawing paper leaving an imprint. Too much paint will cause smearing. Prints of several leaves can be arranged in a graceful pattern on one sheet of drawing paper for framing, or smaller prints can be used for decorating stationary or greeting cards.

*Bright Color Painting.* Something that the more senile patient or one limited in sight can enjoy is painting with bright colors on especially prepared, heavily outlined designs. This gives some feeling of accomplishment, but the worker may have to offer some measure of guidance.

You will find that when each patient works within his capabilities, the entire experience can be satisfying and pleasurable.

If your nursing home has outdoor facilities use them. An art group conducted out-of-doors during the summer on the surrounding grounds can be most enjoyable. Of course, help from nurses' aides and volunteers is necessary for transporting patients in wheelchairs, but the patients' gratitude makes it all worthwhile. Getting the long-term patient outside also helps in lessening the insecurity often felt upon being removed from familiar surroundings.

## Crafts

Needlework projects are endless and the aged women feel very comfortable with them. But let's look at the male patient! He is considered the most difficult challenge for the activities worker. He is often silent and withdrawn and shies away from groups in which he is outnumbered by women, which is almost always the case. There is another reason for his lack of interest. What are the women doing? You guessed it—they are making pot holders and aprons, twisting crepe paper, and stuffing rag dolls. There is nothing in these projects for a man.

I have seen very successful male involvement at the introduction of wood-working projects. Given a separate corner or a table away from the female group, the men work contentedly at sand-papering, shellacking, and painting various pre-cut objects. Before a jig-saw was acquired, the maintenance department consented to cutting out the necessary parts. There was also some light hammering involved in putting together little boxes with hinges and locks.

Also geared for male interests are leather and metal crafts. Even though the projects may be simplified, they require some skill, and care must be taken not to frustrate the participant.

A collage project has been well received. This is especially suggested for the craft worker who "never throws anything away." The materials consist mostly of junk jewelry, wallpaper, samples, bits of yarn, colorful fabrics, bits of string, small boxes, and, in fact, just anything. The balance of the supplies would consist of pieces of cardboard, scissors, and glue. The patients enjoy rummaging for objects to glue to their cardboards. One patient involved in such a project had as a theme a "stop-smoking" assemblage consisting of a small disposable ash tray, a used cigarette, and little clippings denoting the dangers of smoking. Some patients constructed humorous collages and gave them amusing titles. Others made designs—some in very good taste. A few patients became involved to the extent of saving odds and ends in their rooms for future collage projects.

Weaving holds a certain fascination for the aged, not just as an interesting handicraft, but as being reminiscent of an art that was an actual necessity early in their lives. The average table-size loom is good, but for those not capable of handling it there are a number of less cumbersome ones.

### Games

In conducting games, enthusiasm on the part of the leader is the most important ingredient. Money, even when only pennies, adds to the fascination when used in competitive games. Pokeno, a type of card game similar to bingo, has become a close second to bingo in popularity.

Bowling is a very good nursing home game. It can be played by patients with walkers or those confined to wheelchairs. There are inexpensive plastic sets available and the bowling alley can be marked off on a piece of plastic or linoleum. Try to secure teenagers or any physically fit volunteer to act as pinsetters as pinsetting is a strenuous chore.

The National Recreation Association has printed a list entitled "Improvised Games for the Ill and Handicapped Aged." These games are fun and competitive, but simple and involve very little cost. The names are descriptive enough to give you an idea of what they are like; I present a few: bean-bag toss, card flip, bottle-cap pitch, cup-cake bounce.

If the budget allows, there are, in addition, excellent games illustrated in a catalog that can be had by writing to World Wide Games, Inc., Box 450, Delaware, Ohio 43015.

### Idle-Hour Project

Two years ago, I started something called "the Idle-Hour Project." It was brought about by patients' requests for something to do over the long weekends and evenings. Carts were prepared with games, puzzles, scrapbooks, sewing kits, and simple craft materials. These were brought to each room on the infirmary floors every Friday morning. For example, a kaleidoscope was borrowed by a male patient, and the following week he informed us that it served nicely to amuse his great grandson who had visited him. Because requests for reading matter grew a book cart was added. In addition to the regular books, this cart contained paperbacks, magazines, books with large print, and records for talking book machines. On each weekly visit to the infirmary patients, exchanges, new requests, comments, and criticisms were handled. Participation continued to grow, in part due to perseverance and patience of staff, but, even more, because of the individual attention provided and the opportunity to make a choice.

The ambulatory patients who accepted sewing kits usually brought them to the craft session, thus extending their interest.

Scrapbooks and old magazines from which to cut colorful pictures of cats, dogs, food, or of whatever the interest were accepted by a few.

A bed patient interested in the squirrels in a tree outside her window was loaned a pair of binoculars and a book about squirrels. Another expressed an interest in rocks. A small collection—of the type purchased in museums—was left with her along with a magnifying glass and a descriptive booklet.

A few patients with enough artistic talent to paint on their own were furnished with art supplies.

Unless the patient was alert, leaving games—or anything else for that matter—presented the problem of finding someone to help him. This was sometimes accomplished by assigning volunteers on weekends.

During the course of making rounds with the carts, the activities staff did some important listening. This was what they heard:

Mrs. L. might join the discussion group if she can overcome her shyness.

Mrs. C. (who played the piano years ago is now practicing and showing improvement) suggested a washboard, kazoo, and what-have-you orchestra for a talent-night show.

Mrs. H., who ambulates with great difficulty, wants daily walks, and swimming.

The possibilities for similar programs are endless, but it takes a great deal of ingenuity, understanding, and patience to make them successful.

## Music

Music can take many forms. If you are fortunate enough to have a piano on wheels and someone to play it, just add words, in large print, to familiar songs and some lively voices to lead the singing to provide the favorite of all musical programs. In the absence of the piano, sing-a-long records can be used on the talking book machines. Incidentally, these machines can also be used to bring specifically requested records to a patient's room.

### Drama or Role Playing

I don't believe that drama or role playing is very widely practiced in nursing homes. This may be because its application is not very well understood, but it can be a very exciting addition to any program.

The goal is to motivate the elderly to take part in some form of self-expression. Social summaries can help determine which patients, if any, have had experience in any of the performing arts. One should also be on the alert for those who just wait to be coaxed.

The following method has worked well for me: The group is usually composed of those who participate actively and those who just want to watch and enjoy the proceedings. There is a joint effort in forming the outline for a skit or situation. The characters either volunteer or are chosen, and here the activities worker plays the role of director by clarifying each performer's role. The character then decides for himself what he is going to say and how he is going to say it. This is the important part. When the situation is understood, the dialogue comes easily and convincingly. The awkwardness that often results from attempting to memorize a script puts a strain on the proceedings, and, since we are striving for enjoyment, we'll leave the script learning to the more serious.

Briefly, here are a few of the situations that were acted out without props. Two persons, who really don't know each other but neither one will admit it, engage in an amusing but meaningless conversation.

The setting is a department store. A husband, while returning a tie given him as a Christmas gift by his wife, is caught by his wife in the act of being very chummy with the sales girl.

A woman, hiding a neighbor's husband in her apartment, is in a predicament when the neighbor's wife drops in for a cup of coffee and doesn't leave.

Remember, these were situations suggested by the patients. Another device is the use of fake telephones for which a variety of conversations are carried out.

In addition to being a source of amusement, role playing can benefit the patient in a number of ways: Since the patient has too much concern for himself too much of the time, role playing affords him the opportunity to lose himself on occasion; it channels creativity; it has a humanizing influence; it helps release pent-up emotions from institutionalized living; it builds confidence, and proves to the patient that he can do something that he thought he couldn't do; it may shed new light on an otherwise unpopular person.

A final word before leaving the subject of role playing. Staff members can be trained to conduct these sessions and do not necessarily have to have a background in dramatics.

## Education

In a nursing home one would not expect to set up classrooms, but we are often reminded that there is no age limit for the thirst for knowledge. I know of a nursing home patient who is studying Spanish, another who is interested in basic English. Some are constant contributors to a resident publication containing poetry and original articles. The ways are many, but we must be sensitive to them and support them.

## Discussion Groups

Discussion groups are increasingly in evidence in the nursing home setting. It was not too long ago that the assumption was that current issues and world affairs were out of place here. It has been my observation that through radio, television, newspapers, visits from friends and relatives, there is a large degree of awareness of what is going on in the world. A discussion group can be started by merely gathering a few people together and engaging in small talk. The degree of success depends largely upon the personality of the group leader.

## FINAL WORD

The administrator is faced with staggering responsibilities, and there are many departments functioning under his jurisdiction, but, in view of its relative newness, the activities program, in its present role, needs his assurance and support. Something to understand: If the work of the activities department looks easy, it is because its members are working so hard.

Our future goals must be geared to an ever-changing population. The population will be more sophisticated, more demanding, more knowledgeable, and tuned in on the meaningful use of leisure time from years of productive living.

## REFERENCES

1. Ellis, C. B. The aged in American society. Louisiana Commission on the Aging, P.O. Box 4482, Capitol Station, Baton Rouge, Louisiana 70804.
2. Improvised games for the ill and handicapped aged. National Recreation Association, 8 West 8th Street, New York, New York 10011.

3. Life lines. Group Work and Recreation Bulletin, New York State Department of Social Services, 1450 Western Avenue, Albany, New York 12203.
4. Starting a recreation program: In institutions for the ill or handicapped aged. National Recreation Association, 8 West 8th Street, New York, New York 10011.
5. World Wide Games, Inc., Box 450, Delaware, Ohio 43015. Excellent games illustrated in a catalog.

# Organization
# of Nursing Services
# for Geriatric Patients

*Martha Mackay*

**11** The nursing home administrator plays a most important role in our modern, sophisticated, complicated, complex, and automated society. No one has found a way to replace the product of total nursing care and its necessity to be administered by people. Granted, medical science has made great strides in diagnosis, treatment, and prevention in addition to the numerous labor-saving devices. Yet, these are just silent helpers in alleviating some of the nurse's numerous duties and permitting her to devote more time to be where she can do the most good—with her patients.

An added advantage to our position as administrators is the fact that our "product" is never the same, never takes the same course, and remains a challenge from the admission to the discharge of a patient.

The key to nursing home service is *you* as the administrator, what you make of it, how you feel about it, and how you treat the entire situation day-in and day-out. In other words, the administrator is hub of the wheel that makes a facility roll forward to excellence or slip backwards to mediocrity.

In Figure 1, notice the placement of the various departments in a nursing home. As you can see, nursing requires four spokes in the wheel, which should quickly make you realize the importance that it holds in your facility. And please keep in mind always that when you are striving to keep this wheel going, the momentum will come from a superior nursing department.

Prior to organizing nursing services, you, the administrator, must make certain *decisions*, formulate *concepts* of your position, and determine the *goals* of your facility.

You should always keep in mind, when setting up your objectives and goals, the controlling agencies that are effective in your area, for example, the state health department code and the regulations necessary to participate in Medicare.

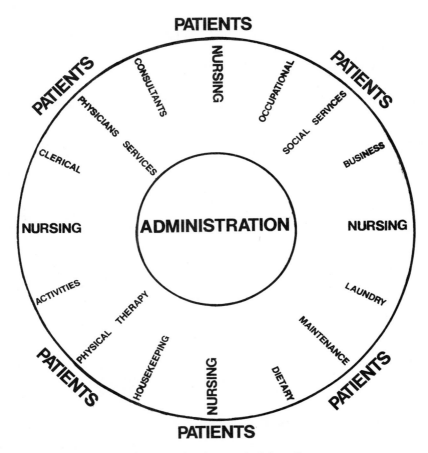

Figure 1.   The "wheel" of nursing home administration.

## FACTORS THAT BRING ABOUT OBJECTIVES

Let us review the factors that will bring about objectives in the organization of nursing services. In outline form these are:

   I. *An understanding of aging and the aged or geriatric process through your recognition of the changes related to aging:*
      A. *Psychological changes:* Compared with younger age group, the memory span of the aged is shorter, the aged are slower to accept changes and new ideas, they have a narrowing of interest, less energy and initiative; they repeat stories—often of old times—and have lessened ability to concentrate.
      B. *Physiological changes:* Decrease in eyesight and hearing, changes in skin, bone, joint, and muscles; increased fatigue upon exertion and susceptibility to systemic diseases caused by decreased circulation.

C. *Social changes:* The needs of the aged increase—the need to love and be loved, need for companionship, recognition, personal achievement, security, and new experiences. Or to sum up, some one to care, something to do, and somewhere to live. Of these, the need for one to *CARE* is the most important.

II. *Knowledge of your facility and its capabilities:* This implies assessing each corner of your building; knowing design, equipment, and utilization factors.

III. *Statement of goals and objectives:* This is an extremely important factor and the one that should receive the greatest amount of consideration. It includes type of care—how much, what kind, what quality, and with what emphasis. The objective is the statement of why your nursing home was created and what is expected of it at all times. These are things that the board, the owners, or yourself will have to decide. If your institution was created as a financial investment (to get the greatest amount of return), then, you, the administrator, will be directly influenced by this fact. If, on the other hand, your facility was created to give high-quality service with a reasonable financial return, you will adjust to fit the pattern as stated. In other words, you must know the purpose for establishment and the expectations. I would like to interject here that I am going to assume that each and every one of you will be working in an institution or facility that was established to give the ultimate in service. Sample objectives of your home might be:

A. To provide continuing *care* for those recovering or suffering from some medical or surgical disorder.

B. To assist patients in reaching optimal physical and emotional health.

C. To provide for the total needs of patients—physical, emotional, and spiritual.

D. To assist the geriatric patient toward an active participation in life.

E. To provide rehabilitative services.

F. To work cooperatively with other community and social agencies.

IV. *Knowledge of leadership and its use to reach your set goals:* As you are aware, there are many types of leadership, but there is one that I would like you to consider for use in your facility. This is called "participative leadership;" in it, decisions result from consultation with your employees. The advantage is that this type of leadership gives employees a voice but still exerts the proper control. The disadvantage is that it requires *EXCELLENT COORDINATION AND COMMUNICATION.*

If you refer to the wheel and to the many services and departments that are included in your facility, you will see the reason why I mention participative leadership. In order to arrive at the ultimate in care, your decisions should come from consultation with your employees. Personally, I feel that you will have a more satisfied group if its members have this type of participation, yet this still gives you the proper control.

V. *Principles of administration:* As a leader in your role as administrator, there are seven principles that should help to make your position easier; they are:

A. *Totality:* This is the most important and the most difficult to practice. It refers to an administrator's ability to continually take into account all aspects of the operation of his home when he makes a decision. In order to achieve true totality, you should think continually of all those involved in the operation of the facility. It is true that the primary interest will *always* be the welfare of the patient, but running a close second to this will be the consideration of your employees and the community. To achieve totality, time in each day should be set aside to manage. Never allow yourself to be so encumbered by routine duties that you lose site of your overall operation. This means that you must learn to know each of your patients and each of your employees, and understand their needs and limitations. The size of your facility should have no bearing at all on this factor.

B. *Delegation:* It is obvious that you cannot devote the time and energy to becoming an expert in all areas of your facility. Therefore, you should learn to select and train your assistants to the degree that they have confidence in their own areas of responsibility and then you should depend upon them to direct and provide the services necessary for the operation of the home. In doing this, you delegate both responsibility and authority, but you should have sufficient knowledge *in* each area to understand how it should function. To implement delegation, each employee and department must have job descriptions; these will be discussed later in this chapter.

C. *Coordination:* The administrator who *delegates* must assume the responsibility to coordinate. He must see that each member of his staff performs the duties assigned to him in a manner that does not conflict with, or duplicate, those assigned to other employees. This, too, can be achieved very well through job descriptions and written operational policies.

D. *Cooperation:* Cooperation goes hand in hand with coordination as well as with understanding, and all are generated from the top— *YOU.* This does not mean wishy-washiness or lack of purpose, but it does mean diplomacy. The way you say something makes a great difference in the way it is accepted and this leads us right into the next principle, communication.

E. *Communication:* Faulty or erratic communication of policies and other information leads to ill-will, confusion, and distrust. Employees who do not know or understand what is expected of them or what is going on around them usually dislike and distrust fellow employees and patients alike. With dislike and distrust in any organization, large or small, hope of achievement is lost. There are six aspects of communication for you to keep in mind: (1) idea, (2) code, (3) sending, (4) receiving, (5) decoding, and (6) idea. To go along with this, think of the following example: *Who* says *what* to *whom* for what *purpose* through what *channel* with what *effect.*

F. *Consistency:* Consistency does not mean inflexibility or arbitrariness, but it does mean that the same combination of factors should always bring the same administrative decision or result. It also means that you should be as objective as possible in reaching your decisions.

G. *Planning:* This principle seems to be the one that is most frequently overlooked. You cannot really establish the principle of planning until you have established each of the other six principles. And to do your planning effectively you must have control of the preceding six items. Underneath all of these principles runs an underlying philosophy which is: "The nursing home is the administrator and the administrator is the nursing home." In other words, the actions of the administrator, the policies of the administrator, and the personality of the administrator are the factors that determine the care in the home. If you want understanding, service, and loyalty in your home, you must give these same qualities to it. Your actions and your examples set the standards of professional competency and proficiency that you want your staff and your home to achieve.

VI. *The administrator's awareness of the difference between hospital and geriatric nursing:* When comparing long-term patients with short-term or acute hospital patients in respect to total nursing personnel, the needs of long-term patients are considerably greater. The principal difference between nursing service for the long-term and that for the short-term patient lies in the use of auxiliary nursing personnel—nurses' aides and orderlies. You are probably thinking that there is no difference—hospitals have aides and orderlies; but nursing homes require more work hours for nurses' aides and orderlies than do hospitals.

What are the reasons why the long-term geriatric patient requires a higher percentage of time of the auxiliary nursing personnel? He has a greater demand for assistance at meals, for bed baths, and for assistance in getting out of bed. He may be incontinent. He may need assistance from auxiliary nursing personnel in recreation programs and in transfer to physical and occupational therapy areas. The nursing personnel must instill a new motivation in the patient and have the time and patience to get him to do for himself, to care for his own needs. The final reason is that *the staff must be attentive in discerning when the patient should be encouraged to do for himself.*

The acute hospital patient usually can be encouraged by the fact that his condition will improve; he will have a favorable attitude toward the nurse because she will be associated with this improvement. Noticeable improvement is also a very positive factor in the morale of acute nursing service personnel. The chronically ill or physically disabled patient can usually look forward to only gradual improvement, but very seldom can hope for a complete cure. Usually he has few family ties or the security of employment; his instability affects his attitude toward himself and those working with him. It is most important that the members of the nursing staff understand the social and psychological implications of chronic illness and be prepared to cope with them. In administering medication, for example, in acute hospitals the nurse can usually *instruct* the patient, whereas, in the long-term facility, often she has to *coax* the patient to take even a simple vitamin pill.

In summary, nursing home nursing consists in total care—giving the best care possible with a great deal of compassion and interest toward and for the patient.

VII. *Administrative understanding of nursing service in its proper perspective:* The very name "nursing home" implies that nursing is the central service. The purpose of administration in the nursing home is to create and maintain an environment that offers both the quality and the quantity of care to correspond to the needs of the patient in the home. It is the administrator's responsibility to provide adequate care for the patients whom he has accepted into the home. In addition, the administrator must make his facility:
  A. Attractive to nurses and paramedical personnel.
  B. Responsive to the medical needs of his patient.
  C. Obvious and reassuring to the public.

### SELECTION OF DIRECTOR OF NURSING SERVICES

Now that you know what you want, where you are going, and what your position is, your next and most important job is the selection of your director of nursing services. This nurse will be the key to your effective operation; her importance cannot be stressed enough.

What are the qualifications, abilities, and personal characteristics that you will be interested in when processing applicants for the position of director of nursing services? In addition to being a registered professional nurse, this person should have:
  1. A desire to work with older people. Basically, a *love* of the aged is required to do the job well.

2. Adequate knowledge and experience relating to her work.
3. Ability to solve problems and make effective decisions.
4. Persuasive qualities and ability to express herself.
5. Drive and a willingness to do whatever is required of her at any given time.
6. Ability to select, appraise, and develop subordinates.
7. Superior ability to counsel others as well as conference leadership qualities.
8. Good health, professional appearance, and good manners.
9. The ability to follow through on a job until its completion.
10. An interest in nursing education for herself and her staff.

The director of nursing should also be:
1. A good organizer who displays sound judgment.
2. Loyal and enthusiastic in matters relating to the facility.
3. Persistent, tactful, and able to get wholehearted cooperation from other people.
4. Able to react to pressure when necessary.
5. Cost conscious and constantly endeavoring to discover new methods to improve present methods of operation.
6. Open-minded and receptive to new ideas.
7. Able to adapt to change.

Now that you know some of the qualities that you are looking for, how do you begin your search? You advertise widely in newspapers, journals relating to nursing homes, and sometimes just by communication with members of the community. Assuming that you have a number of applications, you go over all of them carefully, eliminating the applicants whose credentials do not meet your requirements or needs. In order to obtain the person who will best fill the shoes of your director, you should allow enough time for interviews.

### Interviews

In conducting an interview you should have your qualifications mentally available and know exactly what kind of information you want to acquire from the applicant.

There should be mutual honesty between you and your applicant. You have the right to expect a true presentation of her qualifications. In turn, you and she should know exactly what is expected of her in filling the position she is applying for. You should have a copy of her educational records, experience records, and references available for review. In addition to this, it is important for you to gain an insight into her personality and her background as well as her attitude toward employees and patients (a very important point). Her attitude can easily be determined by asking certain questions such as:

*What are your views on geriatric patients and what do you feel nursing can do for them?* In her answer to this question, you could determine her basic ideas and attitudes toward geriatrics, her nursing techniques, and, in addition, how well and to whom she is going to delegate the authority to care for her aged patients.

*How would you handle an employee who is a person whom you do not want to lose from your staff but somehow manages to stir up trouble by making other peoples' business her business?* This answer should give you evidence about how diplomatic the applicant is and to what extent she is willing to work with this difficult employee. It will also assist you in perceiving what judgments she would make in handling situations of this nature. Hopefully, she would want to find out as much as possible about the situation, talk to those involved in the problem (the employee and his or her superior), and, if the head nurse and/or supervisors are unable to handle the situation effectively, discuss the problem with the employee herself.

In conducting the interview, you should always have in mind the qualifications that the controlling agencies require for this particular staff position. You should contact the proper state and/or federal agencies to make certain that you will be in compliance when you do make your decision.

The applicant will probably ask you many questions about your philosophies, objectives, and goals so that she would know (or, hopefully want to know) exactly where she would stand in your organization.

Another important thing for you to keep in mind during the interview with the applicant is *your attitude* toward nurses and nursing care. If you can give this nurse the impression that you will be satisfied with only the finest type of nursing care in your nursing home, you will, in most instances, immediately eliminate anyone who hasn't the desire or ability to produce this quality care. Remember that if you are *unfortunate* enough to hire a nurse with second-rate ideas, your institution will soon become one with a second-rate reputation.

### Review and References

Following the interview, review and conclusions should be made immediately (or as soon as possible) after the applicant leaves your office. You have a list of the capabilities and requirements she should have and now it is up to you to review these carefully. If these intangibles impress you favorably, then you will proceed to check her references and past experience record. The method of doing this depends on the institution that you are contacting. Some places will not accept phone questions regarding a past employee and some will be more than helpful in giving you any and all information that you request.

This you will have to find out on your own. If possible, it is best to check not only with the personnel office but also to talk with the person who was your applicant's immediate supervisor. If this person happened to be the director of nurses in another facility, then it would be helpful for you to talk with the administrator of that institution.

If many qualified applicants decline your offer, it might be wise to re-evaluate the salary structure. The position you are filling is an important one; since this person is going to have a great deal of responsibility, her salary should be commensurate with her ability. If you plan to attract to your facility capable and responsible personnel, then you must be competitive in your wage scale. It is not too difficult to find out what other local institutions—whether they be hospitals or nursing homes—are paying their employees. You should, at least, try to meet this rate (or offer a little higher rate) if you plan to attract the staff. This is true not only for the director of nurses, but goes right down to the nurses' aides, housekeepers, laundress, and maintenance personnel.

## DELEGATION OF RESPONSIBILITIES

At this point, let us assume that you have your director of nurses and that she is a most capable person, one who is well-qualified to perform the duties of her position. I am also going to assume that many of you are probably thinking at this time that it took so long to get this director of nursing that now you can sleep a little bit easier at night and maybe have time to put your feet up on the desk and be relaxed. You are sadly mistaken! Granted, you do have this capable person who is going to be doing a lot for you, but there are still many things that you and she together have to do before you can even think about taking one patient into your facility.

As you know (or as you should know by now), your operation is rapidly becoming a very complex and skilled management job. Therefore, it would be virtually impossible for you to have the knowledge necessary to direct all areas of your facility competently. For this reason, delegation of responsibilities is considered to be a vital administrative task. You must keep in mind that by deputizing others, you in no way relinquish your control. It is in establishing controls and lines of authority that each department functions well and the staff member measures up to the standards set by you. This represents a trust that every supervisor and department head should know and have—to be granted the authority that rightfully belongs with his or her position. In other words, if you want someone to accept leadership in an area for which he is specifically trained, you should be more than prepared to give him the freedom and authority to function in this role effectively. It also goes without saying that if this person is found unworthy and unable to cope with his position, then you have no alternative but to replace him with someone who can handle this assignment well.

The most effective way for you to maintain this control over your personnel is to define your lines of authority carefully. To do this, you should develop an organizational structure or what is most commonly called an "Organizational Chart" or "Chain of Command." There are numerous ways in which this chart can be set up since it pertains only to your facility, the services available, and how you want your authority to be delegated.

The heads of your various departments are responsible to you and/or your nursing director, but they have several people responsible to them. This relieves you of many day-to-day small and petty problems but still places you in the right perspective at the top of the chain of command. The nursing director and nursing supervisors are placed where they are to establish and maintain a first-class nursing department. Always keep in mind, however, that the organizational chart is a very excellent administrative tool; but, if the persons involved in it are not aware of its purpose and meaning, it might as well be forgotten.

## OPERATIONS OF DEPARTMENT OF NURSING SERVICES

With a director of nursing services in place and having provided her with the opportunity to meet with and work with the other supervisory personnel in your facility, she is now ready to establish and operate a department of nursing for your facility which meet your requirements and those established for your facility.

Through her attendance and contributions at policy meetings, your director of nurses has a very good idea of what you and your facility expect to attain and from these policies she can now develop her department. In order to do this she must have: (1) a statement of philosophy; (2) an established plan of organization; (3) written administrative policies; (4) policies for personnel; (5) a program for providing nursing care; (6) a budget for the operation of nursing services; (7) an estimate of the needs and operations of a system for the control and use of equipment, facilities, and supplies; (8) an effective system for developing and maintaining clinical and administrative records and reports; (9) a program of in-service education for all staff members; and (10) a systematic appraisal program for evaluation of progress toward attaining objectives.

### Statement of Philosophy

A statement of policy should include: *prevention* of disabilities intensified by the aging process, *treatment* of the patient for the needs created by the aging process, and *restoration* of the person to a level consistent with the limitations imposed by the aging process.

In conjunction with the philosophy will be a *statement of objectives:*
1. To provide 24-hour nursing care for illnesses and for the restoration and protection of the physical and emotional well-being of the patient.
2. To make sure that objectives are consistent with those adopted by the entire facility.
3. To ascertain that the objectives of the program for nursing care are coordinated with the objectives of the medical care program.
4. To make certain that plans be translated into short-term and long-range objectives.
5. To make sure that the philosophy, objectives, and short-term and long-range plans are understood by all personnel concerned in addition to being evaluated periodically and revised in terms of changing nursing care requirements.

## Established Plan of Organization

A plan of organization that is consistent with the objectives of nursing care and the overall nursing home organization should be established. This plan defines responsibility, authority, and relationship of all positions within the nursing department. In other words, just as the entire facility has an organizational plan, the nursing services department must have its own organizational plan. The organizational plan must take into consideration:
1. The size of the facility.
2. The structure of the facility (e.g., whether it is a multi-story or a single-floor building).
3. Number of nursing stations.
4. Nursing personnel needed to provide comprehensive nursing care. A good rule of thumb here is to use the following formula: Consider that 50 percent of the patients will require full care or a minimum of four hours of nursing care per day; that 30 percent of the patients will be of an intermediate level and require at least two hours of nursing care per day; and that only 10 percent to 20 percent (and it usually falls closer to the 10 percent) will be limited-care patients and require one hour of nursing care per day. Obviously, these percentages will change as your census changes, but it would behoove the director to set up her organization on this basis.

## Written Administrative Policies

The written administrative policies are set up to clarify for nursing services the overall nursing home policies in which nursing shares responsibility. Examples are: (1) activities program, (2) dental services, (3) dietary services, (4) fire regulations (e.g., drills, emergency plans, extinguishers), and (5) physician services. All of the overall facility policies should be reviewed and those that pertain to nursing in *any* way should be written up and the nursing responsibilities in regard to these defined.

### Personnel Policies

The director of nurses should know and review the personnel policies that are in effect for the entire facility. At this point she knows exactly the personnel she is going to need to run her service efficiently. With her organizational chart in hand, she is now able to ascertain the numbers needed for supervisory nurses, head nurses, staff nurses, licensed practical nurses, nurses' aides, and orderlies.

*Job Description and Job Specification.* The next step is formulation of job descriptions and specifications. Let us first define these two terms so that we will all be thinking along the same lines:

*Job description:* A statement setting forth the characteristics, duties, and responsibilities of a specific job.

*Job specification:* A written record of the minimum hiring requirements or standards which must be met by an applicant for a specific job.

In order to write a good job description and job specification, the person must *know* the job and all aspects that pertain to it. This is another reason why the choice of a qualified director of nursing services is so important; with her past experience, she will be able to effectively write these job descriptions that will guide and direct all members of her nursing service department. It is vitally important that all the employees' main duties and responsibilities be stated explicitly. This will virtually eliminate employees saying, "Well, that's not part of my job."

Let us take a look at a sample job description for one of our nursing positions. For this we will use that of the nurses' aide. Please keep in mind this is just a sample. Your descriptions can be written up in any manner suitable to your facility as long as they cover all the material stated previously. The title would be "Nurses' Aide Job Description."

*General Job Description:* The nurses' aide, as a valuable member of the nursing home staff, is responsible for the comfort and safety of all patients and assists professional and licensed practical nurses with nursing care. After receiving formal and bedside instruction, he/she will be assigned various duties, delegated by the nurse in charge, according to the patients' needs. The nurses' aide is always under the jurisdiction of a nurse and responsible to her for reporting observations and progress. Periodically, he/she will receive a performance evaluation to show his/ her status on the team, the areas in which he/she has improved, and the areas that still require more effort.

*Qualifications:*

  *Age:*       Minimum, 16, but preferably 18 to 20 years of age.

  *Education:* High school diploma or equivalent in experience.

  *Health:*    Good, and able to pass the pre-employment physical examination.

*Knowledge and Abilities:*

1. Knowledge and correct usage of English language.
2. Must be able to:
   a. Understand and follow oral and written directions.
   b. Communicate effectively.
   c. Work and cooperate with all kinds of people.
   d. Make good judgments, knowing own limitations.

*Personality Characteristics:*

1. A genuine liking for older persons.
2. Sincere interest in caring for patients, showing kindness, patience, understanding, and diplomacy in dealing with all staff members and patients.
3. Initiative.
4. Personal desire to perform well.
5. Ability to treat confidental information with utmost reticence.
6. Emotional maturity.

*Appearance:*

Expected always to wear clean uniforms; clean, white duty-shoes; hose; and a "neat" hair style.

*Main Duties and Responsibilities:*

1. To acquaint him/herself with the contents of the personnel manual.
2. To perform as an important member of the nursing staff, report to the nurse in charge, give and receive assistance.
3. To work with accuracy, neatness, and completenesss.
4. To assist with admissions, discharges, and transfer of patients.
5. To answer patients' signal lights and assist if possible, and to seek help if necessary.
6. To observe and report patients' general conditions and any behavioral changes.
7. To give bed baths and tub baths, and assist patients with partial care.
8. To give and/or prepare for good oral hygiene, mouthwash, and/or denture cleaning.
9. To position patients in beds and chairs; assist patients to and from wheelchairs, beds, and stretchers, using proper body mechanics.
10. To collect urine and stool specimens as directed.
11. To measure, record, and report intake and output.
12. To test urine specimens for sugar, acetone, etc.

The above is only a partial listing. Again, my point is, put everything expected of the employee in writing and make certain that he or she has a copy.

*Recruitment.* Now that you know how many personnel you need and what they are going to do, from where are you going to get them? The same thing will hold true here as it did when *you* were looking for your director of nurses; you would advertise in the newspapers. Don't limit the search only to your own community, but canvas outlying areas or communities, but not too distant ones. Also employ word-of-mouth advertising.

*Selection.* Review the applications carefully. If your job descriptions and specifications are written to meet your goals, final selection should be no problem.

*Placement.* A high percentage of the persons applying to you for employment are going to be working mothers. There may be many reasons why these mothers have to work, but the prime one is to supplement the present family income. Therefore, it is assumed that the applicant and her husband and/or her family have agreed upon her seeking employment (an important point to establish before hiring). There is probably a specific shift that is going to work out best for her which will not interfere with her home duties. With this in mind, try to hire the applicant for the shift that she desires. If that shift does not have a vacancy, promise to give her the shift that she desires as soon as there is an opening. You want satisfied and steady employees and by meeting the shift request, you will promote just that.

*Orientation and Training.* From the standpoint of efficient management, a sound orientation and training program is a necessity. This enables employees to adjust to a new work environment and become fully productive quickly, and with a minimum of stress. Too often administrators discourage such programs because they believe, incorrectly, that an effective program requires additional staffing and that success depends upon having teachers or in-service coordinators. However, this training can be successfully done by key planning and the cooperation of your head nurses and general staff under the supervision of your nursing director.

Applicants with previous educational experience (such as registered nurses and practical nurses) do not need a training program but do need a period of guidance and orientation to your facility. Whether you are going to orient or train, you will need a planned outline which should include the following factors:
1. Total time to be devoted to the program.
2. A daily time schedule.
3. Names of those participating in the program.
4. Material in areas to be covered during this period.
5. Tools to be used during the program (i.e., procedure manuals, job descriptions, policy manuals, drug lists, organizational charts, etc.).

A knowledgeable administrator and nursing director may set up a program, but it requires planning and staff support to produce the desired results.

*Health, Welfare, and Safety Programs.* Provision for health, welfare, and safety programs for each employee eventually will save you many dollars, especially compensation insurance ones.

*Maintenance of a Confidential File.* A confidential file should be maintained for each employee. It should contain pertinent data from the date of employment to separation. Included in this file will be:

1. The application for employment.
2. Reports of physical examination and re-examination.
3. Reference checks.
4. Report of attendance.
5. Evaluation forms.

## A Program for Providing Nursing Care

The professional nurse, in cooperation with other members of the nursing staff, develops, implements, and evaluates a written plan of care for each patient. The plan is up-dated as the patient's nursing needs change. It supports the medical care plans and reflects the preventive, supportive, therapeutic, and restorative care needed by the patient.

The written nursing care plan is reflected in the patient's clinical record and Kardex which give evidence of the nursing care provided and the progress made by the patient. An added note here, your staff may be doing marvelous things with the patient, but, without documentation, all progress will go unnoticed.

The professional nurse determines nursing care requirements, assumes those responsibilities requiring professional skill and judgment, and assigns and supervises that care which can be safely performed by the other members of her nursing staff.

Written policies and procedures are established to implement the program of nursing care. This is called "The Patient and Nursing Care Manual," in which is described everything that is performed by the nursing staff for the patient, directly or indirectly. It will include, for example, how to give a bed bath, prevention of pressure sores, application of a posey belt, and the like.

## Budget for the Operation of Nursing Services

The budget developed by the department of nursing services is compatible with defined objectives and organizational plans as well as being coordinated with the total budget of your facility.

### Estimation of Needs and Operations of a System for Control and Use of Equipment, Facilities, and Supplies

If your facility is not large enough to warrant a purchasing agent then some member of the nursing staff, preferably a supervising nurse, should be assigned to manage medical supplies and equipment. In your building there should be a separate room or area to keep this inventory which would include such things as: catheters, medicine cups, dressings, stock drug items, and the like. In most facilities, the utility and drug rooms are not of sufficient size to keep large inventories or for things that nurses as a rule love to hoard. The hoarding tendency probably reverts to hospital training during which there was a limited supply of items such as pillow cases and washcloths and each unit kept a running competition to see who could amass the most. Keeping a good supply is fine for the individual unit, but most difficult for the budget and good inventory control. One way to avoid this is to stock the units with basic supplies which can be replenished as needed by a nurse who is placed in charge of the supplies. Then, when the time comes to order any supplies or equipment for nursing use, this nurse should consult with you before the purchase is made. Too many administrators and/or purchasing agents buy without consultation and with the best price as their guide. This type of practice you will sooner or later regret.

### An Effective System for Developing and Maintaining Clinical and Administrative Records and Reports

There should be a system for reporting to the nursing home administrator and supervisory nursing personnel the progress, activities, and accomplishments of patients. This is one effective way for the administrator to know what has happened to his patients during each shift. A means of effecting this could be the use of a daily nursing report that gives the important patient events that have occurred during the three shifts of the day, besides supplying your business office with an accurate census. These reports are kept at the individual nursing stations, written at the end of each shift, and handed in to your office or the business office every day for your perusal before filing.

There should also be forms for reporting such happenings as accidents and incidents involving patients, personnel, and visitors; employee absences; and the like. All of these are an essential part of your administration tool kit. But again, these are only effective if those expected to use them know the method and importance.

There should also be a system for recording accurate and objective observations of patients in the clinical record. The contents of your health records will be determined basically by the controlling agencies. You must remember that these health care records are a form of communication and, like all types of communication, will be effective only if they are well-documented. They will be of great value not only to those agencies that will survey your facility but also even more important to the patient, administrator, and physicians. They can be one of the most important medical and administrative tools that you have. Always remember that once a patient has left your institution, the only way anyone can evaluate the treatment he received is through the review of this health care record.

**A Program of In-service Education for All Staff Members**
In order for the department of nursing service to participate in a program for in-service education you must:

1. Have a written plan for ongoing in-service education.

2. Make certain that appropriate staff representatives participate in the planning, conducting, evaluating, and revision of the in-service education programs.

3. Plan for nursing staff participation in appropriate patient care discussions and educational programs. This is essential to keep nursing staff members current with changing concepts, to increase their basic knowledge, understanding, and competency, and to further develop their ability to analyze problems.

4. Make provision for nursing participation in community activities and professional organizations.

**Systematic Appraisal Program**
The department of nursing service conducts a systematic appraisal program which evaluates the progress made toward attainment of the established objectives. This must be done by all nursing personnel—formally and informally, consciously and unconsciously, in emergency and routinely—around the clock. All nursing personnel should know the established objective so well that individually, as well as in group session, they will work toward their attainment.

Unconsciously, informally, and routinely, appraisal is made whenever nursing personnel care for or observe the patients and their activities. Consciously and formally, appraisal is made:

1. When the head nurse makes out her daily assignments.
2. When the nurses write the nursing care plan and nurses' notes.
3. When nursing supervisors and/or the director observe nursing activities.
4. At regularly scheduled nurses' aide meetings.
5. At planned, regular meetings with the patient care team. This would include representation from all facility departments—administrator, head nurses, nursing supervisors, director of nursing, therapists, social worker, and dietary, maintenance, and housekeeping personnel. In these meetings, discussions would include:

A. New admissions and the tentative goals for each patient.
B. Patients whose conditions are frequently fluctuating and difficult, in hope of obtaining team idea for possible solutions.
C. Patients pending discharge and the plans for discharge.
D. Problems or situations presented at the last meeting or new ones pertaining to the effective administration of the nursing home. The objective is to keep everyone informed so that goals may be reached smoothly.

Records should be kept of all meetings and copies given to the department heads so that the other staff members such as nurses' aides, dietary aides, maids, and laundry workers will receive the suggestions and/or criticisms that were presented. As far as you, the administrator, are concerned, attendance at these meetings is a must. You should not necessarily lead these meetings, but be there to listen and learn.

### STOP—LOOK AND LISTEN

Now that you have your nursing department organized and operating, how will you determine whether it is and will continue to function properly? *STOP—LOOK* and *LISTEN.* You are probably thinking that's wise advice to heed when you reach a railroad crossing, but what connection does it have with my position as administrator? Believe it or not, a great deal.

Let's take each of these words separately, define their relationship to your position, and then you be the judge.

*STOP* every day and plan to spend time out of your office.

*STOP* to talk to your staff, patients, and visitors. Let them get an idea of who *YOU* are more than the person behind the door marked "Administrator."

*STOP* so that you will be able to *LOOK.*

*LOOK* everyday at the nursing report.

*LOOK* at everything and everyone in your facility when making a daily tour.

*LOOK* at the patients. Do they appear to be clean and content?

*LOOK* to see how many patients are in the physical and recreational therapy areas.

*LOOK* to see how many of your patients go to the dining room and how they get there—the number walking, the number wheeled.

*LOOK* at your staff and their actions at various times during the day.

*LOOK* at the patients' charts; read a nursing summary.

*LOOK* at a patient care plan. Does it state in detail what the patient's activities and needs are?

*LOOK* and *LOOK,* but if you see a situation that you feel should not exist, don't make the unfortunate mistake of immediately criticizing or correcting. If you are disturbed by what an employee does, talk to the employee's supervisor. There may be a good reason for the employee's action.

The ability to *LISTEN* is *MOST* commendable and necessary.

*LISTEN* to your staff whether they are complaining or engaged in light conversation.

*LISTEN* to your patients.

*LISTEN* to the patients' families. They may often feel that you are the only one who can solve *their* problems.

*LISTEN* at every meeting you attend—to new ideas, to old problems. Perhaps they *are* important and *have* meaning.

If you can truly *STOP–LOOK* and LISTEN, then, and only then, will you really determine how your nursing department is functioning.

There is one other key to be considered. That is *SMELL*! If your patients are receiving the proper care, there should not be any offensive odor—not *EVER*. If there is, it should be traced and immediately corrected. Unpleasant odor is one of the *first* signs of neglect.

Society has given us a trust and a mission. This makes us humble, but it also inspires us to the challenge of excellence. We must rise to that challenge.

# Dietary Services: Nutrition for the Geriatric Resident

*Bernice Hopkins*

**12** The total care of the residents in the nursing home includes food service that provides adequate nutrition for each person. One of the Medicare standards specifies:

> The food and nutrition needs of patients are met in accordance with physicians's orders and, to the extent medically possible, meet the dietary allowances of the Food and Nutrition Board of the National Research Council, adjusted for age, sex and activity.

In order to ensure that each resident receives the recommended dietary allowances, the food service must be so organized, with policies and procedures clearly defined, as to provide meals as well as supplemental feedings that the resident will consume. The planning of adequate menus and the service of food, even though attractively presented, is not enough; the food must be eaten to provide adequate nourishment.

It is generally accepted that each nursing home is unique. The physical structure, the philosophy of management, the personnel, and the residents are different, but all have the basic similarities that make the application of general principles for standards of care possible. The *Code of Federal Regulations* provides nursing homes with standards of dietary care.[1] These standards are supplemented by state codes, which are required to be no lower than the federal standards. It is the responsibility of the individual facility to translate these standards to meet the needs of the individual nursing home.

Any time food is served, at mealtime or coffee hour, is a high spot in the day of the resident. It is a time for social contact. The activity of eating has always been a familiar one; it is among the first responses of the infant and continues throughout life. In most nursing homes, one can readily observe the residents waiting for mealtime in anticipation of good food and companionship. The emotional needs of the residents are an important consideration in food services in nursing homes. Recognition of the differences in ethnic backgrounds and regional food patterns form a basis for menu planning.

It is well to remember that the greatest number of residents in nursing homes at this time are members of the age group who, in their homes, were accustomed to eating at a table covered with a cloth, probably a linen one, and set with damask napkins, silverware, and china. Paper plates and paper napkins were used only for picnics. Therefore, when consideration is being given to the use of single service, careful consideration of acceptability to the residents is indicated.

When many of the residents were in their own homes, mealtime was a "family time;" when friends came to call, food was offered—a meal, a cup of coffee, cake or cookies. Is it not possible in planning the food service in a nursing home that some provision can be made for the resident to offer guests the same courtesy that he offered them in his own home?

The resident in a nursing home has relinquished much of his independence. The food service may be of the best, but it cannot be forgotten that the nursing home is not home; one is "eating out." In order to provide food service for a group of people necessitates institutional aspects. The goal of each person responsible for such food service should be to provide the most attractive food possible with as many extras as feasible, thereby aiding the home to make the stay (in most instances their last years) of the residents as pleasant as possible.

## MANAGEMENT AND PERSONNEL

In providing the climate for the development of the food service department, it is expected that the administrator will have in mind the good management practices that result in a well-run department. Organization charts, job descriptions, policies, and procedures to provide good communications are required to have a department in which all personnel will function with efficiency.

### Dietary Supervisor or Consultant

The food service department may be under the management of the facility or of a food contract company. In either situation, the federal and state codes apply in setting the standards for the department. In the *Code of Federal Regulations*[1] it is specified that the dietary service be directed by a qualified person:

> ... Dietary Supervision:—a person designated by the administrator is responsible for the total food service of the facility. If this person is not a professional dietitian, regularly scheduled consultation from a professional dietitian or other person with suitable training is obtained.

The dietitian, whether working in the facility full-time or part-time, functions as a consultant (i.e., he or she works through and with the personnel in the dietary department to provide adequate nutritional care). It is recognized that the role of the consultant in the nursing home is relatively new. Usually the dietitian has been trained in a hospital setting with an orientation to the care of acutely ill patients, as opposed to the care for long-term residents in a nursing home. It appears logical that the most effective consultant will have had a number of years (at least five) of varied experience in the many aspects of dietetics. This background will provide experience and courses upon which to draw to give guidance to the personnel in the dietary service. The consultant offers advice that may be implemented or not; he or she does not have direct authority for the operation of the department.

The administrator should expect that the consulting dietitian will be a member of the American Dietetic Association, registered dietitian (R.D.), or a member of the ADA (although not registered). In those geographic areas of the United States where the number of dietitians is limited, the administrator may find it necessary to select a consultant from those available persons with lesser qualifications. As noted in *Conditions of Participation,* "Other persons with suitable training are graduates of baccalaureate degree programs with major studies in food and nutrition."[1]

There is no specified number of hours per week that a consultant is expected to be in the facility. At the present time, the guidelines being widely used are based upon an article by W. F. Robinson.[2] It is the wise administrator who works out with the consulting dietitian the optimal coverage for the facility to ensure good food service. If a new consultant is employed, it is often of mutual value to the home and the consultant for the consultant to spend a greater number of hours at the beginning of employment than later on. The initial experience will provide the dietitian with an opportunity to become familiar with the facility and the personnel, to evaluate the situation, to get to know the people with whom he or she will be working, and to establish priorities for consultation. There should be a clear understanding between the administrator and the dietitian of what the administrator can expect from the dietitian and what the dietitian can expect from the administrator. The method for reporting the dietitian's visits and progress should be established. A mutually acceptable contract is good business.

The administrator can expect the dietitian to keep abreast with developments in the field of dietetics—to be a catalyst, ever on the alert to improve the dietary care of each resident.

It is well to remember that the dietitian is usually self-employed thereby providing his or her own "fringe benefits" which, understandably, makes the comparison of the salary range with the dietitian in the local hospital invalid. At present, guidelines given by Robinson are the most valid.[2]

Inasmuch as the dietitian is expected to have expertise in all aspects of dietetics as he or she functions as a consultant, it is apparent that adequate supportive personnel is needed to leave time to do those things for which he or she is best qualified.

## Dietetic Supportive Personnel

The American Dietetic Association has designated two categories of supportive personnel in the dietetic field. These are dietetic assistants and dietetic technicians.

A *dietetic technician* is supervised by the dietitian or by the administrator and the consulting dietitian. This person acts as an assistant in providing and assessing the food services. The American Dietetic Association specifies that he should have completed successfully an associate degree program for dietetic technicians that meets with the standards of the Association and should be skilled in food administration or nutrition care.

A *dietetic assistant,* formerly known as a food service supervisor, is supervised by the dietetic technician or the administrator and the consulting dietitian. The American Dietetic Association specifies that he should be a high school graduate, or have had the equivalent educational background, and should have successfully completed a course in food service management or nutrition care that meets with the standards of the Association.

It is realistic to accept the fact that personnel with the qualifications stipulated by the American Dietetic Association may not be available in many geographic areas. It has been found that a cook-manager is filling such a position in many facilities. It frequently is desirable to seek training opportunities for such an employee in a resident course for dietary assistants, or by a correspondence course. Information is usually available from the nutritionist in the state health department as to the availability of such courses.

## DUTIES OF THE DIETETIC TECHNICIAN
## OR FOOD SERVICE MANAGER

The day-to-day manager in the nursing home is the responsible person for food service. He should be expected, with the consultation of the dietitian, to perform the following functions in the dietary department:

1. The planning of menus for regular and modified diets.
2. The purchase of food and supplies.
3. Maintenance of records.
4. The selection, orientation, supervision, and evaluation of the dietary personnel.
5. Supervision of sanitation.
6. Provision of in-service training for personnel.

He should be included in:
1. Review of policies and procedures.
2. Plan for budget.

3. Plans for remodeling or new construction.
4. Selection of new equipment.

The well-trained, motivated manager (in consultation with an able dietitian) should be able to provide good food service for the nursing home. It is considered a good investment on the part of the administrator to encourage and provide for continuing education for the manager at workshops and institutes.

The number of residents, the number of personnel, the design and layout of the facility, the type of menu, and purchasing policies all are determining factors in the number of personnel required in the dietary department.

## MENU PLANNING

Menu planning for the nursing home takes into consideration the same factors as any other food service: the population—its number, ethnic background, age range, sex, and activity; the available equipment; the type of service; and the competency of the personnel.

The value of the cycle menu is well-recognized. A cycle menu is a set of menus to be used for a period of time (usually 3 to 6 weeks) and then repeated. There is no question concerning its efficiency. Once the cycle of menus has been planned, time is saved, purchasing is efficient, and a consistent food cost can be achieved. However, it is important that the dietitian and the manager plan the menus carefully to avoid monotony of repetition. They should remember that most of the residents in a nursing home are captive customers to whom food is of great importance. Therefore, variety and interest must be maintained.

If a selective menu is used in a nursing home it must be carefully planned. The choices of foods must have similar values. It is necessary to observe with care the selections made by the residents to assure adequate ingestion of foods to supply the essential nutrients.

The five-meal-a-day plan has been introduced in some nursing homes. The five small meals are served at intervals during the day and evening. With this plan, attention must be given to the recommended dietary allowances, making certain that there is a reasonably fair distribution of the various nutrients throughout the day. The plan has been reported to be well-received in some homes, but in other homes it has not been acceptable. Because dietary needs (depending upon the facility and its residents' dietetic requirements) may differ slightly, utmost care should be taken to afford the residents of any particular facility the best food service available.

Physiological changes due to the influence of the aging process may affect the resident's eating patterns. The resident may find that the act of eating, though once very enjoyable, now poses a problem. His dentures may not fit or he may choose not to use them. He may have arthritis which inhibits his ability to feed himself. The loss of vision (and general debility) may interfere with his eating ability.

The nutritional needs of the nursing home resident are much the same as when he was younger with the exception of caloric needs, which are lessened due to his decrease in activity. Care should be exercised to maintain the level of proteins and minerals to assure optimal nutrition.

Menus for specific therapeutic diets (ordered by the physician) require expertise and care in preparation. In most situations the diet is provided with more leniency than in an acute care facility.

## Diet Roster

The *diet roster* (Table 1) consists of a list of the individual residents compiled from the residents' charts. It includes the resident's name and the diet, either general or modified, that has been prescribed by a physician. The individual food likes and dislikes may be listed as well as modifications needed because of chewing problems. Also information concerning residents who need help in eating may be included.

The diet roster should be maintained by the person in charge of food service. It must be kept up-to-date, changes being made as often as necessary to keep it current. When a new diet roster is made out the previous roster should be filed as part of dietary records.

A written roster of patients to be served therapeutic, special diets must be prepared each day and this information made available to the employees serving the residents. The daily roster should also be filed as part of dietary records.

## Food Purchase Record

To maintain the *food purchase record* (Table 2), the food invoices for the inventory period are entered on the record when they are received. Breaking the record into food classifications makes it possible to obtain a figure for the amount of money spent for each food group. This enables one to observe shifts in spending that may be throwing food cost out of line. The information from the food purchase record may be transferred directly to a food cost report.

## Special Occasions

The food service manager, with imagination, can provide many interesting functions. If possible, birthday parties should be planned for each individual on *his* day rather than a monthly affair at which all residents having a birthday falling within that particular month are honored. A birthday is a very special day to the individual; show him that you remembered. Many holidays, such as Halloween, Washington's birthday, and Lincoln's birthday, as well as the major holidays, Christmas, Thanksgiving, and New Year's Day,

Table 1. Diet Roster

| Room and Bed Number[a] | Residents' Names | Regular | Soft | Diabetic | Low-salt | Low-fat | Other | Modified As: | Comments (e.g., help needed to eat; chewing problems; food likes and dislikes) Date |
|---|---|---|---|---|---|---|---|---|---|
| 10-4 | Doe, John | X | | | | | | | Extra cream for coffee |
| 10-5 | Smith, George | X | | | | | | | Tea at noon |
| 10-6 | Matthews, Jim | | | X | | | | Diabetic—1400 cal. (70-60-150) | No teeth—chop food |
| 11-4 | Rich, Ellen | X | | | | | | | Needs to be fed |
| 11-5 | Kent, Sally | | | | X | | | No salt added in cooking | |
| 11-6 | Kimble, Elsie | X | | | | | | | |
| 12-1 | | | | | | | | | |
| 12-2 | | | | | | | | | |

[a] List *all* bed numbers consecutively. Include empty beds.
[b] Mark X in proper square for diet order.

Table 2. Food Purchase Record (Selected Examples)

| Accounting Period | | Date *February 1* | | | through *February 28* | |
|---|---|---|---|---|---|---|
| Date of Invoice | Name of Firm | Milk and Ice Cream | Meats, Poultry, Fish, etc. | Fruits and Vegetables Fresh and Frozen and Juices | Groceries, Staples, etc. | Totals |
| February 3 | Whites Dairy | 20.70 | | | | |
| February 8 | Jones | | 25.00 | 18.00 | 17.28 | |
| February 15 | Brown & Sons | | | | | |

lend themselves to extras—special menus with special table or tray decorations. Religious holidays, according to the religions of the residents, should be observed with respect to traditional foods.

The introduction of a cocktail or sherry hour is being well-received in many facilities. The sanction of the physicians caring for the residents is always necessary. There appears in the literature some information that may be helpful to the food service manager in developing this social hour.

## CONCLUSION

Both the consulting dietitian and the day-to-day manager should be acutely aware of each patient's needs. They should know the patient well, be aware of his dietary needs, and realize his physiological limitations and psychological needs. With predetermined vital knowledge of the resident, the nutritional needs should be met adequately.

## REFERENCES

1. The conditions of participation: Extended care facilities. Federal Health Insurance for the Aged (Code of Federal Regulations, Title 20, Chap. III, Part 405). U.S. Department of Health, Education and Welfare, Social Security Administration. U.S. Printing Office, Washington, D.C.
2. Robinson, W. F. 1967. Dietitians' role in the nursing homes and related facilities: guidelines for part-time and consulting service. J. Amer. Diet. Ass. 51: 130—137.

# Environmental Health Control for the Nursing Home

*Alvin Jacobson*

**13** The terms "environment," "environmental pollution," and "environmental control" are now in fashion. Those of us who have been concerned for many years welcome this interest that is being shown by everyone even though it is somewhat belated. I want to share with you some of my thoughts on environmental control as it relates to the nursing home. I will first discuss briefly the relationships between the host, agent, and environment (epidemiology).

For initial consideration are the *hosts* or patients in the nursing home. These people are usually over sixty-five years of age; two-thirds of them are women; about one-half cannot walk alone; one-third are incontinent. They have a variety of conditions leading to a greater frequency for both diseases and accidents than for younger persons. The second concern is the *agent*. This includes the causes of infections and accidents. There are many varieties of *pathogenic* organisms that may be present in the environment, some of which have become resistant to current treatment methods. When penicillin was first introduced, many felt that it was going to provide a cure for any and all diseases; however, experience has shown that many organisms have developed a resistance to the various antibiotics available. The *environment*, the third portion of the triad, deals with the physical plant and its surroundings. In the environment there is a concentration of people—residents, employees, visitors, and others. This concentration of people in the nursing home provides *agents* that may cause infection and/or accidents which, in turn, may result in illness, injury, and even death.

The purpose of environmental control in the nursing home is to eliminate or reduce the *physical, microbiological, chemical,* and *radiological* hazards that may result in infections, accidents, injury, or death. The older people enter the nursing home seeking comfort, convenience, companionship, and security—items which they can no longer maintain for themselves in their own homes. In time, they may also require special nursing care for functions that they are unable to perform for themselves. Many of the residents in the home may be mentally disoriented, at least a part of the time. Some come to

201

the home because of conditions such as cardiovascular disease, arthritis, rheumatism, fractures, or paralysis—states frequently of long duration. It is your responsibility as a nursing home administrator to provide a home or a place for them to come to and live in, where they can be properly cared for during their stay.

It has been suggested by some experts in the field of gerontology that the location, construction, and environment have as much effect upon the health and mental outlook of the patient as does the nursing and medical care that he receives. The relationship between health and housing has long been recognized by environmental health specialists. It can be summed up in four basic principles:

1. Protection of and provision for mental needs.
2. Protection of and provision for physiological needs.
3. Protection against contagion.
4. Protection against accidents.

"Proper care" makes provisions for several considerations such as:

1. Environment for as much independent living as possible, within the limited abilities of the patient.
2. A quality of environment, at the least, equivalent to or better than the patient's private home environment.
3. Provisions for the patient's limitations, such as failing eyesight, hearing, ability to climb stairs, and limited physical energy.
4. Provisions for accommodating the possible physical and mental deterioration of the patient such as, blindness and forgetfulness.

These four basic concepts are applicable to a much greater degree in nursing homes than in domestic housing, and for this reason you, as the administrators, must give greater consideration to these various needs.

## WATER SUPPLY

As a specific for a functional, safe nursing home let us first examine the problem of providing a safe water supply. Generally, the water, whether from a private, community, or public supply, must meet the state health department standard. You must have adequate volumes or quantity of both hot and cold water; the amount may vary from 150 to 200 gallons per patient per day. Some nursing homes require less and some require more than this quantity, depending on programs, type of patients, and allied factors. The water pressure must be adequate to operate all fixtures, on all floors, during the hours of maximum demand. The minimum pressure required is generally between 15 and 25 pounds per square inch of the system. If you have a private supply, an emergency source should be provided; if a public supply is used, you should have two service connections or a loop system to ensure an adequate supply during emergencies. Should the water supply be private, I suggest that you have at least two wells connected to opposite ends of your nursing home for emergency purposes.

All water utensils should be handled properly, cleaned, and disinfected for use by succeeding patients. Ice must be handled and properly stored so as to prevent contamination.

The water supply in some communities is treated to remove minerals that cause scale formation or corosion of the pipes. In some instances, your boiler water may have to be treated to prevent scale formation within the system. Boiler systems should never be connected to the public water supply system because chemicals used in the treatment of the water may be contaminated and in turn contaminate the water supply system of the nursing home. Steam supplies from the boiler should never be used for the cleansing of utensils used in food preparation.

## SEWAGE

The second area of concern is that of sewage. The sewage system should provide quick removal of liquid wastes with a minimum of nuisance. The objectives of sewage disposal systems are: (1) prevention of pollution of water sources, (2) prevention of the possible spread of illness, (3) prevention of odors due to the decomposition of organic material, and (4) prevention of the destruction of acquatic and plant life. The nursing home and you, as the administrator, must also be concerned with the fact that liquid waste from your nursing home may contain the waste from the laundry, which, if you have a private sewage disposal system, may overload the system and result in contamination. If possible, your sewage system should be attached to a municipal disposal system to prevent many and sundry problems.

The disposal of garbage into sewers is very efficient, effective, and sanitary. However, because of inadequate treatment facilities, in many communities the disposal of these wastes into the sewerage systems is prohibited. The municipal sewage treatment plant may become overburdened.

## PLUMBING HAZARDS

The plumbing system consists of water supply lines that furnish water to the various parts of the building and sewer lines that remove wastes and discharge them to the sewers for final disposal. Faults in this system may result in contamination. Some of these are: (1) cross connections that permit the flow of waste materials from a sewer line back into the water supply, (2) back-siphoning causing waste material to be transferred from the waste lines into the water supply lines. Air gaps and vacuum breakers are devices that should be used to prevent contamination of the water supply. Air gaps should be used on the waste lines of autoclaves, instrument washers, and many other fixtures within the nursing home. Vacuum breakers should be used on the discharge line of toilets, bedpan washers, autoclaves, dishwashing machines, garbage grinders, and many other pieces of equipment that have submerged or submersible inlets. You, as the administrator, are responsible. You should have a person on your staff who is totally familiar with these problems and is able to see that they are prevented.

## FOOD SANITATION

Food is not only essential for the promotion and maintenance of health, but also for the morale of the aged and infirm. However, if proper precautions are not taken, it can serve as a vehicle for conveying pathogenetic organisms, bacterial toxins, or poisonous chemcials to the patients, staff members, and visitors. You should be familiar with the fact that some organisms are transmitted through food and cause food-borne disease. In nursing homes, careless handling of food presents more serious problems than in many other situations. Statistics indicate that, in the United States, the average number of patients or persons in a nursing home who are affected by food-borne outbreaks is over one hundred a year. Although food-borne illness is usually nonfatal in a normal population, in a nursing home it is a more serious problem because the patients, or *hosts*, are aged and infirm, and therefore more susceptible to infection and its consequences. You, as the administrator, should also be interested in the economic implications. In a nursing home, a food-borne epidemic will add to the total operating costs because of increased medical and nursing care, lost work by employees, overtime, additional personnel needed, and increasing quantities of drugs and medicines required for treatment of patients and staff members. The problems from the financial standpoint also include possible payment of judgments arising from legal actions. Lastly, you may have hastened the death of a patient and failed in your responsibility.

*What food-borne disease control measures must you pay attention to in your daily food service?* I list the fundamental ones:

1. Only wholesome food from approved sources should be purchased.

2. Food handlers should be free from disease. No person with boils, pimples, or a cold should ever be permitted to prepare or serve food. All employees handling food should maintain a high degree of personal cleanliness. They should conform to good hygienic practices while on duty. They should wash their hands following the use of the toilet, keep their fingernails clean, use hairnets, and always wear clean uniforms.

3. No smoking should be permitted during food preparation because this leads to contamination of the hands and may introduce pathogenic organisms into the food being served and prepared.

4. Pre-employment physical examinations should be required. It is important for the employer to determine that the employees do not have tuberculosis or other communicable disease. In some instances, stool examinations should be required to determine whether the staff members or prospective employees are infected, are carriers of typhoid fever, or are harboring various types of parasites.

5. Adequate facilities should be provided for all of the employees. I cannot stress too strongly the importance of adequate toilet and hand-washing facilities that are, above all, conveniently located. Soap and towels should be provided. Adequate lockers should be available for all employees. However, employees should never be permitted to store food products within those lockers because this attracts insects and rodents.

6. Kitchens should be properly designed and laid out to facilitate a smooth operation flow of foodstuffs from the receiving area to the point of service, while at the same time minimizing hazards. Consultation with dietary and environmental health specialists should be obtained in planning the kitchen arrangement.

7. Consideration should be given to kitchen equipment. A supplier who wants to make a sale will provide good advice. Equipment should be constructed of durable material; it should be nontoxic and smooth-surfaced; no seams or sharp corners should be permitted; and, above all, it should be designed so that any part of it can be easily disassembled for thorough cleaning. All equipment should meet the standards of the National Sanitation Foundation and have the Foundation's seal of approval.

8. Leftovers should be disposed of to prevent food-borne disease.

*The basic principles of good food handling consist in the prevention of contamination.* Some contamination, however, will result under the best of conditions. Microorganisms of certain types are always present. Their growth in food can be prevented by maintaining the food at specified temperatures during any period of storage or holding. High heat generally destroys microorganisms, including pathogenic ones, if the food is held at these high temperatures for a defined period of time. Cold will also destroy them or prevent their growth. Therefore, holding temperature should be either above 140°F. or below 40°F. (Your state's code will probably give specific recommendations.)

### Dish Washing

Dishes should be washed at 140°F. and then given a final rinse at 170°F. or higher for a minimum of thirty seconds. This will destroy any and all pathogenic organisms. Single service disposables have become available and are used by more and more nursing homes and, if handled properly, can eliminate many problems of sanitation. I suggest that you and your food service staff should consider their use, if their cost is not too great. Also to be taken into account is that disposables may add to the cost of solid waste disposal. Sometimes one can't win!

### Housekeeping in the Dining Areas

Dust and dirt accumulating on the floors and ceiling can become contaminated with pathogenic organisms that may be introduced into the food. A good housekeeping program can alleviate or eliminate this potential hazard.

### Lighting

Adequate lighting that permits a view of out-of-the-way corners should be provided to facilitate the cleanliness operation.

### Grease Filters

Frequent inspection and cleaning of grease filters in the exhaust system are another concern. Failure to maintain filters properly could result in grease fires as well as in food contamination.

## SOLID WASTE

Solid waste includes kitchen waste, rubbish, floor sweepings, dressings, soiled articles, and, in some nursing homes, several types of surgical wastes and wastes from laboratory departments, as well as the disposables referred to previously. The handling and storage of solid waste must be done efficiently and in a sanitary manner in order to prevent unpleasant odors and sights, and breeding places for insects and rodents. In addition, good fire control and safety demand that accumulation of solid waste must not be permitted in your nursing home. For temporary storage of waste on the premise of the nursing home, sturdy containers with tight lids or a "dumpster" that holds a minimum of a day's waste material should be provided. If spillage occurs, this should be immediately cleaned up. The use of liners for trash containers kept within the nursing home not only provide a means of sanitation, but also results in less washing and handling of the containers thus helping to reduce noise and depreciation.

The problem of collection and disposal can be facilitated by a public or privately operated community collection system. All waste may be disposed of by means of the collection system except that which is infected or highly contaminated. Contaminated material should be destroyed as rapidly as possible. Generally, it is incinerated on the premises. Incineration provides a very sanitary method of solid waste disposal and many sanitary codes require the incineration of all infectious wastes. The build-up of ashes resulting can usually be disposed of as a fill material.

*Air pollution ordinances* may prohibit the burning of waste. In some areas, garbage may be disposed of by means of a garbage grinder, thus circumventing air pollution. However, the use of this efficient and sanitary method is not permitted in some communities. You doubtless begin to appreciate solutions to the pollution problem as you try to cope with your own waste disposal problems.

## VECTOR CONTROL

Vector control is important in nursing homes because insects, such as flies, mosquitos, fleas, lice, and bugs of various kinds, and rodents may be vectors of disease. These pests may destroy and/or contaminate stored food supplies, posing both a health and an economic problem. Some venomous insects may represent a serious hazard; for instance, the bite of scorpions, spiders, bees, and wasps may result in serious clinical manifestations in the elderly or infirmed patient.

Control of insects and rodents is based on the following principles: (1) Basic sanitation or environmental control in general. This includes keeping the premises free of litter, proper handling of garbage and other solid wastes, and the elimination of breeding areas of the various types of insects and rodents. (2) Protection of persons against insects and rodents. This can be accomplished through screening of windows and doors and rat-proofing of all buildings to remove breeding places for both rats and mice. (3) Avoidance of venomous insects. This is accomplished by the education of patients and staff in the identification of types of venomous insects that may be very hazardous. Pesticides should be last on this list of methods used for control because they are toxic. They should be used only in the breeding areas and must *NOT* be used where they might come in contact with food. Special training of employees in handling pesticides is important. You, as the administrator, must assume the responsibility for this training. The services of an exterminator are satisfactory and sometimes required in coping with insect and rodent problems.

It is essential that vector control be effective. It is advisable to have one employee trained in this area whether or not an exterminator is periodically employed. I suggest a short course in vector control. Such a course is often provided by a local or state health department. I further suggest that you call your health department and seek their assistance in training a staff member.

## LAUNDRY AND HANDLING LINEN

Health hazards may result from the improper handling of contaminated linen. Some basic principles to be followed are: (1) Avoidance of unnecessary agitation of linen that has been soiled. This will help to prevent air contamination. (2) Transportation of dirty linen in closed hampers or bags. (3) Provision of an area for storage of dirty linen or a laundry room. This room or area may also be used for sorting soiled linens. (4) Whenever possible, placing soiled linens in a closed container after sorting and keeping them there until they are put into a washer or sent to a commercial laundry. (5) Prohibiting carts, bags, etc., employed for transportation of dirty linens to be used for clean linens. (6) Provision of separate storage areas for clean linens. These areas should never be used for any other purpose.

Whether you wish to operate your own laundry or use the services of a commercial laundry will depend on local circumstances and the economics involved. The main criterion of a good laundry is the supply of sufficient clean linen at all times.

## HOUSEKEEPING

In a nursing home, housekeeping involves keeping the premises, equipment, and facilities clean and orderly. It has a direct effect on the comfort and morale of the patients as well as on the staff and visitors. Basic determinants of any housekeeping program are: (1) the design and structural characteristics of the building, (2) number and types of patients, (3) medical care offered, and (4) the size and quality of the housekeeping staff. Very few nursing homes are large enough to employ executive or institutional housekeepers. The responsibility of supervising, therefore, falls upon the administrator. Descriptions of the precise methods for the execution of the various tasks are beyond the scope of this chapter. Guidelines for the establishment of work schedules, showing specific tasks for each employee and arranged in successive order for each hour of each day throughout the week, should be developed. Cleaning tasks, plus the use of equipment and supplies employed in their performance, should be *carefully* described. Good cleaning is the first requisite; the second is thorough disinfection. Detergents, disinfectants, and detergent disinfectants are available on the market to facilitate cleaning and disinfection. Dust should be reduced or eliminated because it may be a factor in the spread of pathogenic organisms.

## ACCIDENT PREVENTION

Accident prevention and the promotion of safety consciousness must be emphasized to all employees and residents of the nursing home. A well-planned and well-executed safety program is an essential part of the nursing home operation. For its execution, a sincere interest must be manifested by the administrator and supervisory personnel at all times. Unless the accident problem and types of accidents are thoroughly understood by nursing home personnel, an effective program does not exist. Understanding requires, at least in part, sessions devoted to safety, conducted by trained staff members.

Consultative services and inspections may be available from your insurance company or from the local or state health department.

Remember that the causes of accidents are classified as *environmental* and *human.* Bringing environmental factors under control will not eliminate all accidents. The human factors—sensory, motor, emotional, attitude, age, infirmities, physical condition, and so forth—increase the accident potential in the nursing home.

Accidents may be avoided or reduced in number by many means. Handrails installed along both sides of halls and stairways will help to prevent falls. One-story structures should be provided with ramps for easy access for those using wheelchairs or walkers. There should be sufficient lighting without glare. The use of scatter rugs should be prohibited. All obstacles should be removed from floors, including light cords, ladders, mops, and buckets. Nonskid wax should be used on floors. Washing and mopping should be done along one side of a corridor at a time to allow passage along the side with a dry surface. Grab bars and handrails for tubs, showers, and walls should not only be installed but properly anchored and maintained. Water temperature should be adjusted so that it will be no higher than 120°F. to prevent serious injury by burning (see your state's code). Insensitivity to high temperatures—a characteristic of many elderly or seriously ill patients—could have serious consequences if the water temperature were not controlled.

All staff members should be fully aware that elderly and ill patients need extra assistance to prevent accidents.

Accident reports should be made immediately following an accident. All available information, such as how, where, and why the accident occurred, should be included. Your facility must comply with the Federal Occupational Safety and Health Act of 1971, which specifies the requirements for reporting accidents occurring in a nursing home. All accidents occurring in your facility should be discussed and the causes eliminated as soon as possible to prevent similar accidents in the future.

*Fire safety* must be promoted to prevent injury or loss of life. Every year there are a number of nursing home fires resulting in casualties exceeding those for similar types of institutions such as hospitals, mental institutions, and orphanages. In order to prevent development of the conditions that might result in a fire and to minimize the possibility of death and injury due to fire, four components of fire safety must be recognized. These are: (1) the building, (2) the contents of the building, (3) the people in the building, and (4) provisions for fire detection and control. *No structure can be considered 100 percent fireproof.* Even the most modern nursing home constructed of fire-resistant materials is furnished with some materials that are combustible. In addition, patients, employees, and visitors are wearing clothing that will burn. Linen supplies, food, general supplies, and solid waste are all combustible. *No nursing home is free from fire hazards.* Education of the staff in fire safety is extremely important. A plan must be formulated and every staff member made cognizant of his function if a fire breaks out. Frequent fire drills should be carried out to give every employee an opportunity to fully understand his role (see your state code for the number of drills required).

*A fire safety program is based upon several basic principles:* (1) Prevention of fires through basic cleanliness. (2) Control of cigarette, cigar, and pipe smoking to certain specific areas. (3) Turning in the alarm immediately if fire is detected. (4) Having automatic fire and smoke alarms that are connected directly to the community fire department. (5) When fire occurs, evacuation of patients from the area of immediate danger as soon as possible and further removal as is necessary depending upon the extent of the fire. (6) Isolation of the fire by closing doors and windows. (7) Extinguishing the fire by the use of the proper types of fire extinguishers.

Environmental control in nursing homes involves the control of those factors that may have an effect on the physical, mental, and social well-being of the patients, employees, and visitors. Effort should be concerned not only with the prevention of disease and accidents but also in making the nursing home a cheerful and enjoyable place in which to live, work, and play.

# The Audiologist's Role in a Nursing Home

*Louis M. DiCarlo*

**14** During the last decade the spectacularly incredible progress made in medical science and the development of miracle drugs have lengthened the average life span to such an extent that, in the United States, the geriatric population now numbers approximately 20 million, or 9.9 percent of the entire population. Estimates of the number of persons with bilateral hearing loss approximate 4.5 million of 2.5 percent of our total population. Of this segment, over 55 percent, or 2.5 million, are 65 years of age or older. Approximately 13 percent of this group have bilateral hearing losses of various types and degrees.

The incidence of hearing loss among our senior citizens may be higher than the figures given above if unilateral and nonsignificant hearing losses are computed. On the basis of available statistics, the number of hearing-impaired senior citizens in nursing homes who will require rehabilitative measures exceeds 15 percent, and the number who have unilateral or nonsignificant hearing losses probably adds another 10 percent. All of these individuals will need orientation, understanding, and help in healthy, wholesome management of their hearing problems as well as in their adjustment to the hearing deficit. Traditionally, attention to the needs of individuals with impaired hearing has been restricted to those few who had hearing losses earlier in their life, or who, for various reasons, were still active in their usual occupations.

Many senior citizens are not aware of their hearing difficulties, are confused and bewildered, and attribute their failure to communicate effectively to either ego deficits or the conspiracy of persons and events in their environment. While physiological and psychological research has established reduction of intellectual and sensorineural performance among the aged, to date the results of this research are not conclusive enough to justify the stereotyped profiles of the aged in common traffic.[8] The mythological configuration has evolved from a number of anecdotes and selected cases. Evidence now clearly illustrates that the average aged citizen can continue to lead a meaningful, useful, and creative life. Quality programs of health, education, and welfare are the right of every citizen, especially the aged, for the preservation of integrity and the continuing implementation and utilization of skills. The modern nursing home provides an attractive, well-designed facility, housing both medical and related professional expertise and services, integrated through a unifying principle and devoted to the most effective rehabilitation of aged individuals.

## EFFECTS OF AGING AND OF HEARING LOSS

Physiological and psychological research reveal that passage of time induces sensory and motor changes. These changes not only influence perceptual alterations, but also may generate serious, even destructive, behavioral problems related to distorted perception and incorrect interpretation of events. Physiological research demonstrates actual cell-tissue loss with advancing age. Vision, hearing, and tactile and proprioceptive sensitivity reflect reduced reaction time as well as modified response content. Vision and hearing systems—the information receiving stations—function with varying degrees of inefficacy. Of the two systems, the hearing modality provides the complex arterial network and operations for the development, perpetuation, and execution of those communication skills necessary for the interaction of individuals and groups with each other to permit expression of needs, to provide for thoughtful processes vital in the solution of problems, and to supply the necessary means for dealing with the environment. The hearing mechanism often acts as a barometer of an individual's well-being.

While no unifying, single explanatory principle that delineates the relationship between hearing changes and decrements in physiological, psychological, and social behavior has been formulated, nevertheless considerable evidence is available suggesting that such alterations can be devastating and catastrophic.[1,5,7]

Of the many impairments that afflict the aged population, few can scar the personality with greater unhappiness, cause more real tragedy, and culminate in more maladjustment than hearing impairment. Unless the aged citizen is guided into a program of rehabilitation activities and emotional security, bewilderment, intellectual disillusionment, and emotional frustrations may corrode the core of his behavior. The world of reality is gradually perceived beyond his efforts. People and events lurk with many fancied harms; isolated ideas crystallize to the extent that the individual builds a superstructure to justify his failure. His own inadequacies find expression in patterns of withdrawal and isolation. Because he does not hear, he fails to understand and interpret events around him, leading to inadequate personal reactions. Although hearing loss is not the causal factor, it is, nevertheless, a powerful ingredient in the development of paranoid tendencies and anxieties.

The maximum employment of auditory skills depends upon the attentive process and represents the consummation of the interpretive process. Bocca and Calearo[2] have demonstrated that aged individuals with normal or near-normal auditory sensitivity thresholds manifest serious decoding (understanding) disturbances at the central levels. These people claim that they hear, but they experience severe interpretation difficulties. They are unable to discriminate between phonetic contours. Moreover, attempts to amplify speech often result in discomfort, which the listeners are unable to tolerate, without improving discrimination.

Another very difficult task for the aged is listening to speech signals in a noisy environment. Although it is true that speech is quite resistant to noise levels, for these individuals the noisy background interferes with their ability to hear speech, because noise contaminates and distorts the speech signals.[4] The senior citizen cannot extricate meaning from this combination of speech and noise. The task becomes severely fatiguing so that the individual stops trying to understand, consequently aggravating his frustrations and anxiety.

## CAUSES OF HEARING LOSS

Although presbycusis (hearing loss accompanying old age) is a major causal factor for hearing impairment among the older age groups,[6] other variables are also operative. Some individuals will have hearing losses due to otosclerosis (bony accumulations in the middle ear and cochlea) with marked nerve degeneration. Some will have reduced hearing as a result of otitis media (middle-ear disease). Many elderly individuals have hearing losses due to continuous exposure to excessive noise levels during their working years. A number have pathological retrocochlear disturbances (diseases behind the inner ear involving the nervous system, including brain disturbances) due to acoustic tumors, vestibular (balance) disorders, or anomalies of the brain stem or the brain itself.

Disturbances due to central nervous system conditions, such as retrocochlear lesions, require extensive and meticulous diagnostic procedures that the audiologist employs in cooperation with the otologist and neurologist. Some of these subjects will require medical attention.

## PROGRAMS AND THERAPY

In devising rehabilitation measures for elderly individuals with hearing loss the audiologist effects experiences providing for expression of interests, the adjustments of aspirational levels with capacities planned to permit these individuals to develop realistic self-appraisals so that they can move confidently in their environment. The audiologist's rehabilitation program should embrace means leading to the development of a consciousness of the operative process of social living, helping the aged individual to see his needs clearly and to continue to derive satisfaction from daily living. Without proper guidance, hearing impairment may impose serious restrictions in communications, and, as a consequence, may progress imperceptibly toward total isolation. It is the responsibility of the audiologist to teach the individual avenues of communication leading to optimal operative interactive levels.

## Tests

The audiologist's test battery will permit him to make a proper assessment of the individual's total auditory function. The tests include air- and bone-conduction audiometric configurations, speech reception, discrimination measures, the SISI (short increment sensitivity index), and other tests for recruitment (exaggerated loudness sensation), tone decay, Bekesy test, filtered speech (certain frequencies deleted) test, EDR (electrodermal audiometry, psychogalvanic skin resistance audiometry), EAR (electroencephagraphic auditory response), and typonametry (measures of impedance [resistance] and compliance [elasticity of system]). He will employ other tests deemed necessary, not only for aid in diagnosis, but also for guidance in the preparation for training. He will also provide a time table for testing batteries.

The audiometric configurations provide only a crude index of auditory function at the most primitive level, which represents detection at the peripheral level. Although a wealth of information may be deduced from the audiogram, certain relationships that are valid for a younger population do not correlate significantly in an aged sample. The possession of a threshold of near-functional detection does not guarantee that the auditory processes are intact. The evaluation of the auditory skills involves appraisals of auditory recognition (recognizing gross characteristics of auditory stimuli, e.g., speech as speech without necessarily understanding it), auditory memory span (the ability to carry forward material at the unaware and automatic level for immediate or future use), auditory recall (the ability to remember and reproduce previous auditory stimuli in the absence of such stimuli), auditory synthesis (the ability to be able to construct total meaning of auditory signals in the absence of a number of them because the ear did not hear them), and the ability to capitalize on cue-reduced stimuli (construction of a whole pattern on the basis of one or two elements).

Physiologically and psychologically, hearing remains a relative mode of human response. Individuals with exactly similar hearing configurations vary markedly in their hearing interactions. *On the basis of the test results, the audiologist classifies the audiometric configurations, etiologic background, and extent of hearing loss, as well as personality, intelligence, and other factors, for construction of rehabilitation programs designed to respect the elderly citizen's integrity and involve him in active participation of everyday living.*

## Hearing Aids

Because of the problems involved with amplification, the selection of a proper hearing aid requires testing, trial, and re-evaluation. The hearing aid selection mandates counseling through the entire process. The audiologist will explain the nature and the function of the auditory mechanism in order to provide the individual with a perspective and relate his hearing loss to auditory response. In selection of the hearing aid the problems of gain, output, and type of amplification must be considered. The instrument chosen should not be too difficult to manipulate and should provide its user with hearing gain without discomfort. Binaural hearing amplification (amplification into both ears simultaneously—hearing aid for each ear) may be investigated.

The question of selective amplification will be determined on the basis of test results. Present-day hearing aids not only provide safeguards through gauging, tracking, and limiting impression devices, but also extend the frequency range so that speech may have better quality of voice perception, naturalness in terms of fidelity of reproduction, and quietness as against the concept of blurred speech reception.

Hearing perception of the hearing-handicapped senior citizen may be improved by auditory training. The training must proceed within the framework of the different variables involving loudness perception, discrimination, and tolerance conditions. The first objectives in selection of a hearing aid are to bring to the listener sounds for interpretation and to permit him to discriminate between different phonetic contours.

Periodic otological and audiological reassessment should be a continuous process. The audiologist will test the hearing aid periodically. If examination of the instrument shows deterioration, he will suggest either repair or replacement.

## Lip Reading

Unlike the young, the senior citizen usually has developed linguistic competency. He has a satisfactory vocabulary and is adept at putting words together properly. For the young, lip-reading functions as a vehicle for vocabulary and its effective use. It is an activity that favors early acquisition. Nevertheless, the hearing-handicapped aged individual may be forced to acquire information and consummate communication through more than one modality. Even though modern hearing aids possess high gains and output levels, they cannot be expected to serve as completely adequate substitutes for hearing. As already indicated, amplification may prove insufficient or too difficult for the senior citizen to handle. Making sounds louder does not improve his understanding. The audiologist will program lip-reading experiences to supplement rather than substitute for the hearing impediment. Lip reading will assist in sustaining attention since the individual must give strict attention in attempting to understand thought by this means. It also inculcates a sense of achievement.

The audiologist may design his lip-reading lessons on the basis of actual experience. He may provide instruction on a one-to-one stage until the lipreader attains sufficient proficiency to enter group sessions. In group settings, lip reading acquires a social value and individuals participating in these experiences will appreciate the fact that they are not alone with their handicap. Lip reading as an activity can involve active participation of a group in sharing experiences leading to concentrated attention and dynamic motivation. Because sounds that are hard to hear are easy to "see" and those sounds hard to "see" are easy to hear, lip reading combined with the employment of a hearing aid permits the aged to greater and more efficient understanding of speech and language.

**Auditory Training**
In the beginning of auditory training, after the hearing aid has been selected but not used, the individual with hearing loss should be exposed to all aspects of natural and pleasurable auditory stimuli. This should initiate the first step in the building of a sound consciousness if the individual's auditory discrimination has deteriorated. In the early stages of training, the individual should learn to listen to sounds as natural phenomena. If the material is appropriate, interesting, and meets the person's needs at different levels, sound anticipation, sound curiosity, and the ability to associate sound impressions with sound memories, including the association of experience with auditory stimuli, will be developed.

Adequate auditory training must always be based on learning principles. Motivation must be generated through pleasant experiences and reinforced through repetition—but repetition that involves expressing the thought a different way, providing additional clues, and, if necessary, employing another modality such as writing. Sound presented simultaneously requiring responses will set up patterns of sensory and motor associations that may result in closure for the listener so that he later responds to partial stimuli to replicate the total situation. In listening to music dramatizing a story, the listener first learns the story through attention to the total music pattern. Later on, specific steps in the music will permit him to reconstruct the story.

The next phase in auditory training deals with sound as part of a larger whole. In this phase the individual learns to attribute meaningful values to auditory stimuli. Sounds now are incorporated into his experience and different aspects of meaning will be presented by different dimensions of acoustic frequencies. Work with all auditory stimuli progresses, but emphasis begins moving toward the development of discrimination and identification of speech sounds per se. First, identification and recognition are developed. These aspects are refined as the individual continues training to discriminate between speech sounds, learning contrasts, and detecting similarities in the speech spectra. Work in this phase also is devoted to accent, detection of rhythm patterns, and discrimination between inflection and intensity.

A third and final phase concerns itself with training the individual to listen to speech and other sounds of communication and adjustment stimuli. The aged citizen who will learn to pick out conversation from background and to recognize the meaning of different background sounds in adjusting to his environment. The material will contain speech and other sounds, such as automobile horns, or sirens denoting a speeding fire engine, ambulance, or police vehicle.

A systematic program of auditory training promotes the development of consciousness of sounds present in natural experiences. Auditory training, as does speech and communication training, demands systematic and continuous activity without a hearing aid in the first phase. Hearing and listening are continuous activities during an individual's life. Auditory training, when provided in a meaningful and purposeful manner, will give opportunity for reinforcement and moves toward the implementation of activity in the individual's daily affairs. Only by ensuring continuity and transfer through the utilization of community, group, and individual facilities will the senior citizen develop an attitude, as well as a will, to hear.

The hearing aid is introduced *after* a period of auditory training in order to minimize the danger of acoustic trauma. Increased loudness may introduce distortion of the stimulus as well as discomfort. A well-controlled auditory training program prevents injury and hearing-aid loss resulting from exposure to auditory stimuli. It is recognized that more powerful hearing aids may provide better speech reception if the user's tolerance is raised and his discrimination improved. These objectives are achieved through careful, graduated steps. The first instructions should be presented in a quiet environment to eliminate any distracting stimuli.

A portable hearing aid with individual outlets for ear phones and built-in microphones is useful for training prior to employment of individual hearing aids. The volume control can be situated so that each listener can manipulate it according to his tolerance and discrimination needs.

Outside of the training sessions, through the use of various devices, the elderly may become involved in listening and communication activities. Amplication systems in lecture halls, churches, and other public buildings will permit listening experiences. Signals channeled through an amplifier leading to individually constructed ear inserts allow persons with hearing loss to enjoy television without need of excessive volume. Amplifiers are available for telephones, permitting the person with hearing loss to use the telephone as a means of communication.

If listening has become a pleasant experience for the elderly with hearing loss, transition from the voice to hearing aid should prove to be an easy one since his attitude will be one of wholehearted acceptance of the instrument.

The employment of vision and hearing will consummate the natural integrative relationship between these faculties terminating in the unification of sense responses. The proper employment of vision and hearing permits the person with hearing loss to use his skills with satisfaction and may expedite personality adjustment. Successful use of the hearing aid with simultaneous lip reading adds to the well-being of the elderly by uniting him with his environment and thereby providing him with the indispensible tools for emotional involvement, communication, and integration.

Considerable research now supports the point of view that auditory training, the use of hearing aids, and lip reading contribute not only to the improvement of auditory skills and communication but also in a more satisfactory overall communication performance.[3]

## THE AUDIOLOGIST AS A MEMBER OF THE NURSING HOME TEAM

The cost of administering a program of hearing rehabilitation for the elderly resident of the nursing home is negligible in terms of the total budget. However, in terms of salvaging human self-esteem the program is invaluable. The audiologist plays an important role in the rehabilitation of the elderly with hearing loss. He can prevent deterioration in performance and regression to nonadjustive or maladjustive behavior. He will instruct the members of the different specialties in how to handle the individual with hearing loss in consummating communication. More important, he will alert other members of the team in the prevention of rejection which may prove detrimental to behavior. He will provide extra means of communication to individuals with impaired hearing and will lead them to healthy and worthwhile adjustment. Total health planning and rehabilitation of persons with auditory impairment who reside in a nursing home become effective when all resources—health, education, and welfare—participate in and contribute to the program.

## REFERENCES

1. Birren, J. E., *et. al.* 1963. Human aging: A biological and behavioral study. U.S. Government Printing Office, Washington, D.C.
2. Bocca, E., and C. Calearo. 1956. Aspects of auditory pathology of central origin in aged subjects. Annals of Otolaryngology 55:365—369.
3. DiCarlo, L. M. 1964. The deaf. Prentice-Hall, Englewood Cliffs, N.J.
4. DiCarlo, L. M., and H. Taub. 1972. The influence of compression and expansion on the intelligibility of speech by young and aged aphasics. Journal of Communication Disorders. 5:299—306.

5. International research and education in social gerontology: Goals and strategies. 1972. The Gerontologist. 12:2, Part II.
6. Lindén, G. 1968. Geriatric-audiological problems in modern society. *In* Lindén, G., ed. Almquist and Wiksell, Stockholm.
7. Schaie, K. W. 1968. Theory and methods of research on aging. Virginia University Press, Morgantown, W. Va.
8. Telford, C. W., and J. M. Sawrey. 1972. The exceptional individual. pp. 503-532, Prentice-Hall, Englewood Cliffs, N.J.

# Comprehensive Library Resource Selections for Nursing Home Administrators and Long-term Care Educators

*Norma Wasmuth*

## ADMINISTRATION

A Guide to Medical Care Administration. Medical Care Appraisal—Quality and Utilization. Vol. 1. Washington, D.C.: The American Public Health Association, 1965.

A Guide to Medical Care Administration. Vol. 2. Washington, D.C.: The American Public Health Association, 1965.

Alexander, E. Nursing Administration in the Hospital Health Care System. St. Louis: C. V. Mosby, 1972.

Argyris, C. Diagnosing Human Relations in Organizations: A Case Study of a Hospital. New Haven, Conn.: Yale University Labor and Management Center, 1956.

Argyris, C. Interpersonal Competence and Organizational Effectiveness. Homewood, Ill.: Dorsey-Irwin, 1962.

Arnold, M. Administering Health Systems: Issues and Perspectives. Chicago: Aldine-Atherton, 1971.

Aurner, R. Effective Communication in Business. Cincinnati: South-Western, 1967.

Barnard, C. I. The Functions of the Executive. Cambridge: Harvard University Press, 1968.

Barnard, C. I. Organization and Management. Cambridge: Harvard University Press, 1969.

Blau, P. The Dynamics of Bureaucracy. Chicago: University of Chicago Press, 1955.

Bowers, R. Studies in Behavior in Organizations. Athens, Ga.: University of Georgia Press, 1966.

Buckley, W. F. Sociology and Modern Systems Theory. Englewood Cliffs, N.J.: Prentice-Hall, 1967.

Buckley, W. F. Modern Systems Theory for the Behavior Scientist. Chicago: Aldine, 1968.

Burby, R. Communicating with People: The Supervisor's Introduction to

Verbal Communication and Decision Making. Addison-Wesley Series in Supervisory Training. Reading, Mass.: Addison-Wesley, 1970.

Chapple, E. D., and Sayles, L. The Measure of Management. New York: Macmillan, 1961.

Demone, H. W., Jr., and Harshbarger, D. Handbook of Human Service Organizations. New York: Behavioral Publications, 1973.

Dimock, M. D., and Dimock, G. O. Public Administration. 4th Ed. New York: Holt, Rinehart & Winston, 1969.

Drucker, P. F. The Effective Executive. 1st Ed. New York: Harper & Row, 1967.

Drucker, P. F. The Age of Discontinuity. New York: Harper & Row, 1968.

Durbin, R. L., and Springall, W. H. Organization and Administration of Health Care; Theory, Practice and Environment. St. Louis: C. V. Mosley, 1969.

Dyer, F. C. Executive Guide to Handling People. Englewood Cliffs, N.J.: Prentice-Hall, 1958.

Etzioni, A. The Comparative Analysis of Complex Organizations. New York: The Free Press, 1961.

Famularo, J. Organization Planning Manual. New York: The American Management Association, 1971.

Filley, A. Managerial Process and Organizational Behavior. Oakland, N. J.: Scott, Foresman & Co., 1969.

Garrett, A. Interviewing—Its Principles and Methods. New York: Family Welfare Association of America—Henry Bonnell Fund, 1970.

Georogopoulas, B. S. (ed.). Organization Research on Health Institutions. Arbor, Mich.: University of Michigan Press, 1972.

Gray, G. W., and Braden, W. W. Public Speaking: Principles and Practices. 2nd Ed. New York: Harper & Row, 1963.

Greenblatt, M., Sharaf, M., and Stone, E. Dynamics of Institutional Change. Pittsburgh: University of Pittsburgh Press, 1971.

Griffiths, D. E. Administrative Theory. New York: Appleton-Century-Crofts, 1959.

Gunning, R. Technique of Clear Writing. Revised Ed. New York: McGraw Hill, 1968.

Hage, J., and Aiken, M. Social Change in Complex Organizations. New York: Random House, 1970.

Hardwick, C. Administrative Strategy and Decision Making. Cincinnati: South-Western, 1966.

Hodgkinson, H. Institutions in Transition. New York: McGraw-Hill, 1971.

Hodnett, E. Effective Presentation: How to Present Facts, Figures and Ideas Successfully. New York: Parker, 1967.

Homans, G. The Human Group. New York: Harcourt Brace & World, 1950.

Johns, R. Executive Responsibility. New York: Association Press, 1966.

Katz, D. The Social Psychology of Organizations. New York: John Wiley & Sons, 1966.

Lawrence, P. R. Organization and Environment. Boston: Division of Research, Harvard Business School, 1967.

Learned, E. P., and Ulrich, D. R. Executive Action. Cambridge: Harvard University Graduate School of Business Administration, 1950.

Lee, S. M. Goal Programming for Decision Analysis. Philadelphia: Auerbach Publishers, 1972.

Levinson, H. Exceptional Executive: A Psychological Conception. Cambridge: Harvard University Press, 1968.

Levy, S., and Loomba, N. P. Health Care Administration. Philadelphia: J. B. Lippincott, 1972.

Likert, R. New Patterns of Management. McGraw-Hill, 1961.

Mace, M. The Growth and Development of Executives. Cambridge: Harvard University Graduate School of Business Administration, 1950.

Mace, M. L. Directors: Myth and Reality. Boston: Division of Graduate School of Business Administration, Harvard Business School, 1971.

Managing in Times of Radical Change. New York: The American Management Association, 1971.

March, J. Handbook on Organizations. Chicago: Rand McNally, 1965.

Moss, A., et al. Hospital Policy Decisions: Process and Action. New York: G. P. Putnam's Sons, 1966.

Performance Evaluation: A Manual of Procedures for Association Executives' Self-Evaluation. Washington, D.C.: The American Society of Association Executives, 1970.

Rutstein, D. D. The Coming Revolution in Medicine. Cambridge: M.I.T. Press, 1967.

Sayles, L. R. Human Behavior in Organizations. Englewood Cliffs, N.J.: Prentice-Hall, 1966.

Seashore, S. R. Assessing Organization Performance. Ann Arbor, Mich.: The Foundation for Research on Human Behavior, 1964.

Simon, H. Administrative Behavior: A Study of Decision-Making Processes in Administrative Organizations. 2nd Ed. New York: Macmillan, 1957.

Task Force on Organization of Community Health Services. Health Administration and Organization in the Decade Ahead. Washington, D.C.: The American Public Health Association, 1967.

The Development of Executive Talent. New York: The American Management Association, 1971.

Thompson, J. D. Organizations in Action: Social Science Basis of Administrative Theory. New York: McGraw-Hill, 1967.

Thompson, V. A. Modern Organization. New York: Alfred A. Knopf, 1961.

Townsend, R. Up the Organization: How to Stop the Corporation from Stifling People and Strangling Profits. New York: Alfred A. Knopf, 1970.

Trecker, H. Social Work Administration: Principles and Practices. New York: Association Press, 1971.

Uris, A. Mastery of Management: How to Avoid Obolescence by Preparing for Tomorrow's Management Today. Homewood, Ill.: Dow Jones-Irwin, 1968.

Vanderbilt Sociology Conference. Power in Organizations. Nashville: Vanderbilt University Press, 1970.

Wallace, S. E. Total Institutions. Chicago: Aldine-Atherton, 1971.

Wasmuth, W. and de Lodzia, G. Dynamics of Supervision: Organizational Cases and Intrigues. Columbus, Ohio: Grid, Inc., 1974.

Work in America. Report of a Special Task Force to the Secretary of Health, Education and Welfare. Cambridge: M.I.T. Press, 1973.

## ADMINISTRATION, HOSPITAL

Boston Model City Health Information System Project: Final Report. Cambridge: Massachusetts Institute of Technology, 1971.

Burling, T. The Give and Take in Hospitals: A Study of Human Organization in Hospitals. New York: G. P. Putnam's Sons, 1956.

Coe, R. Planned Change in the Hospital: Case Studies of Organizational Innovations. New York: Praeger, 1970.

Commission of Professional and Hospital Activities. Length of Stay in PAS Hospitals. Ann Arbor, Mich.: The Commission of Professional and Hospital Activities, 1971.

Crul, J. F. Patient Monitoring. Baltimore: Williams & Wilkins, 1970.

Duke University, Graduate Program in Hospital Administration. The Changing Composition of the Hospital System. Durham, N.C.: Duke University Press, 1971.

Essentials of Social Work Programs in Hospitals. Chicago: The American Hospital Association, 1971.

Gilpatrick, E. Occupational Structure of New York City Municipal Hospitals. New York: Frederick A. Praeger, 1970.

Ginzberg, E., and Rogatz, P. Planning for Better Hospital Care. New York: Columbia University Press, 1961.

Greenberg, S. Quality of Mercy: A Report on the Critical Condition of Hospital and Medical Care in the U.S. New York: Atheneum, 1971.

Greenblatt, M. Dynamics of Institutional Change: The Hospital in Transition. Pittsburgh: University of Pittsburgh Press, 1971.

Hamilton, J. A. Decision Making in Hospital Administration and Medical Care: A Casebook. Minneapolis: University of Minnesota Press, 1960.

Jackson, L. G. Hospital and Community. New York: Macmillan, 1964.

Knowles, J. H. Hospitals, Doctors and the Public Interest. Cambridge: Harvard University Press, 1965.

Knowles, J. H. The Teaching Hospital: Evolution and Contemporary Issues. Cambridge: Harvard University Press, 1966.

Larrabee, E. The Benevolent and Necessary Institution: The New York Hospital, 1771–1971. Garden City, N.Y.: Doubleday, 1971.

Letourneau, C. Hospital Administrator. Chicago: Starling Publications, 1969.

McGibony, J. R. Principles of Hospital Administration. 2nd Ed. New York: G. P. Putnam's Sons, 1969.

Neuhauser, D. Relationship between Administration, Activities and Hospital Performance. Chicago: University of Chicago Press, 1971.

Policy Statement on Provision of Health Services. Chicago: The American Hospital Association, 1971.

Public Control of Hospital Operations. Chicago: The Center for Health Administration Studies, 1972.

Rakich, J. S., (ed.). Hospital Organization and Management, A Book of Readings. St. Louis: The Catholic Hospital Association, 1972.

Rowland, V. Evaluating and Improving Managerial Performance. New York: McGraw-Hill, 1970.

Sloane, R. A Guide to Health Facilities—Personnel and Management. St. Louis: C. V. Mosby, 1971.

Study of For-Profit Hospital Chains. Chicago: The American Hospital Association, 1970.

Taylor, C. In Horizontal Orbit: Hospitals and the Cult of Efficiency. New York: Holt, Rinehart & Winston, 1970.

Trussell, R. E. Hunterdon Medical Center. Cambridge: Harvard University Press, 1956.

Willard, H. N., and Kasl, S. V. Continuing Care in a Community Hospital. Cambridge: Harvard University Press, 1973.

## Accreditation

Accreditation Council for Psychiatric Facilities. Accreditation Manual for Psychiatric Facilities. Chicago: The Commission on Accreditation of Hospitals, 1972.

Accreditation Manual for Hospitals; Hospital Accreditation Program. Chicago: The Joint Commission on Accreditation of Hospitals, 1970.

Footnotes to the Accreditation Manual for Hospitals. Chicago: The Joint Commission on Accreditation of Hospitals, 1971.

Hershey, N., and Wheeler, W. Health Personnel, Regulation in the Public Interest: Questions and Answers on Institutional Licensure. Sacramento, Cal.: The California Hospital Association, 1973.

National Forum on Hospital and Health Affairs. Changing Composition of the Hospital System. Durham, N.C.: Duke University Press, 1969.

Standards for Residential Facilities for Mentally Retarded. Chicago: The Joint Commission on Accreditation of Hospitals, 1971.

Standards Manual for Rehabilitation Facilities. Chicago: The Commission on Accreditation of Rehabilitation Facilities, 1971.

U.S. National Institutes of Health. Accreditation and Certification in Relation to Allied Health Manpower. Washington, D.C.: U.S. Government Printing Office, 1971.

## Admitting and Discharge

Murnaghan, J. Hospital Discharge Data: Report of the Conference on Hospital Discharge Abstracts Systems. Philadelphia: J. B. Lippincott, 1970.

The Admitting System: A Special Study in Hospital Systems and Procedures. New York: United Hospital Fund of New York—Training, Research, and Special Studies Division, 1965.

## Automation in Medical Care

DeLand, E. C. Review of Hospital Information Systems. Springfield, Va.: National Technical Information Service, U.S. Department of Commerce, 1970.

Feasibility of a Shared Computer Facility. Bryn Mawr, Pa.: Bryn Mawr Hospital, 1967.

Gabrieli, E. R. Computerization of Clinical Records. New York: Grune & Stratton, 1970.

Mason, E. E., and Bulgren, W. C. Computer Applications in Medicine. Springfield, Ill.: Charles C Thomas, 1964.

Myers, C. Computers in Knowledge-Based Fields. Cambridge: Massachusetts Institute of Technology, 1970.

Provisional Guidelines for Automated Multiphasic Health Testing Services. Rockville, Md.: U.S. Public Health Service, 1970.

Springer, E. Automated Medical Records and the Law. Pittsburgh: Health Law Center, 1971.

Yarnell, S. Acquisition of the Patient Database: A Review of Design Approaches, Performance and Cost of Fifty-five Different Systems. Seattle: Medical Computer Services, 1971.

## Fund Raising

Commission on Foundations and Private Philanthropy. Foundations, Private Giving and Public Policy. Chicago: University of Chicago Press, 1970.

Coulden, J. The Money Givers. New York: Random House, 1971.

Dermer, J. How to Write Successful Foundation Presentations. New York: The Center, 1970.

Haney Associates, Inc. The Health Funds Directory. New York: The Health Funds Institute, 1970.

Projections for the Seventies: A Portrait of American Economy in 1975 and New Challenges and Promises for Fund Raising. New York: The United Community Funds and Councils of America, 1967.

Seymour, H. J. Designs for Fund Raising: Principles, Patterns, Techniques. New York: McGraw-Hill, 1966.

Viewpoints on State and Local Legislation Regulating Solicitation of Funds from the Public. New York: The National Health Council, 1971.

## Governing Board and Trustees

McGibony, J. R. Handbook for Hospital Trustees: A Guide to Service. College Park, Md.: Hospital Publications, 1965.

Statement on the Governing Board and Planning. Chicago: The American Hospital Association, 1970.

Trecker, H. Citizen Boards at Work: New Challenges to Effective Action. New York: Association Press, 1970.

## Medical Administration and Records

Aspen Systems Corporation. Automated Medical Records and the Law. Pittsburgh: Health Law Center, 1971.

Automated Medical Records and the Law. Pittsburgh: Health Law Center, 1971.

Gabrielli, E. R. Computerization of Clinical Records. New York: Grune & Stratton, 1970.

Hayt, E. Legal Aspects of Medical Records. Berwyn, Ill.: Physician's Record Co., 1964.

Keller, D. Psychiatric Record Manual for the Hospital. Pittsburgh: University of Pittsburgh, 1970.

McNabb, B. W. Medical Record Procedures in Small Hospitals. Austin, Tex.: Stick-Warlick Co., 1970.

Psychiatric Patient Records. Washington, D.C.: The American Psychiatric Association, 1971.

Weed, L. L. Medical Records, Medical Education and Patient Care. Chicago: Year Book, 1970.

## Medical Staff

Blumberg, M. S. Trends and Projections of Physicians in the United States. Berkeley, Cal.: Carnegie Commission on Higher Education, 1971.

Duffy, J. C. Emotional Issues in the Lives of Physicians. Springfield, Ill.: Charles C Thomas, 1971.

Eisele, W. The Medical Staff in the Modern Hospital. New York: McGraw-Hill, 1967.

Foreign Medical Graduates in the U.S., 1970. Chicago: The American Hospital Association, 1971.

Friedson, E., and Lorber, J. (eds.). Medical Men and Their Work. Chicago: Aldine-Atherton, 1972.

Geyman, J. P. The Modern Family Doctor and Changing Medical Practice. New York: Appleton-Century-Crofts, 1971.

Gibson, R. N. Studies in Hospital Administration—The Decline of the G.P.: Reasons and Ramifications. Chicago: Center for Health Administration Studies, 1969.

Margulies, H., and Bloch, L. Foreign Medical Graduates in the United States. Cambridge: Harvard University Press, 1969.

Marks, G. Women in White. New York: Charles Scribner's Sons, 1972.

McCleery, R. S. One Life—One Physician: An Inquiry into the Medical Profession's Performance in Self-Regulation. A Report to the Center for Study of Responsive Law. Washington, D.C.: Public Affairs Press, 1971.

Peer Review Manual. Chicago: The American Hospital Association, 1971.

Roemer, M. Doctors in Hospitals: Medical Staff. Baltimore: The Johns Hopkins University Press, 1971.

Schein, C. J. A Surgeon Answers. New York: G. P. Putnam's Sons, 1973.

Statement on the Physician and Planning. Chicago: The American Hospital Association, 1970.

Wilson, D. Lone Woman: The Story of Elizabeth Blackwell, The First Woman Doctor. Boston: Little, Brown, 1970.

## Personnel Administration

Bailey, N. Hospital Personnel Administration. 2nd Ed. Berwyn, Ill.: Physician's Record, 1959.

Developing Personnel. Washington, D.C.: Leadership Resources, Inc., 1968.

Executive Compensation. New York: The Research Institute of America, 1971.

Gilpatrick E. G., and Corliss, P. K. The Occupational Structure of N.Y. City Municipal Hospitals. New York: Frederick A. Praeger, 1970.

Hepner, J. O., Boyer, J. M., and Westerhaus, C. Personnel Administration and Labor Relations in Health Care Facilities. St. Louis: C. V. Mosby, 1969.

Improving Employee-Management Communication Hospitals: A Special Study in Management Practices and Problems. New York: The United Hospital Fund of New York, 1965.

Managing Programs to Employ the Disadvantaged. New York: The National Industrial Corp. Conference Board, 1970.

Manpower Planning: Evolving Systems by Walter S. Wikstrom. New York: National Industrial Corp. Conference Board, Inc., 1971.

New Direction for Wisconsin Inactive Health Personnel. Madison, Wisc: Department of Nursing, Health Sciences Unit, Wisconsin University, 1969.

Otto, C. P., and Glaser, R. O. Management of Training: A Handbook for Training and Development Personnel. Reading, Mass.: Addison-Wesley, 1970.

Salaries and Related Personnel Practices of Voluntary Social and Health Agencies in New York City. New York: The Community Council of Greater New York, 1970.

Salary Ranges of Personnel Employed in State Mental Hospitals and Community Mental Health Centers. Washington, D.C.: The Joint Information Service of the American Psychiatric Association, 1970.

Schifferes, J. J. Healthier Living: A College Text with Readings in Personnel and Environmental Health. 3rd Ed. New York: John Wiley & Sons, 1970.
Selected Training Programs for Physician Support Personnel. Bethesda, Md.: National Institutes of Health, 1970.
The Personnel Man and His Job. Chicago: The American Medical Association, 1971.
U.S. Employment Service. Dictionary of Occupational Titles. Vol. 1. 3rd Ed. Washington, D.C.: U.S. Government Printing Office, 1965.
U.S. Training and Employment Service. Job Descriptions and Organizational Analysis For Hospitals and Related Health Services. Washington, D.C.: U.S. Government Printing Office, 1970.
Wilbur, M. B. Educational Tools for Health Personnel. New York: Macmillan, 1968.

## Planning and Design

Application of Principles of Systems Integration to Design of the "Nursing Tower" Portion of a V.A. Hospital Facility. Washington, D.C.: The U.S. Veterans Administration, 1971.
Barton, A. Communities in Disaster: A Sociological Analysis of Collective Stress Situations. Garden City, N.Y.: Doubleday, 1969.
Gainsborough, H. Principles of Hospital Design. London: Architectural Press, 1964.
Garb, S. Disaster Handbook. New York: Springer, 1969.
Halse, A. O. Use of Color in Interiors. New York: McGraw-Hill, 1968.
Levine, R. The Coupled Pan Space Frame—An Integrated Building System for Hospitals and Other Complex Buildings. Flushing, N.Y.: Xpress, 1971.
Methods of Compensation for Architectural Services. Washington, D.C.: The American Institute of Architects, 1970.
Nellist, I. Planning Buildings for Handicapped Children. Springfield, Ill.: Charles C Thomas, 1970.
Rosenfield, I. Hospital Architecture: Integrated Components. New York: Van Nostrand Reinhold, 1971.
Study of Health Facilities Construction Costs; Report to Congress by Comptroller of U.S. (5 parts.) Washington, D.C.: U.S. General Accounting Office, 1972.
U.S. General Services Administration. Guide for Space Planning and Layout. Washington, D.C.: U.S. Government Printing Office, 1970.
Wheeler, E. Hospital Design and Function. New York: McGraw-Hill, 1964.

## Public Relations

American Society for Hospital Public Relations Directors. Public Relations Essays in Hospital Labor Situations. Chicago: The American Hospital Association, 1972.
Cutlip, S. Effective Public Relations. Englewood Cliffs, N.J.: Prentice-Hall, 1971.
Freidson, E. Patients' Views of Medical Practice. New York: Russell Sage Foundation, 1961.
Hochderffer, J. G. Hospital PR—by Objectives. Fort Wayne, Ind: Public Relations Department, Fort Wayne Hospital, 1971.

## CAREERS

Can They Be Salvaged? A Report of the Health Careers Project. Providence, R.I.: The Rhode Island Council of Community Service, 1970.

Ginzberg, E. Career Guidance: Who Needs It, Who Provides It, Who Can Improve It. New York: McGraw-Hill, 1971.

Hicks, F. New Careers: The Community/Home Health Aide Trainee's Manual. Washington, D.C.: Human Service Press, 1968.

Kirk, W. R. Your Future in Hospital Work. New York: Arco Publ. Co., 1971.

Odgers, R., and Wenberg, B. Introduction to Health Professions. St. Louis: C. V. Mosby, 1971.

Odom, F. Opportunities in Environmental Careers. New York: Vocational Guidance Manuals, 1971.

" . . . People Serving People . . ." Washington, D.C.: U.S. Department of Health, Education, and Welfare, 1970.

Riessman, F. Up from Poverty: New Career Ladders for Non-Professionals. New York: Harper & Row, 1968.

Shatz, E. New Careers: Generic Issues in the Human Services. Washington, D.C.: National Institute for New Careers, 1970.

Zaleznik, D. Orientation and Conflict in Career. Cambridge: Harvard Business School, 1970.

### Dental Health

Brandhorst, O. The American College of Dentists: Its History, Organization, Objectives and How it Functions. Bethesda, Md.: The American College of Dentists, 1970.

Cinotti, W. et al. Applied Psychology in Dentistry. St. Louis: C. V. Mosby, 1964.

Douglas, B. Introduction to Hospital Dentistry. St. Louis: C. V. Mosby, 1970.

Hooley, J. R. Hospital Dental Service. Philadelphia: Lea & Febiger, 1970.

Pelton, D. The Epidemiology of Oral Health. Washington, D.C.: The American Public Health Association, 1969.

## EDUCATION AND TRAINING

A Handbook for Health Care Institutions. Chicago: The Hospital Research and Educational Trust, 1970.

American Association of Junior Colleges. Allied Health Education Programs in Junior Colleges—1970. Bethesda, Md.: National Institutes of Health, 1972.

Anlyan, W. G., et al. The Future of Medical Education. Durham, N.C.: Duke University Press, 1973.

Babbie, E. Science and Morality in Medicine: A Survey of Medical Educators. Berkeley, Cal.: University of California Press, 1970.

Callaghan, D. F. Graduate Education for Hospital and Health Services Administration: A Pattern for the Future. Health Care Research Series No. 16. Iowa City, Iowa: University of Iowa, 1970.

Carnegie Commission. Higher Education Report on Medical Schools. New York: McGraw-Hill, 1970.

Colbert, J., and Hohn, M. Guide to Manpower Training. New York: Behavioral Publications, 1971.

Copley, G., and Lechter, K. Selected Programs for Physician Support Personnel. Bethesda, Md.: National Institutes of Health, Professional Activities Branch of Education, 1971.

Curtis, J. L. Blacks, Medical Schools and Society. Ann Arbor, Mich.: University of Michigan Press, 1971.

Department of Health, Education, and Welfare. Mental Health Training and Public Health Manpower. Washington, D.C.: Superintendent of Documents, 1972.

Evans, L. The Crisis in Medical Education. Ann Arbor, Mich.: University of Michigan Press, 1964.

Fein, R., and Weber, G. I. Financing Medical Education. General Report Prepared for Carnegie Commission on Higher Education and Commonwealth Fund. New York: McGraw-Hill, 1971.

French, R. M. The Dynamics of Health Care. New York: McGraw-Hill, 1968.

Hartman, R. W. Credit for College, Public Policy for Student Loans, A Report for the Carnegie Commission on Higher Education. New York: McGraw-Hill, 1971.

Houser, H. W. Objectives in American Medical Education: A National Survey of Medical Faculty Opinions. Health Care Research Series No. 17. Iowa City, Iowa: University of Iowa, 1971.

Innis, M. Nursing Education in a Changing Society. Toronto: University of Toronto Press, 1970.

Knowles, J. Views of Medical Education and Medical Care. Cambridge: Harvard University Press, 1968.

Lathem, W. Community Medicine: Teaching, Research and Health Care. New York: Appleton-Century-Crofts, 1970.

MacNab, J. The Education of a Doctor. My First Year on the Wards. New York: Simon & Schuster, 1971.

Miller, S. J. Prescription for Leadership: Training for the Medical Elite. Chicago: Aldine, 1970.

Minority Student Opportunities in United States Medical Schools. Washington, D.C.: Association of American Medical Colleges, 1971.

Neleigh, J. R. Training Non-professional Community Project Leaders. New York: Behavioral Publications, 1971.

Popper, H. P. (ed.). Trends in New Medical Schools. New York: Grune & Stratton, 1967.

Purcell, E. (ed.) World Trends in Medical Education. Baltimore: The Johns Hopkins University Press, 1971.

Reader, G. Comprehensive Medical Care and Teaching. Ithaca, N. Y.: Cornell University Press, 1968.

Reform of Medical Education: The Effect of Student Unrest. Washington, D.C.: The National Academy of Sciences, 1970.

Richmond, J. B. Currents in American Medicine: A Developmental View of Medical Care and Education. Cambridge: Harvard University Press, 1969.

Robinson, G. C. Adventures in Medical Education: A Personal Narrative of the Greater Advance of American Medicine. Cambridge: Harvard University Press, 1957.

Roth, D. H., and Prive, D. W. Instructional Television—A Method for Teaching Nurses. St. Louis: C. V. Mosby, 1971.

Schecter, D. S., and O'Farrell, T. M. Universities, Colleges and Hospitals: Partners in Continuing Education. Battle Creek, Mich.: W. K. Kellogg Foundation, 1971.

Selected Training Programs for Physician Support Personnel. Identifying more than 100 programs to help meet critical manpower needs. Health Manpower Data Series. Bethesda, Md.: National Institutes of Health, Professional Activities Branch, 1971.

Sheps, C. G. Medical Schools and Hospitals Interdependence for Education and Service. Evanston, Ill.: Association of American Medical Colleges, 1965.

Tornyay, R. Strategies for Teaching Nursing. New York: John Wiley & Sons, 1971.

U.S. Congress. Senate Committee on Labor and Public Welfare. Physicians Training Facilities and Health Maintenance Organizations. Part 4, Hearings commencing November 17, 1971. Washington, D.C.: U.S. Government Printing Office, 1971.

Wilbur, M. B. Educational Tools for Health Personnel: New York: Macmillan, 1968.

## Health Manpower

Becker, H. S., et al. Boys in White. Chicago: University of Chicago Press, 1961.

Bernstein, L., and Dana, R. Interviewing and the Health Professions. New York: Appleton-Century-Crofts, 1970.

Bredow, M. Medical Assistant: A Guide to Clinical, Secretarial, and Technical Duties. 3rd Ed. New York: McGraw-Hill, 1970.

Financial Aid Programs in Support of Health Occupations. Chicago: The American Hospital Association, 1971.

Gartner, A. Paraprofessionals and Their Performance: A Survey of Education, Health, and Social Service Programs. New York: Praeger, 1971.

Greenfield, H. I. Allied Health Manpower Trends and Prospects. New York: Columbia University Press, 1969.

Grosser, C. (ed.) Nonprofessionals in the Human Services. San Francisco: Jossey-Bass, 1969.

Hartman, G. Health Education, Health Manpower and a System. Iowa City, Iowa: University of Iowa, 1969.

Health Manpower: Adapting in the Seventies; Report of the 1971 National Health Forum, March 15–17, 1971. New York: The National Health Council, 1971.

Merton, R. K., Reader, G. and Kendall, P. The Student Physician. Cambridge: Harvard University Press, 1967.

Michigan University, Bureau of Hospital Administration. Health Manpower Research. Ann Arbor, Mich.: University of Michigan Press, 1967.

New York State Hospital Manpower Survey. Albany: The New York Department of Health, 1970.

Pennell, M. Y. Health Manpower Source Book, Allied Health Manpower Supply and Requirements: 1950–1980. Washington, D.C.: U.S. Government Printing Office, 1970.

Physicians' Assistants Legal Regulation Survey. Pittsburgh: The Health Law Center, Aspens Systems Corporation, 1972.

Public Health Service. Health Manpower: A County and Metropolitan Area Data Book. Washington, D.C.: U.S. Government Printing Office, 1971.

Reiff, R. The Indigenous Nonprofessional. New York: Behavioral Publications, 1965.

Sadler, A. M., Jr. The Physician's Assistant—Today and Tomorrow. New Haven, Conn.: Yale University Press, 1972.

Stryker, R. P. The Hospital Ward Clerk. St. Louis: C. V. Mosby, 1970.

Sturm, H. Technology and Manpower in the Health Service Industry: 1965–1975. Washington, D.C.: U.S. Government Printing Office, 1967.

U.S. Department of Labor. U.S. Manpower in the 1970's: Opportunity and Challenge. Washington, D.C.: U.S. Government Printing Office, 1970.

U.S. Labor Department. Manpower Administration. Nursing Homes and Related Health Care Facilities. Washington, D.C.: U.S. Government Printing Office, 1969.

U.S. Labor Statistics Bureau. Tomorrow's Manpower Needs: National Manpower Projections and a Guide to Their Use as a Tool in Developing State and Area Manpower Projections. Washington, D.C.: U.S. Government Printing Office, 1969.

U.S. National Center for Health Statistics. 1970 Health Resources Statistics: Health Manpower and Health Facilities. Washington, D.C.: U.S. Government Printing Office, 1971.

U.S. National Institute of Mental Health. Non-Professional Personnel in Mental Health Programs, A Survey. Washington, D.C.: U.S. Government Printing Office, 1969.

U.S. President. Manpower Report of the President, and a Report on Manpower Requirements, Resources, Utilization and Training. By the Department of Labor. Washington, D.C.: U.S. Government Printing Office, 1969.

U.S. Public Health Service. State Licensing of Health Occupations. Washington, D.C.: U.S. Government Printing Office, 1967.

Walker, H. Health Manpower: Its Challenge to Organization and Management. St. Louis: C. V. Mosby, 1972.

## ENVIRONMENTAL HEALTH

Accident Control in Environmental Health Programs. Washington, D.C.: The American Public Health Association, 1966.

Directory of Environmental Organizations. New York: The Metropolitan Health Planning Corporation, 1971.

Ewald, W. Environment and Policy. Bloomington, Ind.: Indiana University Press, 1968.

Goldwater, L. J. Mercury: A History of Quicksilver. Baltimore: York Press, 1972.

Hurley, W. Environmental Legislation. Springfield, Ill.: Charles C Thomas, 1971.

Knittel, R. E. Organization of Community Groups in Support of the Planning Process and Code Enforcement Administration. Washington, D.C.: Environmental Control Administration, 1970.

Spiegelman, M. Introduction to Demography. Revised Ed. Cambridge: Harvard University Press, 1968.

Task Force on Environmental Health. Changing Environmental Hazards—

Challenge to Community Health. Washington, D.C.: Public Affairs Press, 1967.

Wolman, A. Water, Health and Society. Bloomington, Ind: Indiana University Press, 1969.

### Air Pollution

Esposito, J. C. Vanishing Air. New York: Grossman, 1970.

Guide to the Appraisal and Control of Air Pollution. Washington, D.C.: The American Public Health Association, 1969.

### Pesticides

Pesticide Residues in Food. Geneva, Switzerland: World Health Organization, 1971.

Safe Use of Pesticides. Washington, D.C.: The American Public Health Association, 1967.

### Water Pollution

Gurnham, C. F. Industrial Waste-Water Control. New York: Academic Press, 1965.

Hopkins, E. S., and Bean, E. L. Water Purification Control. 4th Ed. Baltimore: Williams & Wilkins, 1966.

## FOREIGN HEALTH PROGRAMS

Abel-Smith, B. An International Study of Health Expenditure and Its Relevance for Health Planning. Geneva, Switzerland: World Health Organization, 1967.

Andersen, R. Medical Care Use in Sweden and the United States: A Comparative Analysis of Systems Behavior. Chicago: University of Chicago, 1970.

Bryant, J. Health and the Developing World. Ithaca, N.Y.: Cornell University Press, 1969.

Canadian Department of National Health and Welfare. Illness and Health Care in Canada: Canadian Sickness Survey. Ottowa: Queens Printer and Controller of Stationery, 1960.

Care of the Elderly in Scotland: A Follow-up Report. Edinburgh: The Royal College of Physicians of Edinburgh, 1970.

Eckstein, H. The English Health Services. Cambridge: Harvard University Press, 1958.

Evang, K. Health Service, Society and Medicine. Fairlawn, N. J.: Oxford University Press, 1960.

Field, M. Doctor and Patient in Soviet Russia. Cambridge: Harvard University Press, 1957.

Fry, J. Medicine in Three Societies: A Comparison of Medical Care in the U.S.S.R., U.S.A., and U.K. New York: Elsevier, 1970.

Fry, J., and Farndale, W. J. (eds.). International Medical Care: A Comparison and Evaluation of Medical Care Services throughout the World. Walingford, Pa.: Medical & Technical Publishing Co., 1972.

Geriatric Day Hospital: A Study of Geriatric Day Hospitals in Great Britain and Northern Ireland. London: The King Edward's Hospital Fund, 1970.

Health and Healing: Hospital and Medical Services for South Africa's Devel-

oping Nations. Pretoria, S. Africa: The South African Department of Information, 1969.
Health Services Financing: A Report Commissioned in 1967 by the British Medical Association and Carried Out by an Advisory Panel. London: The British Medical Association, 1970.
Horn, J. S. Away with All Pests: An English Surgeon in People's China: 1954–1969. New York: Monthly Review Press, 1969.
Impact of the Ontario Hospital Labor Disputes Arbitration Act, 1965. Toronto: The Ontario Department of Labor, 1970.
King, M. (ed.) Medical Care in Developing Countries. Fairlawn, N.J.: Oxford University Press, 1966.
Lindsey, A. Socialized Medicine in England and Wales. Chapel Hill, N.C.: The University of North Carolina Press, 1962.
Livingston, A. Social Policy in Developing Countries. New York: Humanities Press, 1969.
National Health Planning in Developing Countries. Geneva, Switzerland: World Health Organization, 1967.
Nuffield, Provincial Hospitals Trust. Screening in Medical Care: Reviewing the Evidence. Fairlawn, N.J.: Oxford University Press, 1968.
Saxon, M. R. British National Health Service: Bad Medicine, Bad Politics, Bad Economics. Aurora, Ill.: Saxon Foundation, 1970.
Schoeck, H. (ed.). Financing Medical Care: An Appraisal of Foreign Programs. Caldwell, Idaho: Caxton Printer, 1962.
Uhr, C. Sweden's Social Security System. Washington, D.C.: U.S. Government Printing Office, 1966.
Weinerman, E. R. Social Medicine in Eastern Europe. Cambridge: Harvard University Press, 1969.
Health Services in the U.S.S.R. Geneva, Switzerland: World Health Organization, 1966.

## GERONTOLOGY AND GERIATRICS

de Beauvoir, S. The Coming of Age. New York: G. P. Putnam's Sons, 1972.
Birren, J. E. Handbook of Aging and the Individual. Chicago: University of Chicago Press, 1960.
Blumenthal, H. T. (ed.). Cowdry's Arteriosclerosis–A Survey of the Program. 2nd Ed. Springfield, Ill.: Charles C Thomas, 1967.
Boston Society for Gerontologic Psychiatry. Normal Psychology of the Aging Process. New York: International Universities Press, 1963.
Britton, J. H. Personality Changes in Aging. New York: Springer, 1972.
Burgess, E. Aging in Western Societies. Chicago: University of Chicago Press, 1960.
Burr, H. T. Psychology Functioning of Older People. 3rd Ed. Springfield, Ill.: Charles C Thomas, 1971.
Busse, E. W. Sexual behavior in old age. in E. W. Busse and E. Pfeiffer (eds.), Behavior and Adaptation in Late Life. Boston: Little, Brown, 1969.
Busse, E., and Pfeiffer, E. Behavior and Adaptation in Late Life. Boston: Little, Brown, 1970.
Busse, E., and Pfeiffer, E. Mental Illness in Later Life. Washington, D.C.: The American Psychiatric Association, 1973.

Cowdry, E. V. Problems of Aging: Biological and Medical Aspects. Baltimore: Williams & Wilkins, 1952.

Cowdry, E. V. The Care of the Geriatric Patient. St. Louis: C. V. Mosby, 1968.

Cumming, E., and Henry, W. E. Growing Old: The Process of Disengagement. New York: Basic Books, 1961.

Curtin, S. R. Nobody Ever Died of Old Age. Boston: Little, Brown, 1972.

Curtis, H. J. Biological Mechanisms of Aging. Springfield, Ill.: Charles C Thomas, 1966.

Goulet, L. R., and Baltes, P. B. Life-Span Developmental Psychology: Research and Theory. New York: Academic Press, 1970.

Guidelines. Durham, N.C.: The Duke University Information and Counseling Service for Older Persons, 1970.

Harris, R. The Management of Geriatric Cardiovascular Disease. Philadelphia: J. B. Lippincott, 1970.

Health in the Later Years of Life. An overview of health status of sixty-two million Americans aged forty-five or older. Washington, D.C.: U.S. Government Printing Office, 1972.

Homburger, F. Medical Care and Rehabilitation of the Aged and Chronically Ill. 2nd Ed. Boston: Little, Brown, 1964.

Interdisciplinary Workshop on Transportation and Aging. Transportation and Aging; Selected Issues Based on Proceedings of Workshop in D.C. Washington, D.C.: U.S. Government Printing Office, 1971.

International Association of Gerontologists. Biological Aspects of Aging. 5th Congress, San Francisco, 1966. New York: Columbia University Press, 1962.

Jaeger, D., and Simmons, L. W. The Aged Ill: Coping with Problems in Geriatric Care. New York: Appleton-Century-Crofts, 1970.

Kaplan, O. (ed.). Mental Disorders in Later Life. Stanford, Cal.: Stanford University Press, 1956.

King, F., and Herzig, W. F. Golden Age Exercises. New York: Crown Publishers, 1968.

Leeds, M., and Shore, H. (eds.). Geriatric Institutional Management. New York: G. P. Putnam's Sons, 1964.

Loether, H. Problems of Aging. Belmont, Cal.: Dickenson Publ. Co., 1969.

Lorhan, P. H. Recreation in Gerontology. Springfield, Ill.: Charles C Thomas, 1964.

Margolin, R. J., and Boldin, G. Dynamic Programming in the Rehabilitation of the Aging. Boston: Department of Rehabilitation and Special Education, Northeastern University, 1967.

McKeown, F. Pathology of the Aged. London: Butterworth and Co., 1965.

Moe, M. I. For Patient's Sake; a Book for All Personnel Who Care for the Aged. Minneapolis: Geriatric Care, 1972.

Neilsen, M. Home Aide Service and the Aged: A Controlled Study. Washington, D.C.: National Technical Information Service, 1970.

Newton, K., and Anderson, H. Geriatric Nursing. St. Louis: C. V. Mosby, 1966.

Osterbind, C. C. (ed.). Health Care Services for the Aged: Problems of Effective Delivery and Use. University of Florida Institute of Gerontology Series No. 19. Gainesville, Fla.: University of Florida Press, 1970.

Paillat, P. M., and Bunch, M. E. Age, Work and Automation. New York: Karger-Phiebig, 1970.

Palmore, E. Normal Aging—Reports from the Duke Longitudinal Study 1955—1969. Durham, N.C.: Duke University Press, 1970.

Pfeiffer, E. Alternatives to Institutional Care for Older Americans: Practice and Planning. Durham, N.C.: Duke University, 1972.

Post, F. The Clinical Psychiatry of Late Life. Oxford, N.Y.: Pergamon Press, 1965.

Prehoda, R. W. Extended Youth: The Promise of Gerontology. New York: G. P. Putnam's Sons, 1968.

President's Task Force on Aging. Toward a Brighter Future for the Elderly. Washington, D.C.: U.S. Government Printing Office, 1970.

Public Health Service. Working with Older People—A Guide to Practice. Vols. 1—4. Washington, D.C.: U.S. Government Printing Office, 1970.

Riley, M. W., Riley, J. W., Jr., Johnson, M. et al. Aging and the Professions. New York: Russell Sage Foundation, 1969.

Riley, M. W., Johnson, M., and Foner, A. Sociology of Age Stratification. New York: Russell Sage Foundation, 1972.

Rosenberg, G. S. The Worker Grows Old. San Francisco: Jossey-Bass, 1970.

Rubin, I. Sexual Life in Later Years. New York: Sex Information and Education Council of the United States, 1970.

Rudd, J., and Margolin, R. Maintenance Therapy for the Geriatric Patient. Springfield, Ill.: Charles C Thomas, 1968.

Shanas, E., et al. Older People in the Industrial Societies. New York: Atherton Press, 1968.

Shock, N. A. Classified Bibliography of Gerontology and Geriatrics Supplements. Stanford, Cal.: Stanford University Press, 1963.

Simon, A. et al. Aging in Modern Society. Washington, D.C.: The American Psychiatric Association, 1968.

Simpson, I. H. Social Aspects of Aging. Durham, N.C.: Duke University Press, 1972.

Talland, G. A. Human Aging and Behavior: Recent Advances in Research and Theory. New York: Academic Press, 1968.

The Golden Years—A Tarnished Myth. New York: The National Council on the Aging, 1970.

Tibbitts, C. Handbook of Social Gerontology. Chicago: University of Chicago Press, 1960.

Townsend, C. Old Age: The Last Segregation. New York: Bantam Books, 1971.

U.S. Congress, Senate Special Committee on Aging. Mental Health Care and the Elderly: Shortcomings in Public Policy. Washington, D.C.: U.S. Government Printing Office, 1971.

U.S. Congress, Special Committee On Aging. Economics of Aging: Toward a Full Share in Abundance. Washington, D.C.: U.S. Government Printing Office, 1969.

U.S. Department of Health, Education and Welfare. Why Men Stop Working at or Before Age 65. Preliminary Findings from the Survey of New Beneficiaries. Report No. 3. Social Security Administration. Washington, D.C.: U.S. Government Printing Office, 1971.

U.S. Social and Rehabilitation Service. Report of the National Protective

Services Project for Older Adults. Washington, D.C.: U.S. Government Printing Office, 1971.

U.S. Social Security Administration. Amounts reimbursed by State and County under Health Insurance for the Aged. Washington, D.C.: U.S. Government Printing Office, 1971.

Wolff, K. Geriatric Psychiatry. Springfield, Ill.: Charles C Thomas, 1963.

Wolk, R. L., and Rochelle, B. The Gerontological Apperception Test (GAT). New York: Behavioral Publications, 1971.

Youmans, E. G. Older Rural Americans: A Sociological Perspective. Lexington, Ky.: University of Kentucky Press, 1967.

## GRANTS

Advisory Commission on Intergovernmental Relations. Special Revenue Sharing: An Analysis of the Administration's Grant Consolidation Proposals. Washington, D.C.: U.S. Government Printing Office, 1971.

Financial Aid Programs in Support of Health Occupations: A Guide for Auxiliaries. Chicago: The American Hospital Association, 1971.

Major Federal Aid Programs for Hospitals. Chicago: The American Hospital Association, 1970.

Survey of Grant-Making Foundations with Assets over $500,000. New York: The Public Service Materials Center, 1970.

The Health Funds Directory: Sources of Governmental and Foundation Aid. Cambridge: Health Funds Institute, 1969.

Urgo, L. A. Manual for Obtaining Foundation Grants. Boston: Robert J. Corcoran Co., 1971.

U.S. Health Facilities Planning and Construction Service. Publications of the Health Facilities Planning and Construction Service, Hill Burton Programs. Washington, D.C.: U.S. Government Printing Office, 1970.

U.S. National Institute of Mental Health. The Comprehensive Community Mental Health Center: Grants for Construction and Staffing. Washington, D.C.: U.S. Government Printing Office, 1969.

U.S. President's Commission on Heart Disease, Cancer and Stroke. A National Program to Conquer Heart Disease, Cancer and Stroke: Report to the President. Washington, D.C.: U.S. Government Printing Office, 1964—1965.

## HEALTH ASSOCIATIONS

Burrow, J. G. American Medical Association: Voice of American Medicine. Baltimore: The Johns Hopkins Press, 1963.

Cray, E. In Failing Health: The Medical Crisis and the A.M.A. New York: Bobbs-Merrill, 1970.

Directory of National Voluntary Health Organizations. Chicago: The American Health Association, 1962.

Dulles, F. R. The American Red Cross: A History. New York: Harper & Row, 1950.

Goulden, J. The Money Givers. New York: Random House, 1971.

Harris, R. A Sacred Trust. Baltimore: Penguin Books, 1966.

Knopf, S. A. A History of the TB Association. New York: National Tuberculosis and Respiratory Diseases Association, 1922.

Shanahan, R. History of Catholic Hospital Associations, 1915–1965. St. Louis: The Catholic Hospital Association, 1965.
Shryock, R. H. National Tuberculosis Association, 1904–1954. History Series 8. New York: National Tuberculosis and Respiratory Disease Association, 1957.
Wasserman, C. S., and Wasserman, P. Health Organizations of the U.S., Canada and Internationally. 2nd Ed. Ithaca, N.Y.: Cornell University Press, 1965.

## HOSPITAL AND CENTRALIZED SERVICES

### Dietary

Coble, M. C. A Guide to Nutrition and Food Service for Nursing Homes and Homes for the Aged. Washington, D.C.: U.S. Government Printing Office, 1971.
Martin, E. A. Nutrition in Action. 3rd Ed. New York: Holt, Rinehart & Winston, 1971.
Robinson, C. H. Normal and Therapeutic Nutrition. New York: Macmillan, 1972.
Smith, E. E. Handbook on Quantity Food Management. 2nd Ed. Minneapolis: Burgess, 1970.
Turner, J. The Chemical Feast. (Ralph Nader Study Group Report on Food Production and the F.D.A.) New York: Grossman, 1970.
U.S. Public Health Services, Division of Hospital and Medical Facilities. Hospital Dietary Services: A Planning Guide. Washington, D.C.: U.S. Government Printing Office, 1966.

### Engineering and Maintenance

Paul, R. (ed.). Hospital and Institutional Engineering and Maintenance Journal Articles. Flushing, N.Y.: Medical Examination, 1970.
Management Engineering for Hospitals. Chicago: The American Hospital Association, 1970.

### Housekeeping

Housekeeping Manual for Health Care Facilities. Chicago: The American Hospital Association, 1969.
U.S. Public Health Service. Care and Cleaning of Housekeeping Equipment and Storage Room in Health Facilities: A Programmed Course for Housekeeping Personnel. Washington, D.C.: U.S. Government Printing Office, 1971.
Work Manual of Executive Housekeeper in the Hospital. Huntington, Ind.: The Huntington Laboratories, 1967.

### Pharmacy

Black, H. J. Impact of Unit Dose Pharmacy Service on the Time Involvement of Registered Nurses with Medication Activities. Iowa City, Iowa: University of Iowa, 1971.
Brands, Generics, Prices and Quality: The Prescribing Debate after a Decade. Washington, D.C.: The Pharmaceutical Manufacturers Assocation, 1971.

Brodie, D. C. Drug Utilization and Drug Utilization Review and Control. Rockville, Md.: Health Service and Mental Health Administration, Department of Health, Education and Welfare, 1970.
Challenge to Pharmacy in the Seventies: Proceedings of an Invitation Conference on Pharmacy Manpower, San Francisco, November 10–12, 1970. Rockville, Md.: U.S. Public Health Service, 1971.
Govoni, L. E., et al. Drugs and Nursing Implications. New York: Appleton-Century-Crofts, 1965.
Halberstam, M. The Pills in Your Life. New York: Grosset & Dunlap, 1972.
Keller, B. G., and Smith, M. C. Pharmaceutical Marketing. Baltimore: Williams & Wilkins, 1969.
Krantz, J. C., et al. The Pharmacologic Principles of Medical Practice. 7th Ed. Baltimore: Williams & Wilkins, 1969.
National Academy of Sciences. Report on Over-the-counter Drugs and Drug Efficacy Study Information Control. Rockville, Md.: Bureau of Drugs, Federal Drug Administration, 1972.
Reference Manual on Hospital Pharmacy. Chicago: The American Hospital Association, 1970.
Role of the Hospital in International Drug Monitoring: Report on W.H.O. Meeting, Geneva, November 18–23, 1968. Geneva, Switzerland: The World Health Organization, 1969.
Smith, M. C., and Knapp, D. A. Drugs and Medical Care. Baltimore: Williams & Wilkins, 1972.
The Merck Index: An Encyclopedia of Chemicals and Drugs. 8th Ed. Rahway, N.J.: Merck and Co., 1968.
Walker, H. D. Market Power and Price Levels in the Ethical Drug Industry. Bloomington, Ind.: Indiana University Press, 1971.

## Religion

Apostolate to the Sick. St. Louis: The National Association of Catholic Chaplains, 1967.
Kelly, G. A. Medico-Moral Problems. St. Louis: Catholic Hospital Association of the United States and Canada, 1958.
Manual on Hospital Chaplaincy. Chicago: The American Hospital Association, 1970.

## Safety

Colling, R. L. Hospital Security and Safety Journal Articles. Flushing, N.Y.: Medical Examination, 1970.
Electric Hazards in Hospitals: Proceedings of a Workshop Held April 4–5, 1968. Washington, D.C.: The National Academy of Sciences, 1970.
International Commission on Radiological Protection. Protection of the Patient in X-Ray Diagnosis. New York: Pergamon Press, 1970.
Iskrant, A. Accidents and Homicide. Cambridge: Harvard University Press, 1968.
Manual for the Safe Use of Electricity in Hospitals. Boston: The National Fire Protection Association, 1971.
Nursing Home Fires and Their Cures. (Reprints from articles in Fire Journal). Boston: The National Fire Protection Association, 1972.

Standard for Essential Electrical Systems for Hospitals. Boston: The National Fire Protection Association, 1970.
Standard for Nonflammable Medical Gas Systems. Boston: The National Fire Protection Association, 1970.
Walter, C. W. Electric Hazards in Hospitals. Washington, D.C.: The National Academy of Sciences, 1970.

## Sanitation

Environmental Sanitation. Chicago: The American Hospital Association, 1968.
Lawrence, C. Disinfection, Sterilization and Preservation. Philadelphia: Lea & Febiger, 1968.
Roberts, R. B., (ed.). Infections and Sterilization Problems. Boston: Little, Brown, 1972.
U.S. Public Health Service. Principles of Infection Control in Health Facilities: A Programmed Course for Housekeeping Personnel. Washington, D.C.: U.S. Government Printing Office, 1971.

## Volunteer and Auxillary Services

Stanton, E. Clients Come Last: Volunteers and Welfare Organizations. Beverly Hills, Cal.: Sage Publications, 1972.
Swanson, M. T. Your Volunteer Program: Organization and Administration of Volunteer Programs. Ankeny, Iowa: Volunteer Coordinators Program, 1970.

## Auxiliaries and Volunteer Services

Arthur, J. Retire to Action: A Guide to Voluntary Service. Nashville: Abingdon Press, 1969.
David, A. A Guide to Volunteer Services. New York: Cornerstone Library, 1970.
Kurtz, H. Effective Use of Volunteers in Hospitals. Springfield, Ill.: Charles C Thomas, 1970.
Kurtz, H. Effective Use of Volunteers in Hospitals and Agencies. Springfield, Ill.: Charles C Thomas, 1971.
Manual on Volunteer Services in Homes for the Aging and Nursing Homes. Austin, Tex.: The Texas Association of Homes for the Aging, 1970.
Schindler-Rainman, E. The Volunteer Community: Creative Use of Human Resources. Washington, D.C.: The National Training Laboratory Learning Resources, 1971.
SERVE: Older Volunteers in Community Service: A New Role and New Resource. New York: The Community Service Society of New York, 1971.
Statement on the Role of the Auxiliary on the Health Care Team. Chicago: The American Hospital Association, 1970.
State of the Art of Volunteering in Rehabilitation Facilities. Washington, D.C.: Goodwill Industries of America, 1971.

## HOSPITAL ORGANIZATION AND MANAGEMENT

Alford, B. Hospital Electronic Data Processing. Flushing, N.Y.: Medical Examination, 1970.

Belinkoff, S. Introduction to Inhalation Therapy. Boston: Little, Brown, 1969.

Bowley, C. C., (ed.). Blood Transfusion: A Guide to the Formation and Operation of a Transfusion Service. Geneva, Switzerland: World Health Organization, 1971.

Brown, E. Newer Dimensions of Patient Care. Part 1: The Use of the Physical and Social Environment of General Hospital for Therapeutic Purposes. New York: Basic Books, 1961.

Brown, E. Newer Dimensions of Patient Care, Part 2: Improving Staff Motivation and Competence in the General Hospital. New York: Basic Books, 1962.

Brown, E. Newer Dimensions of Patient Care, Part 3: Patients as People. New York: Basic Books, 1964.

Campbell, Sister Janice. Orientation Program for Patients. St. Louis: Washington University Press, 1970.

Cripwell, M. Complete Handbook for Professional Ambulance Personnel. Baltimore: Williams & Wilkins, 1970.

Dale, E. Management: Theory and Practice. New York: McGraw-Hill, 1965.

Dale, E. and Michelon, L. C. Modern Management Methods. Cleveland: World Book, 1966.

DeKornfeld, T. Inhalation Therapy Procedure Manual. 2nd Ed. Springfield, Ill.: Charles C Thomas, 1970.

Emergency Care and Transportation of the Sick and Injured. Chicago: The American Academy of Orthopaedic Surgeons, 1971.

Emergency Care: The Hospital Emergency Dept. in an Emergency Care System. Chicago: The American Hospital Association, 1972.

Erkert, C. Emergency-Room Care. 2nd edition. Boston: Little, Brown, 1971.

Haimann, T. Supervisory Management for Hospitals and Related Health Facilities. St. Louis: The Catholic Hospital Association, 1965.

Haire, M. Psychology in Management. 2nd Ed. New York: McGraw-Hill, 1964.

Innovations in Hospital Management. Chicago: The American Hospital Association, 1969.

Johnson, R. The Theory and Management of Systems. 2nd Ed. New York: McGraw-Hill, 1967.

MacEachern, M. Hospital Organization and Management. 3rd Ed., revised. Chicago: Physician's Record, 1957.

Management Engineering for Hospitals. Chicago: The American Hospital Association, 1970.

Mathieu, R. Hospital and Nursing Home Management: An Instructional and Administrative Manual. Philadelphia: W. B. Saunders, 1971.

Metzger, N. et al. Labor-Management Relations in the Health Services Industry—Theory and Practice. Washington, D.C.: Science and Health Publications, 1972.

Musser, A. W. Blood Banking and Immunohematology Journal Articles. Flushing, N.Y.: Medical Examination, 1970.

Newell, J. E. Laboratory Management. Boston: Little, Brown, 1972.

Noble, J. H., Jr., et al. (eds.). Emergency Medical Services: Behavioral and Planning Perspectives. New York: Behavioral Publications, 1973.

Outpatient Health Care—The Role of Hospitals. Chicago: The American Hospital Association, 1969.

Postmortem Procedures. Chicago: The American Hospital Association, 1970.

Public Health Service. 1970 Special Hospital Services for Cardiovascular Disease Patients. Vol. 1, General Services. Vol. 2, Surgical Services. Washington, D.C.: Superintendent of Documents, 1971.

Raphael, W. Patients and Their Hospitals. London: King's Fund Books, 1973.

Richards, M., and Neelander, W. (eds.) Readings in Management. 2nd Ed. Cincinnati: South-Western, 1963.

Rosenfeld, L. S. Ambulatory Care: Planning and Organization. Springfield, Va.: National Technical Information Service, 1971.

Scott, W. G. Organization Theory: A Behavioral Analysis for Management. Homewood, Ill.: Irwin, 1967.

Strauss, G. and Sayles, L. R. Personnel: The Human Problem of Management. Englewood Cliffs, N.J.: Prentice-Hall, 1967.

Stryker, R. The Hospital Ward Clerk. St. Louis: C. V. Mosby, 1970.

Teamster Comprehensive Care Program at Montefiore Hospital. Teamsters Joint Council No. 16. New York: The Teamsters Joint Council, 1969.

Wheeler, K. E. The Four-Day Week; an AMA Research Report. New York: The American Management Association, 1972.

The Unit Management Concept in Hospital Patient Care. St. Louis: The Catholic Hospital Association, 1969.

U.S. Atomic Energy Commission. How to Get a License to Use Radioisotopes. Washington, D.C.: U.S. Government Printing Office, 1969.

U.S. Public Health Service. Hospital Outpatient and Emergency Activities: Functional Programming Guidelines. Washington, D.C.: U.S. Government Printing Office, 1971.

Young, J. A., and Crocker, D. Principles and Practice of Inhalation Therapy. Chicago: Medical Publishers, 1970.

## Economics of Medical Care

Anderson, O. W. The Uneasy Equilibrium: Private and Public Financing of Health Services in the U.S., 1875–1965. New Haven, Conn.: College and University Press, 1968.

Avnet, H. Physician Service Patterns and Illness Rates. New York: Group Health Insurance, Inc., 1967.

Axelrod, D. J. The Economics of Health and Medical Care: Proceedings. Conference on the Economics of Health and Medical Care, University of Michigan, 1962.

Berki, S. E. Hospital Economics. Lexington, Mass.: Lexington Books-D. C. Heath, 1972.

Bureau of Public Health Economics. Medical Care Chart Book. 3rd Ed. Ann Arbor, Mich.: Michigan University Press, 1968.

Capital Financing in Health Care Industry. Chicago: The American Hospital Association, 1970.

Chadwick, J. et al. Cost and Operations Analysis of Automated Multiphasic Health Testing. Springfield, Va.: National Technical Information Service, 1970.

Columbia University, School of Public Health and Administrative Medicine. Attitudes Utilization and Out-of-pocket Costs for Health Services: Report of Interview with Selected Teamster Families. New York: Columbia University Press, 1967.

Committee on the Costs of Medical Care. Medical Care for the American People. Washington, D.C.: U.S. Public Health Service, 1970.

Falk, I. S. The Incidence of Illness and the Receipt and Cost of Medical Care Among Representative Families. Chicago: University of Chicago Press, 1933.

Falk, I. S., Rorem, C. R., and Ring, M. D. The Costs of Medical Care: A Summary of Investigations on the Economic Aspects of the Prevention and Care of Illness. New York: Arno Press, 1972.

Fein, R. The Doctor Shortage: An Economic Diagnosis. Washington, D.C.: The Brookings Institute, 1967.

Feldstein, M. S. The Rising Cost of Hospital Care. Washington, D.C.: Information Resources Press, 1971.

Fendall, N. Auxiliaries in Health Care. Baltimore: The Johns Hopkins University Press, 1972.

Ginzberg, E., and Oston, M. Men, Money, and Medicine. New York: Columbia University Press, 1969.

Glaser, W. A. Paying the Doctor: Systems of Remuneration and Their Effects. Baltimore, Md.: The Johns Hopkins University Press, 1970.

Greenfield, H. The Medical Care Price Index, Health Information Foundation Research Series No. 7. New York: The Health Information Foundation, 1959.

Hallan, J. Economic Cost of Kidney Disease and Related Diseases of the Urinary System. Washington, D.C.: U.S. Government Printing Office, 1970.

Harris, S. The Economics of American Medicine. New York: Macmillian, 1964.

Health Care Delivery in the 1970's—Report, Findings and Recommendations of Sub-Committee on Health Care Delivery of the Committee on Medical Economics. New York: The Health Insurance Association of America, 1969.

Herman, W. R. Catastrophic Illnesses and Costs. Washington, D.C.: U.S. Government Printing Office, 1971.

Hirsh, B. Business Management of a Medical Practice. St. Louis: C. V. Mosby, 1964.

Horowitz, L. A. Medical Care Prices Fact Sheet. Washington, D.C.: U.S. Government Printing Office, 1969.

Kaiser Foundation Medical Care Program. Oakland, Cal.: The Kaiser Foundation Hospitals, 1970.

Klarman, H. E. The Economics of Health. New York: Columbia University Press, 1965.

Klarman, H. E. Empirical Studies in Health Economics: Proceedings of the 2nd Conference on the Economics of Health. Baltimore: The Johns Hopkins University Press, 1970.

Kreps, J. M. Lifetime Allocation of Work and Income. Durham, N.C.: Duke University Press, 1971.

LeSourd, D. Benefit-Cost Analysis of Kidney Disease Programs. Washington, D.C.: U.S. Government Printing Office, 1969.

Munts, R. Bargaining for Health: Labor Unions, Health Insurance, and Medical Care. Milwaukee, Wisc.: University of Wisconsin Press, 1967.

Nader, R. and Blackwell, K. You and Your Pension. New York: Viking Press, 1973.

National Policies and Programs for the Financing of Medical Care. Chicago: The Center for Health Administration Studies, 1971.

Nourse, A. E. The Management of a Medical Practice. Philadelphia: J. B. Lippincott, 1963.

Problems in Paying for Services of Supervisory and Teaching Physicians in Hospitals under Medicare. Washington, D.C.: U.S. General Accounting Office, 1971.

Report of Special Committee on Provision of Health Services: Ameriplan—a Proposal for Delivery and Financing of Health Services in the U.S. Chicago: The American Hospital Association, 1970.

Somers, A. Health Care in Transition: Directions for the Future. Chicago: Hospital Research and Education Trust, 1971.

Somers, A. R. (ed.). The Kaiser-Permanente Medical Care Program. New York: Commonwealth Fund, 1971.

Somers, H. M., and Somers, A. R. Doctors, Patients and Health Insurance: The Organization and Financing of Medical Care. Washington, D.C.: The Brookings Institute, 1961.

Tanzer, M. The Sick Society: An Economic Examination. Chicago: Holt, Rinehart & Winston, 1971.

U.S. Congress, Senate Committee on the District of Columbia. The Medical Services Retirement Benefits, Healing Arts Practice, Employment of Minors, and Police Band Hearings. Washington, D.C.: U.S. Government Printing Office, 1971.

U.S. Congress, Senate Committee on Government Operations. Health Activities: Federally Expenditures and Public Purposes. Washington, D.C.: U.S. Government Printing Office, 1970.

U.S. General Accounting Office. Problems in Paying for Services of Supervisory and Teaching Physicians in Hospitals under Medicare. Washington, D.C., U.S. General Accounting Office, 1971.

U.S. Public Health Service. Selected References on Group Practices. Washington, D.C.: U.S. Government Printing Office, 1967.

Weisbrod, B. Economics of Public Health: Measuring the Economic Impact of Diseases. Philadelphia: University of Pennsylvania Press, 1961.

Yost, E. The U.S. Health Industry: The Costs of Acceptable Medical Care by 1975. New York: Frederick A. Praeger, 1969.

## Financial Management

Accounting Manual for Long-Term Care Institutions. Chicago: The American Hospital Association, 1968.

Berman, H. J., and Weeks, L. E. Financial Management of Hospitals. Research Series No. 6. Ann Arbor, Mich.: The University of Michigan, 1971.

Bookkeeping Procedures and Business Practices for Small Hospitals. Chicago: The American Hospital Association, 1969.

Budgeting Procedures for Hospitals. Chicago: The American Hospital Association, 1971.

Fay, C. Managerial Accounting for the Hospitality Service Industries. Dubuque, Iowa: William C. Brow, 1971.

Herkimer, A. Concepts in Hospital Financial Management. Old Ridge, N.J.: Alfa Associates, 1970.

Internal Control and Internal Auditing for Hospitals. Chicago: The American Hospital Association, 1969.

Safeguarding the Hospital's Assets: A Compilation of Articles on Every
   Aspect of Internal Control. Chicago: The Hospital Financial Management
   Association, 1971.
Seawell, L. Hospital Accounting and Financial Management. Berwyn, Ill.:
   Physician's Record, 1964.
Seawell, L. Introduction to Hospital Accounting. Chicago: Hospital Financial
   Management Association, 1971.
Standards of Accounting and Financial Reporting for Voluntary Health and
   Welfare Organizations. New York: National Health Council and National
   Social Welfare Assembly, 1964.
Survey of Hospital Charges. Chicago: The American Hospital Association,
   1970.
Taylor, P. J. Management Accounting for Hospitals. Philadelphia: W. B.
   Saunders, Co., 1964.
"Group Practice" Guidelines to Forming or Joining a Medical Group. Chi-
   cago: The American Association of Medical Clinics, 1970.
McCall, W. Group Practice and Prepayment of Medical Care. Washington,
   D.C.: Public Affairs Press, 1966.
Somers, A. The Kaiser-Permanente Medical Care Program: Proceedings of
   Symposium Sponsored by Kaiser-Permanente Medical Care Program. New
   York: The Commonwealth Fund, 1971.
Williams, G. Kaiser-Permanente Health Plan: Why It Works. Oakland, Cal.:
   The Kaiser Foundation, 1971.

## Group Practice
Bush, A. S. Group Practice: Planning and Implementing a Community-wide
   Prepayment Plan for Health Services. New York: The New York State
   Health Planning Commission, 1971.
Gintzig, L. Prepaid Group Practice: An Analysis as a Delivery System; The
   Reports and Comparisons of Selected Aspects of Several Prepaid Group
   Practice Plans. Washington, D.C.: Department of Health Care Administra-
   tion of The George Washington University, 1972.

## Health Maintenance Organizations
Benyak, J. M. (ed.). HMO Source Book. 1973 Ed. Pittsburgh: The Health
   Law Center, Aspen Systems Corporation, 1973.
Carey, S. C. Health Maintenance Organizations: An Introduction and Survey
   of Recent Developments, Washington, D.C.: Lawyers' Committee for Civil
   Rights under Law, 1972.
HMO Sourcebook: A Digest of State Laws Affecting the Prepayment of
   Medical Care, Group Practice and HMO's. Pittsburgh: The Health Law
   Center, Aspens Systems Corporation, 1973.
Holley, R. Legal Context for the Development of Health Maintenance Organi-
   zations. Minneapolis: The American Rehabilitation Foundation. 1971.
Roy, W. R. Proposed Health Maintenance Organization Act of 1972. Washing-
   ton, D.C.: Washington Science and Health Communications Group, 1972.

## Social Security and Health Insurance
A List of Worthwhile Life and Health Insurance Books. 1971 Ed. New York:
   The Health Insurance Institute, 1971.

Altmeyer, A. J. The Formative Years of Social Security. Madison, Wisc.: University of Wisconsin Press, 1966.

Anderson, O., and May, J. The Federal Employee Health Benefits Program 1961–1968: A Model for National Health Insurance. Chicago: University of Chicago, 1971.

Columbia University, School of Public Health and Administrative Medicine. Military Medicare: The Physician-Service Component of the Civilian Health and Medical Program of the Uniformed Services. New York: Columbia University, 1969.

Dickerson, O. Health Insurance. 3rd Ed. Homewood, Ill.: Richard D. Irwin, 1968.

Eilers, R. Regulations of Blue Cross and Blue Shield Plans. Homewood, Ill.: Richard D. Irwin, 1963.

Eilers, R., and Moyerman, S. National Health Insurance. Proceedings of the Conference on National Health Insurance. Homewood, Ill.: Richard E. Irwin, 1971.

Elling, R. H. National Health Care: Issues and Problems in Socialized Medicine. Chicago: Aldine-Atherton, 1971.

Faulkner, E. J. Health Insurance. New York: McGraw-Hill, 1960.

Fisher, P. Prescription for National Health Insurance: A Proposal For the U.S. Based on Canadian Experience. New York: North River Press, 1972.

Follmann, J. F. Insurance Coverage for Mental Illness. New York: The Association Press, 1970.

Foundations of Life and Health Insurance. Austin, Tex.: The University of Texas Bureau of Business Research, 1971.

Hirshfield, D. S. The Lost Reform (The Campaign for Compulsory Health Insurance in U.S. from 1932–1943). Cambridge: Harvard University Press, 1970.

Impact of the Advent of Medicare on Hospital Costs. New York: The Hofstra University School of Business, 1970.

MacIntyre, D. Voluntary Health Insurance and Rate Making. Ithaca, N.Y.: Cornell University Press, 1962.

Medicare-Medicaid Guide, Law, Regulations, Explanations. Chicago: Commerce-Clearing House, 1968.

Mehr, R. Principles of Insurance. Homewood, Ill.: Richard D. Irwin, 1966.

Mullins, J. E. Current Concepts in Medical Practice. St. Louis: C. V. Mosby, 1965.

Nagi, S. Z. Disability and Rehabilitation. Legal, Clinical, and Self-Concepts and Measurement. Columbus: Ohio State University Press, 1970.

Pauly, M. V. National Health Insurance: An Analysis. Washington, D.C.: American Enterprise Institution for Public Policy Research, 1971.

Problems in Providing Proper Care to Medicaid and Medicare Patients in Skilled Nursing Homes. Report to Congress by Comptroller of U.S. Washington, D.C.: U.S. General Accounting Office, 1971.

Roemer, M. I., (ed.). Health Insurance Plans: Studies in Organizational Diversity. Los Angeles: School of Public Health, University of California, 1970.

Roemer, M. I. Organization of Medical Care Under Social Security. New York: International Labour Office, 1969.

Schiltz, M. E. Public Attitudes Toward Social Security, 1935–1965. Washington, D.C.: U.S. Government Printing Office, 1970.

Schottland, C. I. The Social Security Program in the United States. 2nd Ed. New York: Appleton-Century-Crofts, 1970.

Skidmore, M. J. Medicare and the American Rhetoric Reconciliation. Birmingham: University of Alabama Press, 1970.

U.S. Advisory Council on Public Welfare. Having the Power, We Have the Duty—Report to the Secretary of H.E.W. Washington, D.C.: U.S. Government Printing Office. 1966.

U.S. Congress, House of Representatives Commission on Ways and Means. Report on Social Security Amendments of 1970. H.R. 91-1096. 91st Congress, 2nd session. Washington, D.C.: U.S. Government Printing Office, 1970.

U.S. Congress, House Ways and Means Committee. National Health Insurance Proposals. Parts 1–14. Washington, D.C.: U.S. Government Printing Office, 1972.

U.S. Congress, Senate. Special Committee on Aging. Cutbacks in Medicare and Medicaid Coverage. Part 1. Hearings . . . held May 10, 1971. Washington, D.C.: U.S. Government Printing Office, 1971.

U.S. Congress, Senate Committee on Finance. Social Security Amendments of 1971. Hearings commencing July 27, 1971. Washington, D.C.: U.S. Government Printing Office, 1971.

U.S. Department of Health, Education and Welfare. Analysis of Health Insurance Proposals, Introduced in the 92nd Congress. Washington, D.C.: U.S. Government Printing Office, 1971.

U.S. Department of Health, Education and Welfare. Report of the Task Force on Medicaid and Related Programs. Washington, D.C.: U.S. Government Printing Office, 1970.

U.S. National Clearinghouse for Mental Health Information. Mental Health Benefits of Medicare and Medicaid. Washington, D.C.: U.S. Government Printing Office, 1969.

U.S. Social Security Administration Office of Research and Statistics. Financing Mental Health Care under Medicare and Medicaid. Washington, D.C.: U.S. Superintendent of Documents, 1971.

U.S. Social Security Administration Office of Research and Statistics. Health Insurance for the Aged; Amounts Reimbursed by State and County, 1969. Washington, D.C.: U.S. Government Printing Office, 1971.

U.S. Social Security Administration. Reimbursement Incentives for Hospital and Medical Care, Objectives and Alternatives. Washington, D.C.: U.S. Goverment Printing Office, 1968.

Ways to Reduce Payments for Physician and X-Ray Services to Nursing Home Patients Under Medicare and Medicaid. Washington, D.C.: U.S. General Accounting Office, 1971.

Witkin, E. Impact of Medicare. Springfield, Ill.: Charles C Thomas, 1971.

## LEGAL ASPECTS

Automated Medical Records and the Law. Pittsburgh: The Health Law Center, Aspen Systems Corporation, 1971.

Bridgman, R. F., and Roemer, M. I. Hospital Legislation and Hospital Systems. Geneva, Switzerland, World Health Organization 1973.

Callehan, D. Abortion: Law, Choice, and Morality. New York: Macmillan, 1970.

Campbell, A., and Campbell, V. Moral Dilemmas in Medicine. Baltimore: Williams & Wilkins, 1972.

Carlson, R. J. Planning and Law: Planners and Lawyers. Minneapolis: The American Rehabilitation Foundation Health Services Research Center, 1969.

Chayet, N. L. Legal Implications of Emergency Care. New York: Appleton-Century-Crofts, 1969.

Creighton, H. Law Every Nurse Should Know. Philadelphia: W. B. Saunders, 1970.

Curry, A. S. Methods of Forensic Sciences. Vols. 3—4. New York: Wiley-Interscience, 1964.

Derbyshire, R. C. Medical Licensure and Discipline in the United States. Baltimore: The Johns Hopkins Press, 1969.

Fox, R. The Medicolegal Report: Theory and Practice. Boston: Little, Brown, 1969.

Goodman, R. M., and Goldsmith, L. S. Modern Hospital Liability—Law and Tactics. New York: Practicing Law Institute, 1972.

Grad, F. P. Public Health Law Manual. Washington, D.C.: The American Public Health Association, 1965.

Group Practice and the Law. Pittsburgh: The Health Law Center, Aspen Systems Corporation, 1971.

Hassard, H. Medical Malpractice: Risks, Protection, Prevention. Oradell, N.J.: Medical Economic Book Division, 1966.

Hayt, E. Law for Hospital Auxiliaries. Albany: Hospital Educational Research Fund, 1964.

Hayt, E. Legal Aspects of Medical Records. Berwyn, Ill.: Physician's Record, 1964.

Holly, R. Legal Context for the Development of Health Maintenance Organizations. Minneapolis: Health Services Research Center, Institute Interdisciplinary, American Rehabilitation Foundation.

Hurley, W. D. Environmental Legislation. Springfield, Ill.: Charles C Thomas, 1971.

Kinzer, D. M. Laws on Order: Confessions of a Lobbyist. Chicago: Modern Hospital Press, 1971.

Leach, G. The Biocrats ("Ethics and the New Medicine"). New York: McGraw-Hill, 1970.

Lesnik, M. J., and Anderson, B. Nursing Practice and the Law. Philadelphia: J. B. Lippincott, 1962.

Long, R. H. The Physician and the Law. 3rd Ed. New York: Appleton-Century-Crofts, 1968.

Lundquist, F. Methods of Forensic Science. Vol. 1. New York: Wiley-Interscience, 1962.

McBride, E. D. Disability Evaluation. 6th Ed. Philadelphia: J. B. Lippincott, 1963.

McCleery, R. One Life—One Physician: An Inquiry into the Medical Profession's Performance in Self-Regulation. Washington, D.C.: Ralph Nader's Center for Responsive Law, 1970.

Meyers, D. The Human Body and the Law: A Medico-Legal Study. Chicago: Aldine, 1970.

Moritz, A. R., and Stetler, D. J. Handbook of Legal Medicine. 2nd Ed. St. Louis: C. V. Mosby, 1964.

Morris, R. C. and Moritz, A. R. Doctor and Patient and the Law. St. Louis: C. V. Mosby, 1972.

Murchison, I. A., and Nichols, T. Legal Foundations of Nursing Practice. New York: Macmillan, 1970.

Needham, R. A. Nursing Homes, Legal and Business Problems. New York: Practicing Law Institute, 1969.

Nick, W. V. Malpractice Literature Index. Columbus, Ohio: Legal Medicine Press, 1971.

Nursing Home Law Manual. Pittsburgh: The Health Law Center, Aspen Systems Corporation, 1970.

Physicians' Assistants Legal Regulation Survey. Pittsburgh: The Health Law Center, Aspen Systems Corporation, 1972.

Problems in Hospital Law. Pittsburgh: The Health Law Center, Aspen Systems Corporation, 1970.

Robitscher, J. B. Pursuit of Agreement: Psychiatry and the Law. Philadelphia: J. B. Lippincott, 1966.

Sagall, E. L. The Heart and the Law: A Practical Guide to Medicolegal Cardiology. New York: Macmillan, 1968.

Sagall, E. L. The Law and Clinical Medicine. Philadelphia: J. B. Lippincott, 1970.

Shindell, S. The Law in Medical Practice. Pittsburgh: University of Pittsburgh, 1966.

Summary of Labor Agreements with Various Hospitals Throughout U.S. Denver, Col.: The Mountain States Employers Council, Inc., 1968.

Szasz, T. Law, Liberty and Psychiatry. New York: Macmillan, 1963.

Tracy, J. E. The Doctor as a Witness. 2nd Ed. Philadelphia: W. B. Saunders, 1965.

University Health Law Center. Hospital Law Manual. Four volumes with quarterly supplements. Pittsburgh: University of Pittsburgh, Health Law Center, 1959–current.

U.S. Congress. Senate Committee on Government Operations. Medical Malpractice: The Patient Versus the Physician. Washington, D.C.: U.S. Government Printing Office, 1969.

Waltz, J. R. Medical Jurisprudence. New York: Macmillan, 1971.

Wasmuth, C. Law for the Physician. Philadelphia: Lea & Febiger, 1966.

Watnabe, T. Atlas of Legal Medicine. Philadelphia: J. B. Lippincott, 1968.

Wecht, C. H. Exploring the Medical Malpractice Dilemma. Mt. Kisco, N.Y.: Futura, 1972.


## LIBRARY SERVICES

Annan, G. Handbook of Medical Library Practice, Medical Library Center of New York. Washington, D.C.: The Medical Library Association, 1970.

Classification of Health Care Institutions. Chicago: The American Hospital Association, 1968.

Current Medical Terminology. 3rd Ed. Chicago: The American Medical Association, 1966.

Davies, P. Medical Terminology in Hospital Practice: A Guide for All Those Engaged in Professions Allied to Medicine. New York: William Heinemann Medical Books, 1969.

Dennis, R., and Doyle, J. M. The Complete Handbook for Medical Secretaries and Assistants. Boston: Little, Brown, 1971.
Donovan, F. Prepare Now for a Metric Future. New York: Weybright and Talley, 1970.
Essentials for Patients' Libraries; A Guide. New York: The United Hospital Fund of New York, 1966.
Frenay, Sister Agnes Clare. Understanding Medical Terminology. 5th edition. St. Louis: The Catholic Hospital Association, 1969.
Golann, S. Coordinate Index Reference Guide to Community Mental Health. New York: Behavioral Publications, 1969.
Guidebook for Catholic Health Care Facilities. St. Louis: The Catholic Hospital Association, 1969.
Standards for Library Service in Health Care Institutions. Chicago: The Association of Hospital and Institutional Libraries, 1970.
Steem, E. B. Medical Abbreviations. 2nd Ed. Philadelphia: Davis Publications, 1968.

## Bibliographies
Altman, I. et al. Methodology in Evaluating the Quality of Medical Care: An Annotated Bibliography, 1955–1968. Pittsburgh: Pittsburgh University Press, 1969.
Division of Medical Care Administration. Nursing Care for the Aged: An Annototated Bibliography for Nurses. By M. I. Brown, et al. Washington, D.C.: U.S. Government Printing Office, 1967.
Dunaye, T. Health Planning Applications of Operations Research and Systems Analysis. Monticello, Ill.: The Council of Planning Librarians, 1971.
Levy, S. and Loomba, N. P. Health Care Administration: A Selected Bibliography. Philadelphia: J. B. Lippincott, 1972.
Leyasmeyer, E., and Whitmarsh, L. A. Continuing Education in the Health Professions: An Annotated Bibliography. St. Paul: Northlands Regional Medical Program, Inc., 1969.
Meyer, J. K. Bibliography on the Urban Crisis: The Behavior, Psychological, and Sociological Aspects of the Urban Crisis. Bethesda, Md.: National Institute of Mental Health, 1969.
Pfeiffer, E. Bibliography on Sexual Behavior in Old Age. Boston: Little, Brown, 1969.
Planning and Regional Planning—What are They? Monticello, Ill.: The Council on Planning Librarians, 1971.
Shock, N. W. Classified Bibliography of Gerontology and Geriatrics. Supplements 1 and 2, 1949/55, 1956/61. Stanford, Cal.: Stanford University Press, 1963.
Starkweather, D. Health Facility Combinations and Mergers: An Annotated Bibliography. Chicago: American College of Hospital Administrators, 1970.
U.S. National Communicable Disease Center. Annotated Bibliography on In Service Training in Mental Health for Staff in Residential Institutions. Washington, D.C.: U.S. Government Printing Office, 1969.
U.S. Public Health Service. Community Care of the Mentally Ill: A Selected Annotated Bibliography. Washington, D.C.: U.S. Government Printing Office, 1966.

U.S. Public Health Service. Selected Bibliography of Regional Medical Pro-
grams. Washington, D.C.: U.S. Government Printing Office, 1969.
U.S. Veterans Administration, Medical and General Reference Library. We
Call it Bibliography: An Annotated Bibliography on Bibliotherapy and the
Adult Hospitalized Patient. Washington, D.C.: Veterans Administration,
1967.

## Cumulative Indices

Cumulative Index of Hospital Literature, 1960–1964. Chicago: The American
Hospital Association, 1966.
Henderson, V. Nursing Studies Index. Philadelphia: J. B. Lippincott, 1963.
Hospital Literature Index. Chicago: The American Hospital Association.
Index to Dental Literature. Chicago: The American Dental Association.
Annual.
National Library of Medicine. Index Medicus. Washington, D.C.: U.S. Govern-
ment Printing Office. Annual.
Nick, W. Malpractice Literature Index. Columbus, Ohio: Legal Medicine
Press, 1971.
U.S. Division of Research Grants, National Institutes of Health. Research
Grants Index. Two-Volume Annual. Washington, D.C.: U.S. Government
Printing Office, 1961.

## Directories

American Medical Directory: 1, Alpha Index of Physicians; 2 and 3, Geo-
graphical Register of Physicians. Chicago: The American Medical Associa-
tion, 1971.
Directory. Alexandria, Va.: The American Association of Medical Clinics,
1971.
Directory: A Register of Physicians of the United States and Canada. Chi-
cago: The American Medical Association, 1971.
Directory of Accredited Allied Medical Education Programs. Chicago: The
American Medical Association, 1969–1970.
Directory of Environmental Organization. Cleveland: The Metropolitan
Health Planning Corporation, 1971.
Directory of Health Sciences Libraries in the U.S. Chicago: The American
Medical Association, 1970.
Dybwad, R. International Directory of Mental Retardation Resources. Wash-
ington, D.C.: President's Committee on Mental Retardation, 1971.
Haney Associates, Inc. The Health Funds Directory. W. Concord, Mass.:
Health Funds Institute, 1970.
Hospitals: Guide Issue. Chicago: The American Hospital Association Annual.
National Ambulance and Medical Services. Directory. Westfield, Mass.: The
National Ambulance and Medical Services Association, 1971.
The AHA Guide to the Health Care Field, 1972 Ed. Chicago: The American
Hospital Association, 1972.
U.S. Administration on Aging. Senior Centers in the United States. Washing-
ton, D.C.: U.S. Government Printing Office, 1970.
U.S. Bureau of Apprenticeship and Training. Directory for Reaching Minority
Groups. Washington, D.C.: U.S. Government Printing Office, 1970.

U.S. National Clearinghouse for Poison Control Centers. Directory of Poison Control Centers. Washington, D.C.: U.S. Government Printing Office, 1970.

U.S. National Institute of Mental Health. Mental Health Directory. Washington, D.C.: Superintendent of Documents, 1971.

U.S. Office of Economic Opportunity Community Action Programs. Directory of Comprehensive Neighborhood Health Services Programs. Washington, D.C.: U.S. Government Printing Office, 1971.

U.S. Public Health Service. Directory of Local Health and Mental Health Units. Washington, D.C.: U.S. Government Printing Office, 1969.

U.S. Public Health Services. Directory of Selected Community Health Services Funded under Section 314(e) of Public Health Service Act. Rockville, Md.: Mental Health Association, 1970.

World Directory of Post-Basic and Post-Graduate Schools of Nursing. 1st Ed. Geneva, Switzerland: World Hospital Organization, 1965.

World Directory of Schools of Public Health. Geneva, Switzerland: World Health Association.

## LONG-TERM CARE

Blumberg, J. Nursing Care of the Long-Term Patient. New York: Springer, 1971.

Winds of Change. Chicago: The American Hospital Association, 1971.

Winter, K. Institutional Care for the Long-Term Patient. Ann Arbor, Mich.: University of Michigan, 1958.

### Extended Care

Griffith, J. R. A Reappraisal of the McPherson Experiment in Progressive Patient Care. Ann Arbor, Mich.: University of Michigan, 1970.

Illinois State Department of Public Health. Training Manual for Rehabilitation Programs in a Nursing Home and an Extended Care Facility. Springfield, Ill.: Rehabilitation Education Service, 1967.

Loebs, S. Traverse City Affiliation in Extended Care. Ann Arbor, Mich.: University of Michigan, 1969.

Transfer Agreements between Extended Care Facilities and Hospitals. Chicago: The American Hospital Association, 1966.

### Home Care

Hurtado, A. V., et al. Home Care and Extended Care in a Comprehensive Prepayment Plan. Chicago: Hospital Research and Educational Trust, 1972.

Nielsen, M. Home Aide Service and the Aged. Springfield, Va.: National Technical Information Service, 1970.

The Hospital and the Home Care Program. Chicago: The American Hospital Association, 1973.

Utilization Review Guidelines for Home Health Agencies. New York: The National League for Nursing, 1971.

## Nursing Homes

Braverman, J. Nursing Home Standards: A Tragic Dilemma in American Health. Washington, D.C.: The American Pharmaceutical Association, 1970.

City of New York, Board of Hospitals. Hospital Code—Part 1—Proprietary Nursing Homes. New York: The City Record, 1970.

Coggeshall, J. H. Management of Retirement Homes and Long Term Care Facilities. St. Louis: C. V. Mosby, 1973.

Cohen, J. B. Stroke Patients in Nursing Homes: A Preliminary Study of their Potential for Rehabilitation. San Francisco: California Commission on Regional Medical Programs, 1971.

Commission on Chronic Illness. Care of the Long-Term Patient. Cambridge: Harvard University Press, 1973.

George Washington University, Department of Health Care Administration. A Study of Nursing Homes and Related Facilities. Washington, D.C.: George Washington University Press, 1969.

Greenberg, D. U.S. Guide to Nursing Homes. New York: Grosset & Dunlap, 1970.

Hooper, L. Care of the Nursing Home Patient. Boston: Little, Brown, 1967.

Jacobs, H. L. Nursing and Retirement Home Administration. 1st Ed. Washington, D.C.: U.S. Government Printing Office, 1966.

Lucas, C. Recreational Activity Development for the Aging in Homes, Hospitals, and Nursing Homes. Springfield, Ill.: Charles C Thomas, 1962.

Mathieu, R. Hospital and Nursing Home Management: An Instructional and Administrative Manual. Philadelphia: W. B. Saunders, 1971.

McQuillan, F. Fundamentals of Nursing Home Administration. Philadelphia: W. B. Saunders, 1967.

Moss, A. L. Nursing Homes and Related Health Care Facilities. U.S. Training and Employment Service. Washington, D.C.: U.S. Government Printing Office, 1969.

Needham, R. A. Nursing Homes: Legal and Business Problems. New York: Practicing Law Institute, 1969.

Nursing Home Fact Book. Washington, D.C.: The American Nursing Home Association, 1971.

Nursing Homes and Their Patients. Albany: New York State Department of Health, 1970.

Nursing Homes for the Aged: The Agony of One Million Americans. Washington, D.C.: The Center for Study of Responsive Law, 1970.

Rogers, W. General Administration in the Nursing Home. Waco, Tex.: Davis Brothers, 1971.

Routh, T. Choosing a Nursing Home: The Problems and Their Solutions. Springfield, Ill.: Charles C Thomas, 1970.

Routh, T. Nursing Homes—A Blessing or a Curse. Springfield, Ill.: Charles C Thomas, 1970.

Schneeweiss, S. and Davis, S. Nursing Home Administration. Baltimore: University Park Press, 1974.

Stotsky, B. The Nursing Home and the Aged Psychiatric Patient. New York: Appleton-Century-Crofts, 1970.

Thomas, W. C. Nursing Homes and Public Policy Drift and Decision in New York State. Ithaca, N.Y.: Cornell University Press, 1970.
U.S. Congress, Senate Special Committee on Aging. Alternatives to Nursing Home Care: A Proposal. Washington, D.C.: Highlights, 1972.
U.S. Division of Health Resources Statistics. Nursing Homes: A County and Metropolitan Area Data Book. Washington, D.C.: U.S. Government Printing Office, 1970.
U.S. National Center for Health Statistics. Arrangements for Physicians Services to Residents in Nursing and Personal Care Homes. Washington, D.C.: U.S. Government Printing Office, 1970.
U.S. National Institutes of Health, Division of Nursing. Nursing Home Research Study: Quantitative Measurement of Nursing Services. Washington, D.C.: U.S. Government Printing Office, 1970.

**Progressive Patient Care**

Griffith, J., Weeks, L., and Sullivan, J. The McPherson Experiment. Ann Arbor, Mich.: University of Michigan Press, 1969.
Weeks, L., and Griffith, J. Progressive Patient Care. Ann Arbor, Mich.: University of Michigan Press, 1969.

## MEDICAL CARE PLANNING

American Assembly. The Health of Americans. Englewood Cliffs, N.J.: Prentice-Hall, 1970.
American Journal of Public Health and the Nation's Health, Vols. 1 and 2. Medical Care in Transition. Reprints from the American Journal of Public Health 1949–1962. Washington, D.C.: U.S. Department of Health, Education and Welfare, no date.
Anderson, O. W. Health Care: Can There Be Equity? The United States, Sweden, and England. New York: John Wiley & Sons, 1972.
An Introduction to Foundations for Medical Care. Chicago: Blue Cross, 1971.
Arnold, M. F., Blankenship, L. V., and Hess, J. Administering Health Systems: Issues and Perspectives. Chicago: Aldine-Atherton, 1971.
Bird, K. T. Teleconsultation: A New Health Information Exchange System. Springfield, Va.: National Technical Information Service, 1971.
Bloomfield, J. The Patient Returns to the Community: A Guide for a Voluntary Service Program in the Community. Washington, D.C.: U.S. Government Printing Office, 1966.
Chase, A. The Biological Imperatives: Health, Politics, and Human Survival. New York: Holt, Rinehart & Winston, 1971.
Davies, L. Facilities and Equipment for Health Services: Needed Research. New York: Milbank Memorial Fund, 1967.
Drucker, P. F. The Age of Discontinuity. New York: Harper & Row, 1968.
Edwards, M. H. Hazardous to Your Health: A New Look at the Health Care Crisis in America. New Rochelle, N.Y.: Arlington House, 1972.
Ehrenreich, B. The American Health Empire: Power, Profits and Politics. New York: Random House, 1971.
Expanding the Supply of Health Services in the 1970's. Report of the National Congress on Health Manpower. Chicago: The American Medical Association, 1971.

Family Planning: A Guide for State and Local Agencies. Washington, D.C.: The American Public Health Association, 1968.

Health Crisis in America. New York: The American Public Health Association, 1970.

Helicopter Ambulance Service to Emergencies–Project Haste. Minneapolis: The Minnesota Department of Health, 1971.

Improving our Nation's Health Care System: Proposals for the Seventies. Washington, D.C.: The U.S. Chamber of Commerce, 1971.

Jarett, I. M. Foundations for Medical Care: Managerial, Organizational System Development Aspects; A Statement of Observations and Recommendations. Springfield, Ill.: School of Medicine, Southern Illinois University, 1972.

Kane, R. L. Federal Health Care (with Reservations!). New York: Springer, 1972.

Kennedy, E. M. In Critical Condition: The Crisis in America's Health Care. New York: Simon & Schuster, 1972.

Knowles, J. Hospitals, Doctors and the Public Interest. Cambridge: Harvard University Press, 1965.

Local Health Official's Guide to Occupational Health. New York: The American Public Health Association, 1968.

Mechanic, D. Public Expectations and Health Care: Essays on the Changing Organization of Health Services. New York: John Wiley & Sons, 1972.

National Urban Coalition. Counterbudget: A Blueprint for Changing National Priorities. New York: Praeger, 1971.

Policy Statement on Provision of Health Services. Chicago: The American Hospital Association, 1971.

Report of a Conference on Care of Chronically Ill Adults. Chicago: The American Hospital Association, 1971.

Report of a Special Committee on the Provision of Health Services. Chicago: The American Hospital Association, 1970.

Reuther, W. The Organization, Costs and Quality of Medical Care in the U.S. Detroit: United Automobile Workers Union, 1968.

Ribicoff, A. A. The American Medical Machine. New York: Saturday Review Press, 1972.

Rushmer, R. F. Medical Engineering: Projections for Health Care Delivery. New York: Academic Press, 1972.

Schorr, D. Don't Get Sick in America. Nashville: Aurora Pub. Co., 1970.

Schulberg, H. Program Evaluation in the Health Fields. New York: Behavioral Publications, 1970.

Somers, A. Health Care in Transition: New Direction for the Future. New York: Hospital Research Educational Trust, 1971.

Stevens, R. American Medicine and the Public Interest. New Haven, Conn.: Yale University Press, 1971.

Strickland, S. P. U.S. Health: What's Wrong and What's Right. New York: Universe Books, 1972.

Symposium on Health. The Recognition of Systems in Health Services. Arlington, Va.: Operations Research Society of America, 1969.

Thomas, C., and Schwartz, J. L. Medical Plans and Health Care: Consumer Participation in Policy Making with a Special Section on Medicare. Springfield, Ill.: Charles C Thomas, 1968.

Titmuss, R. The Gift Relationship: From Human Blood to Social Policy. London: George Allen & Unwin, 1970.

Training in National Health Planning. Geneva, Switzerland: The World Health Organization, 1970.

Tripodi, T. Social Program Evaluation. Itasca, Ill.: F. E. Peacock, 1971.

U.S. Congress, House Commission on Ways and Means. Basic Facts on the Health Industry. Washington, D.C.: U.S. Government Printing Office, 1971.

U.S. Department of Health, Education and Welfare. Towards a Comprehensive Health Policy for the 1970's. Washington, D.C.: U.S. Government Printing Office, 1971.

U.S. Public Health Service. Ethical Issues in Health Care. By J. Carmody. Washington, D.C.: U.S. Government Printing Office, 1970.

White, R. L. Right to Health: The Evolution of an Idea. Iowa City, Iowa: Graduate Program in Hospital and Health Administration, University of Iowa, 1971.

Wolstenholme, G. Teamwork for World Health. Baltimore: Williams & Wilkins, 1971.

## Area Wide and Comprehensive Planning

Bjorn, J. C. Problem Oriented Private Practice of Medicine. Chicago: Modern Hospital Press, 1970.

Boothe, W. Consumer Participation in Comprehensive Health Planning. Monticello, Ill.: The Council of Planning Librarians, 1969.

Brown, D. R. Areawide Hospital Planning Process. Springfield, Va.: National Technical Information Service, 1971.

Community Health, Inc. Toward an Approval Program for Area Wide Health Planning Agencies; Report of a Conference at Detroit. New York: The Corporation, 1969.

Silver, G. A. Family Medical Care: A Report on the Family Health Maintenance Demonstration. Cambridge: Harvard University Press, 1963.

Task Force on Comprehensive Personal Health Service. Comprehensive Health Care: A Challenge to American Communities. Washington, D.C.: Public Affairs Press, 1967.

Towards a Comprehensive Health Policy for the 1970's. Washington, D.C.: U.S. Department of Health, Education and Welfare, 1971.

## Community Planning

Anderson, C. L. Community Health. St. Louis: C. V. Mosby, 1969.

Beigel, A. The Community Mental Health Center: Strategies and Programs. New York: Basic Books, 1972.

Buell, B. et al. Community Planning for Human Services. New York: Columbia University Press, 1952.

Coleman, J. Community Conflict. New York: The Free Press, 1957.

Community Organization, Planning and Community Development. (Some common and destructive elements; a collection of papers). New York: The Council on Social Word Education, 1961.

Comprehensive Community Services for Alcoholics. Washington, D.C.: The U.S. National Institute of Mental Health, 1970.

Conant, R. The Politics of Community Health. Washington, D.C.: The American Public Health Association, 1968.

Confrey, E. A., (ed.). Administration of Community Health Services. Chicago: International City Managers' Association, 1961.

Cox, F. M., et al. Strategies of Community Organization: A Book of Readings. Itasca, Ill.: F. E. Peacock, 1970.

Cross, J. N. Guide to the Community Control of Alcoholism. Washington, D.C.: The American Public Health Association, 1968.

Form, W. Community in Disaster. New York: Harper & Row, 1958.

Kotz, A. Health and Community. New York: The Free Press, 1965.

Meyer, R. J. Getting It All Together: Problems, Priorities and Funding for Community Health Programs. Washington, D.C.: Department of Health, Education and Welfare, 1970.

Morris, R. Feasible Planning for Social Change. New York: Columbia University Press, 1966.

National Commission on Community Health Services. Health is a Community Affair; Report. Cambridge: Harvard University Press, 1966.

Parks, R. B. Community Health Services for New York City: A Case Study in Urban Medical Delivery. New York: Frederick A. Praeger, 1968.

Rhodes, W. Behavioral Threat and Community Response. New York: Behavioral Publications, 1972.

Ross, M., and Lappin, B. W. Community Organization, Theory, Principles and Practices. 2nd Ed. New York: Harper & Row, 1967.

Schindler-Rainman, E. The Volunteer Community: Creative Use of Human Resources. Washington, D.C.: National Training Laboratory Learning Resources, 1971.

The Community Mental Health Centers Programs—Improvements Needed in Management. Washington, D.C.: U.S. General Accounting Office, 1971.

Zusman, J. Organizing the Community to Prevent Suicide. Springfield, Ill.: Charles C Thomas, 1971.

## Neighborhood Planning

Chenault, W. W. Consumer Participation in Neighborhood Comprehensive Health Care Centers. Springfield, Va.: National Technical Information Service, 1971.

Richardson, W. C. Ambulatory Use of Physicians' Services in Response to Illness Episodes in Low-Income Neighborhood. Chicago: Center for Health Administration Studies, 1971.

## MEDICINE AND PUBLIC HEALTH

Alexander, F. Psychosomatic Medicine. New York: W. W. Norton, 1950.

Alvariz, W. C. Little Strokes. Philadelphia. J. B. Lippincott, 1966.

American Public Health Association. Vital and Health Statistics Monographs: Cardiovascular Disease in the United States. Cambridge. Harvard University Press, 1971.

Babbie, E. R. Science and Morality in Medicine: A Survey of Medical Educators. Berkeley, Cal.: University of California Press, 1970.

Baker, F., et al. (ed.). Industrial Organizations and Health. New York: Barnes & Noble, 1969.

Baldry, P. E. The Battle against Heart Disease. New York: Cambridge University Press, 1971.

Beecher, H. Research and the Individual: Human Studies. Boston: Little, Brown, 1970.

Belinkoff, S. Emphysema and Chronic Bronchitis. Boston: Little, Brown, 1971.

Brim, O. The Dying Patient. New York: Russell Sage Foundation, 1970.

Brook, S. M. The V.D. Story: Medicine's Battle against the Scourge of Venereal Disease. Cranbury, N.J.: A. S. Barnes, 1971.

Brooke, B. N. Understanding Cancer. New York: Holt, Rinehart & Winston, 1973.

Brown, W. et al. Syphillis and Other Venereal Diseases in the United States. Cambridge: Harvard University Press, 1970.

Burris, D. S. The Right to Treatment: A Symposium. New York: Springer, 1969.

Burton, L. E., and Smith, H. H. Public Health and Community Medicine. Baltimore: Williams & Wilkins, 1970.

Campion, R. The Invisible Worm. New York: Macmillan, 1972.

Cardiovascular Diseases. Monograph. San Francisco: The American Public Health Association, 1962.

Catastrophic Illness in the Seventies: Critical Issues and the Complex Decisions. New York: Cancer Care, Inc. of The National Cancer Foundation, 1971.

Clark, D. and MacMahon, B. Textbook of Preventive Medicine. Boston: Little, Brown, 1967.

Clarke, E. Modern Methods in the History of Medicine. London: Athlorie Press, 1971.

Cheraskin, E. New Hope for Incurable Diseases. Jericho, N.Y.: Exposition Press, 1971.

Coe, R. M. and Brehm, H. P. Preventive Health Care for Adults; A Study of Medical Practice. New Haven, Conn.: College & University Press, 1972.

Committee for Radiation Therapy Studies. Prospect for Radiation Therapy in the U.S. Bethesda, Md.: National Institutes of Health, 1968.

Control of Communicable Diseases in Man. 10th Ed. Washington, D.C.: The American Public Health Association, 1965.

Coser, R. Life in the Ward. East Lansing, Mich.: Michigan State University Press, 1962.

Crichton, M. Five Patients: The Hospital Explained. New York: Alfred A. Knopf, 1970.

Cutler, A. Four Minutes to Life. New York: Cowles, 1970.

DeVise, P. Slum Medicine: Chicago's Apartheid Health System. Chicago: University of Chicago, 1969.

Downing, A. B. Euthanasia and the Right to Death. New York: Humanities Press, 1970.

Dublin, L. I. Factbook on Man from Birth to Death. 2nd Ed. New York: Macmillan, 1965.

Dubos, R. Mirage of Health: Utopias, Progress and Biological Change. Garden City, N.Y.: Doubleday, 1961.

Dubos, R. Man, Medicine and Environment. New York: Praeger, 1968.

Duffy, J. Epidemics in Colonial America. Baton Rouge, La.: Louisiana State University Press, 1971.

Entralso, P. L. Doctor and Patient. New York: McGraw-Hill, 1969.

Fox, J. P., et al. Epidemiology: Man and Disease. New York: Macmillan, 1970.

Galdston, I. Medicine and the Other Disciplines. New York: International Universities Press, 1973.

Galdston, I. Medicine in Transition. Chicago: University of Chicago Press, 1965.

Galdston, I. On the Utility of Medical History. New York: International Universities Press, 1973.

Gerber, A. The Gerber Report, The Shocking State. New York: David McKay, 1971.

Geyman, J. The Modern Family Doctor and Changing Medical Practice. New York: Appleton-Century-Crofts, 1971.

Goerke, L., and Stebbins, E. Mustard's Introduction to Public Health, New York: Macmillan, 1968.

Goodman, R. M. The Face in Genetic Disorders, St. Louis: C. V. Mosby, 1970.

Guidelines for Cancer Care: Organization, Personnel Facilities. Chicago: The American College of Surgeons, 1970.

Haagard, H. W. Devils, Drugs and Doctors, New York: Harper & Row, 1929.

Hanlon, J. Principles of Public Health Administration. 4th Ed. St. Louis: C. V. Mosby, 1964.

Harvard University School of Public Health. Political Science and Public Health; Report of the Harvard University School of Public Health. Rockville, Md.: Community Health Service, Health Services and Mental Health Administration, 1971.

Henry Ford Hospital. Pain. Boston: Little, Brown, 1966.

Hunter, D. The Diseases of Occupations. Boston: Little, Brown, 1969.

Jellinek, E. The Disease Concept of Alcoholism. New Haven, Conn.: Hillhouse Press, 1960.

Jones, B. (ed.). Health of Americans. Englewood Cliffs, N.J.: Prentice-Hall, 1970.

Kelly, G. A. Medico-Moral Problems. St. Louis: Catholic Hospital Association of the United States and Canada, 1958.

Kessler, I. Community As an Epidemiologic Laboratory. Baltimore: The Johns Hopkins University Press, 1970.

Kubler-Ross, E. On Death and Dying. New York: Macmillan, 1969.

Labby, D. H. Life or Death Ethics and Options. Portland, Ore. Reed College, 1968.

Leavell, H. R. Textbook of Preventive Medicine. New York: McGraw-Hill, 1953.

Leavell, H. R. Preventive Medicine for the Doctor in His Community. 3rd Ed. New York: McGraw-Hill, 1965.

Local Health Official's Guide to Occupational Health. New York: The American Public Health Association, 1968.

Longmore, D. Machines in Medicine: The Medical Practice of the Future. Garden City, N.Y.: Doubleday, 1970.

McCready, B. W. On the Influence of Trades, Professions, and Occupations in the U.S. in the Production of Disease. New York. Arno Press, 1943.

MacKenzie, R. Clinical Rheumatology. Philadelphia: J. B. Lippincott, 1970.

MacKenzie, R. Risk. New York: Viking Press, 1971.

MacMahon, P. I. Epidemiologic Methods. Boston: Little, Brown, 1960.
Magraw, R. M. Ferment in Medicine: A Study of the Essence of Medical Practice and of Its New Dilemmas. Philadelphia: W. B. Saunders, 1966.
Marshall, C. L. and Pearson, D. Dynamics of Health and Disease. New York: Appleton-Century-Crofts, 1972.
Mason, M. Clinical Rheumatology. Philadelphia: J. B. Lippincott, 1970.
Masters, W. H. Human Sexual Inadequacy. Boston: Little, Brown, 1970.
Maxey, K. F., and Sortwell, P. Rosenau's Preventive Medicine and Public Health. New York: Appleton-Century-Crofts, 1965.
May, J. M. The Ecology of Human Disease. Chicago: MD Publications, 1968.
Miller, B. F., and Galton, L. Freedom from Heart Attacks. New York: Simon & Schuster, 1972.
Miller, G. Moral and Ethical Implications of Human Organ Transplants. Springfield, Ill.: Charles C Thomas, 1971.
National Stroke Congress: Rehabilitation Management Prevention. Proceedings. Springfield, Ill.: Charles C Thomas, 1964.
Oliver, W. Stalkers of Pestilence. College Park, Md.: McGrath, 1971.
Palmore, E. Prediction of Life Span. Lexington, Mass.: Heath Lexington Books, 1971.
Public Health Service, Department of Health, Education and Welfare. 1970 Special Hospital Services for Cardiovascular Disease Patients. Washington, D.C.: Superintendent of Documents, 1971.
Ramsey, P. The Patient as a Person: Explorations in Medical Ethics. New Haven, Conn.: Yale University Press, 1970.
Rogers, F. Studies in Epidemiology: Selected Papers of Morris Greenberg, M.D. New York: G. P. Putman's Sons, 1965.
Rosen, G. A History of Public Health. New York: MD Publications, 1958.
Roueche, B. Annals of Epidemiology. Boston: Little, Brown, 1967.
Russell Sage Foundation Bulletin. Sociology and the Field of Public Health. New York: The American Sociological Association, 1971.
Rutstein, D. D. The Coming Revolution in Medicine. Cambridge: M.I.T. Press, 1967.
Schoenberg, B. Loss and Grief: Psychological Management in Medical Practice. New York: Columbia University Press, 1970.
Sigerist, H. Civilization and Disease. College Park, Md.: McGrath, 1971.
Sigerist, H. Medicine and Human Welfare. College Park, Md.: McGrath, 1971.
Sinacore, J. S. Health: A Quality of Life. New York: Macmillan, 1968.
Smith, H. L. Ethics and the New Medicine. Nashville: Abingdon Press, 1970.
Smith, R. At Your Own Risk: The Case Against Chiropractice. New York: Trident Press, 1969.
Snow, J. On the Mode of Communication of Chlorea. Radford, Va.: Commonwealth Fund Press, 1936.
Stevens, R. American Medicine and the Public Interest. New Haven, Conn.: Yale University Press, 1971.
Strauss, A. Where Medicine Fails. Chicago: Aldine, 1970.
Strickland, S. P. Politics, Science and Dread Disease. Cambridge: Harvard University Press, 1972.
Taylor, G. R. The Biological Time Bomb, New York: World Publ. Co., 1968.
Thorner, R. Principles and Procedures in the Evaluation of Screening for Disease. Washington, D.C.: U.S. Government Printing Office, 1971.

Thornwald, J. The Patients. New York: Harcourt Brace Javanovich, 1972.

Titmuss, R. The Gift Relationship: From Human Blood to Social Policy. New York: Pantheon Books, 1971.

Torrey, E. F. Ethical Issues in Medicine: The Role of the Physician in Today's Society. Boston: Little, Brown, 1968.

Tunley, R. The American Health Scandal. New York: Harper & Row, 1966.

U.S. Congress, House Committee on Education and Labor. Black Lung Benefits. Washington, D.C.: U.S. Government Printing Office, 1971.

U.S. Congress, Senate Committee on Labor and Public Welfare. Conquest of Cancer Act, 1971. Washington, D.C.: U.S. Government Printing Office, 1971.

U.S. Congress, Senate Subcommittee on Health of the Elderly. Hearings on Detection and Prevention of Chronic Disease Utilizing Multiphasic Health Screening Techniques. Washington, D.C.: U.S. Government Printing Office, 1966.

U.S. National Heart Institute. Cardiac Replacement: Medical, Ethical, Psychological and Economic Implications. Washington, D.C.: U.S. Government Printing Office, 1969.

U.S. Public Health Service. Automated Multiphasic Health Testing Bibliography. Washington, D.C.: U.S. Government Printing Office, 1970.

U.S. Public Health Service. Provisional Guidelines for Automated Multiphasic Health Testing Services. Washington, D.C.: H.S.M.H.A., 1970.

Wallach, J. Interpretation of Diagnostic Tests: A Handbook Synopsis of Laboratory Medicine. Boston: Little, Brown, 1972.

Warbasse, J. The Doctor and the Public. College Park, Md.: McGrath, 1971.

Wolff, H. G. Stress and Disease. Springfield, Ill.: Charles C Thomas, 1968.

Zimmerman, C. Techniques of Patient Care: A Manual of Bedside Procedures for Students, Interns and Residents. Boston: Little, Brown, 1972.

## Acupuncture

Austin, M. Acupuncture Therapy. New York: ASI Publishers, 1972.

Duke, M. Acupuncture. New York: Pyramid House, 1972.

## Housing

Guide for Health Administrators in Housing Hygiene. Washington, D.C.: The American Public Health Association, 1967.

## Multiphasic Screening

Gelman, A. Multiphasic Health Testing/Screening Systems. Rockville, Md.: National Technical Information Services, 1970.

U.S. Department of Health, Education and Welfare and Mental Health Administration. Multiphasic Health Testing Systems: Reviews and Annotations. Washington, D.C.: U.S. Government Printing Office, 1971.

## Thanatology and Euthansia

Gould, J. (ed.). Your Death Warrant? The Implications of Euthanasia—A Medical, Legal and Ethical Study. Worcester, England: Fowler-Wright Books, 1971.

Kutscher, A. H., and Kutscher, L. G. Religion and Bereavement: Counsel for the Physician, Advice for the Bereaved, Thoughts for the Clergyman. New York: Health Sciences Publ. Corp., 1972.

Lasagna, L. Life, Death, the Doctor. New York: Alfred A. Knopf, 1968.

Scott, F. G. Confrontations of Death: A Book of Readings and Suggested Method of Instruction. Cornwallis, Ore.: Continuing Education Publications, 1971.

Verwoerdt, A. Communication with the Fatally Ill. Springfield, Ill.: Charles C Thomas, 1966.

Weisman, A. Dying and Denying—A Psychiatric Study of Terminality. New York: Behavioral Publications, 1972.

Weisman, A. D. and Kastenbaum, R. The Psychological Autopsy. New York: Behavioral Publications, 1968.

Williams, R. H. (ed.). To Live and To Die: When, Why, and How. New York: Springer-Verlag, 1973.

Zborowski, M. People in Pain. San Francisco: Jossey-Bass, 1969.


## MENTAL HEALTH

Albee, G. W. Mental Health Manpower Trends. New York: Basic Books, 1959.

Alvarez, A. The Savage God. New York: Random House, 1972.

American Psychiatric Association. Remotivation: Basic Facts About a Useful Nursing Home Program. Washington, D.C.: Smith Kline & French Laboratories, no date.

Anderson, D. B., and McClean, L. J. Identifying Suicide Potential. New York: Behavioral Publications, 1971.

Arieti, S. American Handbook of Psychiatry. New York: Basic Books, 1966.

Barry, A. Bellevue is a State of Mind. New York: Harcourt Brace & World, 1971.

Barten, H. H. Brief Therapies. New York: Behavioral Publications, 1971.

Baumeister, A. Residential Facilities for the Mentally Retarded. Chicago: Aldine, 1970.

Belsasso, G. Psychiatric Care of the Underprivileged, No. 088692. Boston: Little, Brown, 1972.

Bernstein, N. Diminished People: Problems and Care of the Mentally Retarded. Boston: Little, Brown, 1972.

Bindman, A. (ed.) Perspectives in Community Mental Health. Chicago: Aldine, 1969.

Bond, D. D., et al. Psychiatry and Applied Mental Health. Chicago: Year Book Medical Publishers, 1971.

Bovkoven, J. Moral Treatment in Community Mental Health. New York: Springer, 1972.

Caplan, G. Principles of Prevention Psychiatry. New York: Basic Books, 1964.

Carter, J. W., Jr. Research Contributions from Psychology to Community Mental Health, New York: Behavioral Publications, 1968.

Caudill, W. The Mental Hospital as a Small Society. Cambridge: Harvard University Press, 1958.

Choron, J. Suicide. New York: Charles Scribner's Sons, 1972.

Clausen, J. A. Sociology and the Field of Mental Health. New York: Russell Sage Foundation, 1956.

Cleland, C. C. Mental Retardation: Approaches to Institutional Change. New York: Grune & Stratton, 1969.

Coles, R. Erik H. Erikson: The Growth of His Work. Boston: Little, Brown, 1970.

Collins, W. J. Out of the Depths: The Story of a Priest-Patient in a Mental Hospital. Garden City, N.Y.: Doubleday, 1971.

Dunham, H. W., and Weinberg, S. The Culture of the State Mental Hospital. Detroit: Wayne State University Press, 1960.

Favazza, A. R. Guide for Mental Health Workers. Ann Arbor, Mich.: University of Michigan Press, 1970.

Glasscote, R. et al. The Community Mental Health Center: An Interim Appraisal. Washington, D.C.: Joint Information Service of The American Psychological Association and The American Medical Association, 1969.

Glasscote, R. Halfway Houses for the Mentally Ill: A Study of Programs and Problems. Washington, D.C.: Joint Information Service of The American Psychiatric Association, 1971.

Goffman, E. Asylums. Garden City, N.Y.: Doubleday, 1961.

Golann, S.E. Coordinate Index Reference Guide to Community Mental Health. New York: Behavioral Publications, 1969.

Gottesfeld, H. The Critical Issues in Community Mental Health. New York: Behavioral Publications, 1972.

Greenblatt, M. From Custodial to Therapeutic Patient Care in Mental Hospitals. New York: Russell Sage Foundation, 1955.

Greenblatt, M. Dynamics of Institutional Change: The Hospital in Transition. Pittsburgh: University of Pittsburgh Press, 1971.

Grunebaum, H. The Practice of Community Mental Health. Boston: Little, Brown, 1970.

Gurin, G. et al. Americans View Their Mental Health. New York: Basic Books, 1960.

Harvard Medical School. Community Mental Health and Social Psychiatry: A Reference Guide. Cambridge: Harvard University Press, 1962.

Hollingshead, A. B., and Redlick, F. C. Social Class and Mental Illness. New York: Basic Books, 1960.

Jarvis, E. The Insanity and Idiocy in Massachusetts (Report of the Commission on Lunacy, 1855). Cambridge: The Commonwealth Fund, Harvard University Press, 1971.

Joint Commission on Mental Health. Action for Mental Health. New York: Basic Books, 1961.

Joint Commission on Mental Health of Children. Crisis in Child Mental Health: Challenge for the 1970's. New York: Harper & Row, 1970.

Kaplan, O. J. Mental Disorders of Later Life. Stanford, Cal.: Stanford University Press, 1956.

Kastenbaum, R. Contributions to the Psychology of Aging. New York: Springer, 1966.

Kline, N. S., et al. (eds.). Modern Problems of Pharmacopsychiatry. Vol. 3, Depression, Its Diagnosis and Treatment, Lithium, The History of Its Use in Psychiatry. New York: Karger-Phiebig, 1969.

Lamb, R. H. (ed.). Handbook of Community Mental Health Practices. San Francisco: Jossey-Bass, 1969.

Lamb, R. H., et al. Rehabilitation in Community Mental Health. San Francisco: Jossey-Bass, 1971.

Leedy, J. Compensation in Psychiatric Disability and Rehabilitation. Springfield, Ill.: Charles C Thomas, 1971.

Leininger, M. Contemporary Issues in Mental Health Nursing. Boston: Little, Brown, 1972.

Lester, G. The Gamble with Death. Englewood Cliffs, N.J.: Prentice-Hall, 1971.

Mechanic, D. Mental Health and Social Policy. Englewood Cliffs, N.J.: Prentice-Hall, 1969.

Mental Health Services and the General Hospital. Chicago: The American Hospital Association, 1970.

Mental Health Problems of Aging and Aged. World Health Organization Technical Report. Geneva, Switzerland: The World Health Organization, 1959.

Monroe, R. et al. Psychiatry, Epidemiology and Mental Health Planning. Washington, D.C.: The American Psychiatric Association, 1967.

Morris, G. The Mentally Ill and the Right to Treatment. Springfield, Ill.: Charles C Thomas, 1970.

Morrissey, J. R. The Case for Family Care of Mentally Ill. Monograph No. 2. New York: Behavioral Publications, 1967.

Neugeboren, B. Psychiatric Clinics: A Typology of Service Patterns. Metuchen, N.J.: Scarecrow Press, 1970.

Post, F. The Clinical Psychiatry of Late Life. London: Pergamon Press, 1965.

Raphael, W. Psychiatric Hospitals Viewed by Their Patients. London: King Edward's Hospital Fund for London, 1972.

Reiff, R. and Reissman, F. The Indigenous Non-Professional: A Strategy of Change in Community Action and Community Mental Health Programs. Monograph 1. New York: Behavioral Publications, 1965.

Roberts, L. M., et al. Comprehensive Mental Health: The Challenge of Evaluation. Madison, Wisc.: University of Wisconsin Press, 1968.

Robinson, A. M. Working with the Mentally Ill. 4th Ed. Philadelphia: J. B. Lippincott, 1971.

Rosen, G. Madness in Society: Chapters in the Historical Sociology of Mental Illness. Chicago: University of Chicago Press, 1968.

Scheibe, K. College Students on Chronic Wards. Monograph No. 5. New York: Behavioral Publications, 1969.

Scheidemandel, P. Mentally Ill Offender; A Survey of Treatment Programs. Washington, D.C.: Joint Information Service of The American Psychiatric Association and National Association for Mental Health, 1969.

Shore, M. F. Mental Health and the Community: Problems, Programs, and Strategies. New York: Behavioral Publications, 1969.

Slotkin, E. J. Mental Health Related Activities of Companies and Unions. New York: Behavioral Publications, 1971.

Sobey, F. The Non-Professional Revolution in Mental Health. New York: Columbia University Press, 1970.

Soddy, K. Mental Health in a Changing World. Philadelphia: J. B. Lippincott, 1965.

Squire, M. Current Administrative Practices for Psychiatric Services. Springfield, Ill.: Charles C Thomas, 1970.

Susser, M. Community Psychiatry: Epidemiologic and Social Themes. New York: Random House, 1968.

Szasz, T. S. Law, Liberty and Psychiatry. New York: Macmillan, 1963.

Thomas, A., and Sillen, S. Racism and Psychiatry. New York: Brunner-Mazel, 1972.

Tulipan, A. B., and Feldman, S. Psychiatric Clinics in Transition. New York: Brunner/Mazel, 1969.

Ulett, G. A., and Goodrich, D. W. A Synopsis of Contemporary Psychiatry. St. Louis: C. V. Mosby, 1969.

Ullmann, L. P. Institution and Outcome: A Comparative Study of Psychiatric Hospitals. New York: Pergamon Press, 1967.

Ullman, M. Behavioral Changes in Patients Following Strokes. (Publication 479, American Lecture Series.) Springfield, Ill.: Charles C Thomas, 1962.

U.S. National Institute of Mental Health. Mental Health Consultation to Programs for Children; a Review of Data Collected from Selected U.S. Sites. Washington, D.C.: U.S. Government Printing Office, 1970.

U.S. National Institute of Mental Health. Mental Health Directory. Washington, D.C.: U.S. Government Printing Office, 1971.

U.S. National Institute of Mental Health. Non-Professional Personnel in Mental Health Programs—A Survey. Washington, D.C.: U.S. Government Printing Office, 1969.

U.S. President's Committee on Mental Retardation. A First Report to the President on the Nation's Progress and Remaining Great Needs in the Campaign to Combat Mental Retardation. Washington, D.C.: U.S. Government Printing Office, 1967.

U.S. President's Committee on Mental Retardation. Residential Services for the Mentally Retarded; An Action Policy Proposal. Washington, D.C.: U.S. Government Printing Office, 1970.

U.S. President's Task Force on the Mentally Handicapped. Action Against Mental Disability. Washington, D.C.: U.S. Government Printing Office, 1970.

Weiner, L. Home Treatment: Spearhead of Community Psychiatry. Pittsburgh: University of Pittsburgh Press, 1967.

What Are the Facts about Mental Illness in the U.S.? Washington, D.C.: National Committee Against Mental Illness, 1966.

Whittington, H. C. Psychiatry in the American Community. New York: International Universities Press, 1973.

Wolff, K. Social and Cultural Factors in Mental Health and Mental Illness. Springfield, Ill.: Charles C Thomas, 1971.

Zuk, G. H. Family Therapy—A Triadic Based Approach. New York: Behavioral Publications, 1972.

## Alcoholism

Comprehensive Community Services for Alcoholics. Washington, D.C.: National Institute of Mental Health, 1970.

Cross, J. N. Guide to the Community Control of Alcoholism. Washington, D.C.: The American Public Health Association, 1968.

Strachan, J. G. Alcoholism: Treatable Illness. Vancouver, Can.: Mitchell Press, 1971.

Strachan, J. G. Practical Alcholism Programming. Vancouver, Can.: Mitchell Press, 1971.

**Drug Abuse**

Ball, J. C., and Chambers, C. D. (eds.). The Epidemiology of Opiate Addiction in the United States. Springfield, Ill.: Charles C Thomas, 1970.

Bloomquist, E. R. Marijuanna: The Second Trip. Beverly Hills, Cal.: Glencoe Press, 1971.

Brill, L., and Lieberman, L. Major Modalities in the Treatment of Drug Abuse. New York: Behavioral Publications, 1972.

Epstein, S. Drugs of Abuse. Cambridge: M.I.T. Press, 1971.

Smith, D. E., et al. The Free Clinic: A Community Approach to Health Care and Drug Abuse. Beloit, Wisc.: Stash Press, 1972.

U.S. Congress, Commission on Government Operations. The Safety and Effectiveness of New Drugs: Advertising and Promotion of Prescription Drugs. Hearings . . . held May 4, 1971. Washington, D.C.: U.S. Government Printing Office, 1971.

U.S. Congress, House Commission Government Operations. The Safety and Effectiveness of New Drugs: Standards for Evaluating Drug Effectiveness and Enforcement Problems, Hearings . . . held May 5, 1971. Washington, D.C.: U.S. Government Printing Office, 1971.

U.S. Congress, House Commission on Government Operations. The Safety and Effectiveness of New Drugs: Marketing of Fixed Combination Drugs and Unapproved New Drugs; Implementation of Drug Officacy Findings, Hearings . . . held May 26, 1971. Washington, D.C.: U.S. Government Printing Office, 1971.

**NURSING**

Alexander, E. et al. Nursing Service Administration: Principles and Practice. St. Louis: C. V. Mosby, 1962.

Alexander, E. Nursing Administration in the Hospital Health Care System. St. Louis: C. V. Mosby, 1972.

ANS's Facts About Nursing 1970–1971. New York: The Department of Research and Statistics, American Nursing Association, 1972.

Black, H. Impact of Unit Dose Pharmacy on the Time Involvement of Registered Nurses W. Medication Activities. Iowa City, Iowa: University of Iowa, 1971.

Brown, E. L. Nursing in the Future. New York: Russell Sage Foundation, 1948.

Brown, E. L. Nursing Reconsidered. A Study of Change. Philadelphia: J. B. Lippincott, 1970.

Cohn, H., et al. Manual for Nurses in Family and Community Health. Boston: Little, Brown, 1969.

Cooper, S. S. Contemporary Nursing Practice: A Guide for the Returning Nurse. New York: McGraw-Hill, 1970.

Creighton, H. Law Every Nurse Should Know. Philadelphia: W. B. Saunders, 1970.

DeYoung, C., and Tower, M. Nurses' Role in Community Mental Health Centers: Out of Uniform and Into Trouble. St. Louis: C. V. Mosby, 1971.

Eckelberry, G. K. Administration of Comprehensive Nursing Care: The

Nature of Professional Practice. New York: Appleton-Century-Crofts, 1971.

Eng, E. Staff Development in a Hospital Nursing Service. New York: National League for Nursing, 1972.

Friesen No-Nursing Concept: Its Effects on Nurse Staffing. Ann Arbor, Mich.: Chix Systems, Inc., 1970.

Geitgey, D. A. Handbook for Head Nurses. 2nd Ed. Philadelphia: F. A. Davis, 1971.

Handel, D. Studies in Hospital Administration: Nurses and Collective Bargaining. Chicago: Center for Health Administration Studies, 1969.

Heckel, R. V. Psychology—The Nurse and the Patient. St. Louis: C. V. Mosby, 1967.

Innis, M. Nursing Education in a Changing Society. Toronto: University of Toronto Press, 1970.

Kallin, E. L. Textbook of Public Health Nursing. St. Louis: C. V. Mosby, 1967.

King, I. Toward a Theory for Nursing: General Concepts of Human Behavior. New York: John Wiley & Sons, 1971.

Leininger, M. Contemporary Issues in Mental Health Nursing. Boston: Little, Brown, 1972.

Lesnik, M. J. Nursing Practice and the Law. 2nd Ed. Philadelphia: J. B. Lippincott, 1962.

Lewis, E. P., et al. Changing Patterns of Nursing Practice: New Needs, New Roles. Contemporary Nursing Series. New York: American Journal of Nursing Company, 1971.

Mayers, M. G. A Systematic Approach to the Nursing Care Plan. New York: Appleton-Century-Crofts, 1972.

Miller, C. Nurses and the Law. Danville, Ill.: Interstate Printers and Publishers, 1970.

Murchison, I. Legal Foundations of Nursing Practice. New York: Macmillan, 1970.

National Commission for the Study of Nursing and Nursing Education. Abstract for Action. New York: McGraw-Hill, 1970.

Newton, K., and Anderson, H. Geriatric Nursing. St. Louis: C. V. Mosby, 1966.

Norton, D. By Accident or Design? A Study of Equipment Development in Relation to Basic Nursing Problems. Edinburgh, Scotland: E. & S. Livingstone, 1970.

Nursing Personnel in Hospitals, 1968. Bethesda, Md.: National Institutes of Health, Division of Nursing, 1970.

Phaneuf, M. C. The Nursing Audit: Profile for Excellence. New York: Appleton-Century-Crofts, 1972.

Practical Approaches to Effective Functioning of the Department of Nursing Service; a Guide for Administrators of Nursing Service. Chicago: The American Hospital Association, 1972.

Price, E. M. Staffing for Patient Care: A Guide for Nursing Service, Based on a Research Report. New York: Springer, 1970.

Shanks, M. D. Administration in Nursing. New York: McGraw-Hill, 1970.

Shanks, M. D. The Theory and Practice of Nursing Service Administration. New York: McGraw-Hill, 1970.

Stryker, R. P. Back to Nursing: A Guide to Current Practice for Active and Inactive Nurses. 2nd Ed. Philadelphia: W. B. Saunders, 1971.

Survey of Registered Professional Nurses Employed in Hospitals in N.Y. State. Albany: State University of N.Y., 1965.

Use of Managerial Tools in Evaluating and Improving the Quality of Nursing Care: A Survey of Selected Hospitals in New Jersey. New York: The National League of Nursing, 1970.

U.S. Public Health Service. Community Health Nursing for Working People. Revised Ed. Washington, D.C.: U.S. Government Printing Office, 1970.

Willig, S. H. The Nurse's Guide to the Law. New York: McGraw-Hill, 1970.

Zeitz, A. N. Associate Degree Nursing: A Guide to Program and Curriculum Development. St. Louis: C. V. Mosby, 1969.

## REHABILITATION

Agronovitz, A., and McKeown, M. R. Aphasia Handbook for Adults and Children. Springfield, Ill.: Charles C Thomas, 1964.

A Guide for Activity Programs. Madison, Wisc.: The Wisconsin State Board of Health, 1962.

American Standard Specifications for Making Buildings and Facilities Accessible to, and Usable by, the Physically Handicapped. New York: The American Standards Association, 1961.

A Step-by-Step Guide to Personal Management for Blind Persons. New York: The American Foundation for the Blind, 1970.

Burris, D. S. The Right to Treatment. New York: Springer, 1972.

Chronic Disease and Rehabilitation: A Program Guide for State and Local Health Agencies. New York: The American Public Health Association, 1960.

Conference on Delivery of Health Care in Relation to Stroke, October 7, 1970 proceedings. Chicago: The Chicago Heart Association, 1970.

Continuity in Care for Impaired Older Persons. New York: The Community Service Society, 1964.

Corliss, E. L. Hearing Aids. NBS monograph No. 117. Washington, D.C.: U.S. Government Printing Office, 1970.

Disabled Housewives in Their Kitchen: A Series of One-Day Conferences. London: The Disabled Living Foundation, 1970.

Homburger, F., and Bonncer, C. Medical Care and Rehabilitation of the Aged and Chronically Ill. 2nd Ed. Boston: Little, Brown, 1964.

Koestler, F. A. The Patient's Role in Overcoming Chronic Disabilities. New York: Rehabilitation Workshop, 1968.

Lamb, H. R. et al. Rehabilitation in Community Mental Health. San Francisco: Jossey-Bass, 1971.

Leedy, J. J. Compensation in Psychiatric Disability and Rehabilitation. Springfield, Ill.: Charles C Thomas, 1971.

Margolin, R. J., and Bolden, G. Dynamic Programming in the Rehabilitation of the Aging. Boston: Department of Rehabilitation and Special Education, Northeastern University, 1967.

Nelson, N. Workshops for the Handicapped in the U.S. Springfield, Ill.: Charles C Thomas, 1971.

Rusk, H. A. A World to Care For. (Autobiography). New York: Random House, 1972.

Rusk, H. A. Rehabilitative Medicine. St. Louis: C. V. Mosby, 1971.
Safilios-Rothschild, C. Sociology and Social Psychology of Disability and Rehabilitation. New York: Random House, 1970.
Standards Manual for Rehabilitation Facilities. Chicago: The Commission on Accreditation of Rehabilitation Facilities, 1968.
Stroke and Its Rehabilitation. New York: The American Public Health Association, 1965.
Sussman, M. B. (ed.) Sociology and Rehabilitation. Washington, D.C.: The American Sociological Association, 1965.
U.S. Department of Health, Education and Welfare, Social and Rehabilitative Service. Questions and Answers on Title XIX: Medical Assistance. Washington, D.C.: U.S. Government Printing Office, 1968.
Black, B. J. Principles of Industrial Therapy for the Mentally Ill. New York: Grune & Stratton, 1970.
Button, W. H. Sheltered Workshops in the U.S.: an institutional overview. *In* W. H. Button (ed.), Rehabilitation, Sheltered Workshops and the Disadvantaged. Ithaca, N.Y.: New York School of Industrial and Labor Relations, Cornell University, 1970.
Goodwill Industries of America, Inc. State of the Art of Volunteering in Rehabilitation Facilities. Washington, D.C.: U.S. Government Printing Office, 1971.
Nelson, N. Worshops for the Handicapped in the United States: An Historical and Developmental Perspective. Springfield, Ill.: Charles C Thomas, 1971.
Smolkin, C., and Cohen, B. S. New Directions in Vocational Rehabilitation: The Stroke Patient. Baltimore: Sinai Hospital of Baltimore, Inc., 1971.

### Physical Therapy

Occupational Therapy—Manual on Administration. New York: The American Occupational Therapy Association, 1965.
Physical Therapy Service: A Guide to Organization and Management. Chicago: The American Hospital Association, 1965.

## RESEARCH AND TRENDS

Aguilera, D. et al. Crisis Intervention—Theory and Methodology. St. Louis: C. V. Mosby, 1970.
Beecher, H. Research and the Individual: Human Studies. Boston: Little, Brown, 1970.
Brooks, C. M. (ed.). The Changing World and Man: The Cultural and Social Environment of Man. Baltimore: Garamond/Pridemark Press, 1970.
Caro, F. Readings in Evaluation Research. New York: Russell Sage Foundation, 1971.
Cochran, W. G. Sampling Techniques. New York: John Wiley & Sons, 1963.
Fox, D. J. Fundamentals of Research in Nursing. New York: Appleton-Century-Crofts, 1970.
Freeman, H. E. Social Research and Social Policy. Englewood Cliffs, N.J.: Prentice-Hall, 1970.
Health Insurance for the Aged: Number of Hospital and Extended Care Facility Admissions by State, Fiscal Year 1970. Washington, D.C.: Social Security Administration, Office of Research and Statistics, 1971.

Kent, D. P. Research Planning and Action for the Elderly. New York: Behavioral Publications, 1971.

Koldin, L. C. The Welfare—Or How to Get Wealthy on Welfare. New York: Exposition Press, 1971.

Lathem, W. Community Medicine: Teaching, Research and Health Care. New York: Appleton-Century-Crofts, 1970.

Length of Stay in PAS Hospitals (U.S., Pre- and Post-Medicare). Ann Arbor, Mich.: The Commission on Professional and Hospital Activities, 1969.

National Center for Health Services Research and Development. Catalog of Health Services Research: Abstract of Public and Private Projects, 1967—1970. Rockville, Md.: Health Services and Mental Health Administration, Public Health Service, U.S. Department of Health, Education and Welfare, 1971.

PAS and MAP Brochure. Ann Arbor, Mich.: The Commission on Professional and Hospital Activities, 1969.

Progress: Health Services Research Center on Planning. Minneapolis: The American Rehabilitation Foundation, 1969.

Reagan, C. E. Ethics for Scientific Research. Springfield, Ill.: Charles C Thomas, 1971.

Reference Data on the Profile of Medical Practice. Chicago: The American Medical Association, 1971.

Research Series No. 28—The Relationship between Administrative Activities and Hospital Performance. Chicago: The University of Chicago Center for Health Administration Studies, 1971.

Selected Data on Charge Patterns in Short-Stay General Hospitals Under Medicare. Washington, D.C.: Social Security Administration, Office of Research and Statistics, 1971.

U.S. Department of Health, Education and Welfare. Inter-Organizational Research in Health Proceedings of Conference. Washington, D.C.: U.S. Government Printing Office, 1971.

U.S. Health Services and Mental Health Administration. An Index to Clinical Research in the Federal Health Programs Service. Washington, D.C.: U.S. Government Printing Office, 1970.

U.S. National Institute of Mental Health. 1970 Census Data Used to Indicate Areas with Different Potentials for Mental Health and Related Problems. Washington, D.C.: U.S. Government Printing Office, 1971.

U.S. National Institutes of Health. Nursing Home Research Study: Quantitative Measurement of Nursing Services. Washington, D.C.: U.S. Government Printing Office, 1970.

Utilization Review Using PAS and MAP. Ann Arbor, Mich.: The Commission on Professional and Hospital Activities, 1969.

## SOCIOLOGY IN MEDICINE

Andersen, R. and Anderson, O. W. A Decade of Health Services: Social Survey Trends in Use and Expenditure. Chicago: University of Chicago Press, 1967.

Barclay, G. W. Techniques of Population Analysis. New York: John Wiley & Sons, 1958.

Bierstedt, R. A Design for Sociology: Scope, Objectives and Methods. Philadelphia: American Academy of Political and Social Science, 1969.

Blackwell, E. Essays in Medical Sociology. New York: Arno Press, 1902.

Bloom, S. W. The Doctor and His Patient: A Sociological Interpretation. New York: Basic Books, 1963.

Brock, M. G. Social Work in the Hospital Organization. Toronto: University of Toronto Press, 1969.

Bruce, M. The Coming of the Welfare State. New York: Schocken Books, 1966.

Crawford, C. Health and the Family: A Medical Sociological Analysis. New York: Macmillan, 1971.

deGrazia, S. Of Time, Work, Leisure. New York: Anchor-Doubleday, 1964.

DeGroot, L. (ed.). Medical Care: Social and Organizational Aspects. Springfield, Ill.: Charles C Thomas, 1966.

Dreitzel, H. P. Social Organization of Health. New York: Macmillan, 1971.

Demographic Aspects of the Black Community. New York: The Milbank Memorial Fund, 1970.

Dubos, R. Man Adapting. New Haven, Conn.: Yale University Press, 1965.

Erasmus, C. J. Man Takes Control: Cultural Development and American Aid. Minneapolis: University of Minnesota Press, 1968.

Ferkiss, V. C. Technological Man: The Myth and the Reality. New York: George Braziller, 1969.

Field, M. Patients are People: A Medical-Social Approach to Prolonged Illness. 3rd Ed. New York: Columbia University Press, 1967.

Freeman, H. Handbook of Medical Sociology. 1st Ed. Englewood Cliffs, N.J.: Prentice-Hall, 1963.

Freeman, H. Handbook of Medical Sociology. 2nd Ed. Englewood Cliffs, N.J.: Prentice-Hall, 1972.

Freidson, E. Patient's Views of Medical Practice. New York: Russell Sage Foundation, 1961.

Friedson, E. The Hospital in Modern Society. New York: The Free Press, 1963.

Friedson, E. Professional Dominance: The Social Structure of Medical Care. New York: Atherton Press, 1970.

Garcia, J. D. The Moral Society: A Rational Alternative to Death. New York: Julian Press, 1971.

Glaser, W. Social Settings and Medical Organization. New York: Atherton Press, 1970.

Goldston, I. Man's Image in Medicine and Anthropology. New York: International University Press, 1963.

Gordon, G. A., et al. Disease, Individual and Society. Chicago: College and University Press, 1968.

Harrington, M. The Other America. New York: Macmillan, 1962.

Heer, D. M. Social Statistics and the City. Cambridge: Harvard University Press, 1968.

Inkeles, A. What is Sociology? An Introduction to the Discipline Profession. Englewood Cliffs, N.J.: Prentice-Hall, 1964.

Irelan, L. M. Low Income Life Styles. Washington, D.C.: U.S. Government Printing Office, 1966.

Jackson, J. Professions and Professionalization. New York: Cambridge University Press, 1970.

Jaco, E. G. Ecological Aspects of Patient Care and Their Relation to Hospital

Organization: An Appraisal. Riverside, Cal.: Department of Sociology, University of California, 1970.

Jaco, E. G. Patients, Physicians and Illness; Source Book. New York: The Free Press, 1958.

Jacques, E. Work, Creativity and Social Justice. New York: International Universities Press, 1970.

Kaluger, G. Psychology and Sociology—An Integrated Approach to Understanding Human Behavior. St. Louis: C. V. Mosby, 1969.

Kaplan, N. Science and Society. Chicago: Rand McNally, 1965.

King, C. W. Social Movements in the United States. New York: Random House, 1956.

Knutson, A. L. Individual, Society, and Health Behavior. New York: Russell Sage Foundation, 1965.

Leighton, A. Explorations in Social Psychiatry. New York: Basic Books, 1957.

Lindsey, G. Handbook of Social Psychology. Reading, Mass.: Addison-Wesley, 1954.

Lowry, N. Community Structure and Change. New York: Macmillan, 1960.

Marsh, D. C. The Future of the Welfare State. Baltimore: Penguin Books, 1964.

Marshall, T. H. Social Policy. London: Hutchinson University, 1965.

Mead, M. Culture and Commitment; A Study of the Generation Gap. New York: Doubleday, 1969.

Mechanic, D. Medical Sociology; A Selective View. New York: The Free Press, 1968.

Miller, S. M. Social Class and Social Policy. New York: Basic Books, 1968.

Morais, H. M. The History of the Negro in Medicine. New York: Publishers Co., 1967.

Norman, J. C. Medicine in the Ghetto. Des Moines: Meredith Corp., 1969.

Read, M. Culture, Health and Disease. Philadelphia: J. B. Lippincott, 1966.

Rosengren, W. R. Hospitals and Patients. New York: Atherton Press, 1969.

Rosengren, W. R. Organization and Clients; Essays in the Sociology of Service. Columbus, Ohio: Charles E. Merrill, 1970.

Russell Sage Foundation Bulletin. Sociology and the Field of Public Health. Washington, D.C.: The American Sociological Association, 1971.

Schooler, D. Science, Scientists and Public Policy. New York: The Free Press, 1971.

Shryock, R. H. Medicine and Society in America, 1660–1860. New York: New York University Press, 1960.

Shuval, J. T. Social Functions of Medical Practice. San Francisco: Jossey-Bass, 1970.

Silverstein, H. (ed.). The Social Control of Illness. New York: Thomas Y. Crowell, 1968.

Stacey, M. Hospitals, Children and Their Families. New York: Fernhill House, 1970.

Stern, B. Society and Medical Progress. College Park, Md.: McGrath, 1971.

Strickland, S. P. Politics, Science, and Dread Disease. A Short History of United States Medical Research Policy. Cambridge: Harvard University Press, 1972.

Sudnow, D. Passing On: The Social Organization of Dying. Englewood Cliffs, N.J.: Prentice-Hall, 1967.

Taylor, C. In Horizontal Orbit: Hospitals and the Cult of Efficiency. New York: Holt, Rinehart & Winston, 1970.
Tawney, R. H. Equality. London: George Allen and Unwin, 1964.
The One-Worker Social Service Department. St. Louis: The Catholic Hospital Association, 1969.
Titmuss, R. M. Commitment to Welfare. New York: Pantheon Books, 1968.
Toffler, A. Future Shock. New York: Random House, 1970.
Trecker, H. Social Work Administration: Principles and Practices. New York: Association Press, 1971.
U.S. Bureau of the Census. 200 Million Americans. Washington, D.C.: U.S. Government Printing Office, 1967.
U.S. Department of Health, Education and Welfare. Why Men Stop Working At or Before Age 65: Preliminary Findings from the Survey of New Beneficiaries. Washington, D.C.: Social Security Administration, 1971.
U.S. Indian Health Service. Indian Health Trends and Services. Washington, D.C.: U.S. Public Health Service, 1970.
Verson, G. Sociology of Death: An Analysis of Death-Related Behavior. New York: Ronald Press, 1970.
Wallace, S. E. Total Institutions. Chicago: Aldine-Atherton, 1971.
Whiteleather, M. Seven Polarizing Issues in America Today. Philadelphia: American Academy of Political Science, 1971.
Wilson, R. N. Sociology of Health: An Introduction. New York: Random House, 1970.
Wolff, K. Social and Cultural Factors in Mental Health and Mental Illness. Springfield, Ill.: Charles C Thomas, 1971.

**Poverty**

Bullough, B. Poverty, Ethnic Identity and Health Care. New York: Appleton-Century-Crofts, 1972.
Lerner, B. Therapy in the Ghetto: Political Impotence and Personal Disintegration. Baltimore: The Johns Hopkins University Press, 1972.

## STATISTICS

Brackett, J. C. Retired Couples Budget for a Moderate Living Standard. Washington, D.C.: U.S. Government Printing Office, 1968.
Cancer Control and Registry Report. Albany: The New York Department of Health, 1970.
Facts on the Major Killing and Crippling Diseases in U.S. Today. New York: The National Health Education Commission, Inc., 1971.
Hill, A. B. Principles of Medical Statistics. New York: Oxford University Press, 1966.
Kilpatrick, S. J., Jr. Statistical Principles in Health Care Information. Baltimore: University Park Press, 1973.
Length of Stay in PAS Hospitals, United States. Ann Arbor, Mich.: The Commission on Professional and Hospital Activities, 1971.
Lewis, A. E. Biostatistics. New York: Van Nostrand Reinhold, 1966.
Mainland, D. Elementary Medical Statistics. Philadelphia: W. B. Saunders, 1963.
Manual of the International Statistical Classification of Diseases, Injuries and Courses of Death. Geneva, Switzerland, World Health Organization, 1968.

National Research Council—Committee on Trauma. Accidental Death and Disability: The Neglected Disease of Modern Society. Washington, D.C.: U.S. Government Printing Office, 1970.

Tuberculosis Statistics: States and Cities. Washington, D.C.: The U.S. National Center for Disease Control, 1971.

U.S. Bureau of Labor Statistics. Industry Wage Survey; Nursing Homes and Related Facilities. Washington, D.C.: U.S. Government Printing Office, 1965.

U.S. Bureau of Labor Statistics. The Negroes in the U.S.: Their Economic and Social Situation. Washington, D.C.: U.S. Government Printing Office, 1966.

U.S. Division of Health Resources. Hospitals—A County and Metropolitan Area Data Book. Washington, D.C.: U.S. Government Printing Office, 1970.

U.S. National Center for Health Statistics. An Aid in Planning Comprehensive Health Statistics. Washington, D.C.: U.S. Government Printing Office, 1969.

U.S. National Center for Health Statistics. Charges for Care in Nursing Homes, U.S. April—September 1968 (P.H.S. Pub. No. 1000, Series 12, No. 14). U.S. Health Services and Mental Health Administration Publication No. 72-1037. Washington, D.C. U.S. Government Printing Office, 1972.

U.S. National Center for Health Statistics. Development and Evaluation of an Expanded Hearing Loss Scale Questionnaire. Washington, D.C.: U.S. Government Printing Office, 1970.

U.S. National Center for Health Statistics. Health Resource Statistics. Washington, D.C.: U.S. Government Printing Office, 1971.

U.S. National Center for Health Statistics. Natality Statistics Analysis. Washington, D.C.: U.S. Government Printing Office, 1970.

U.S. National Center for Health Statistics. Need for Dental Care Among Adults, United States, 1960—1962. Washington, D.C.: U.S. Government Printing Office, 1970.

U.S. National Center for Health Statistics. 1970 Health Resources Statistics: Health Manpower and Health Facilities. Washington, D.C.: U.S. Government Printing Office, 1971.

U.S. National Center for Health Statistics. Origin, Program and Operation of the U.S. National Health Survey. Washington, D.C.: U.S. Government Printing Office, 1963.

U.S. National Institute of Mental Health. Staffing Patterns in Mental Health Facilities, 1968. Washington, D.C.: U.S. Government Printing Office, 1970.

U.S. National Institute of Mental Health. Statistics in Mental Health Pro-

U.S. National Institute of Mental Health. Statistics in Mental Health Programs. Washington, D.C.: U.S. Government Printing Office, 1970.

U.S. Public Health Service. Hospital; A County and Metropolitan Area Data Book—Data Compiled from the 1967 Master Facility Inventory. Washington, D.C.: U.S. Government Printing Office, 1970.

U.S. Public Health Service. Nursing Homes; A County and Metropolitan Area Data Book. Washington, D.C.: U.S. Government Printing Office, 1970.

U.S. Social Security Administration. Net Income for Hospitals. Washington, D.C.: Office of Research and Statistics, 1970.

# Index